"I love this book! I loved reading it cover to cover: I was awed, and compelled, and interested, and emotional throughout the whole book. I loved learning this complex subject by seeing things so clearly laid out. This is the language course we missed in school—the one that will help us make sense of the kids we haven't understood!

"Marge has done an amazing job of taking an abstract subject, one that depends on other abstract subjects, and making it readable, understandable, and doable. Marge's style feels like a natural conversation with the reader—which makes the reader want to take part in the conversation and do the exercises she has laid out. Marge's book motivates us, teaches us, and tells us how to become the support to children that we want to be!

"This is a reference book I will return to again and again because the words are so powerful and important for understanding our kids, recognizing how far they have come when they mitigate, and knowing how to help them continue towards developing generative language.

"Thank you, Marge! This is such an essential book for every SLP and every parent of a child who uses echolalia!"

Leslie Wellauer, M. A., CCC-SLP, Private Practice, Park City, UT

"This book is a blessing for parents and SLPs! It gives us permission to focus on language development, which we are uniquely educated to appreciate and support. By her careful review of the literature, Marge reminds us that the documentation of children with ASD developing natural language is not new, and has been seen across time, children, and environments. But in our current educational climate, we are rarely afforded the time and permission to support students in the ways we know will matter to them as individuals with great potential. As a public school SLP, I so often hear parents and teachers recognizing the limitations of "functional language programs," passionately protesting: "But there's so much more in there!" Now, with the principles of NLA explained and illustrated, we can outline programs of true language development for our students so they can express their own intentions—and find their own authentic voices. Thank you! The book is marvelous!"

Kjersten Sandin, M. S., CCC-SLP, Mukwonago, WI

"Natural Language Acquisition has changed the way I approach kids' language treatment! As a hospital-based SLP, I find parents to be so in touch with their kids that I give them the theory and they provide me examples! This book feels very personal, but it's bigger than that: it is profound and awe-inspiring. Because of the Communication Development Center, there are people all over the country who are carrying seeds of change with them. I feel like a seed that has been watered, and I find that I am talking to my colleagues and families all the time about this exciting, but natural, approach. There is a movement afoot that is fueled by Marge's work."

Kristen Powell Lee, M. S., CCC-SLP, Indianapolis, IN

"As an SLP, I can feel parents' uneasiness trying to carry out techniques that "teach" communication skills while trying to honor their personal relationship and bond with their own child. It has been a joy to share Natural Language Acquisition with parents and witness their excitement the first time they participate in a meaningful and reciprocal conversation with their child with ASD. This book empowers parents and SLPs to fully appreciate and honor the language their children have, provides strategies and tools to facilitate further language development, and provides opportunities for families to experience mutually fulfilling and exciting communicative interactions. Approaching language development from the NLA perspectives facilitates understanding of the physical, environmental, and emotional supports for each child as well as an appreciation of their unique strengths. And there is nothing that warms the heart and motivates the spirit like seeing a child experience success."

Jessica Schmidt, M.S., CCC-SLP, Creative Perspectives Autism Centers of Colorado, Englewood, CO

"Marge has brought together decades of research and clinical insight to develop this comprehensive look at the patterns of language development through which kids on the autism spectrum progress. Marge's work will revolutionize your thinking about your child's language and help you understand the depth of meaning behind it!"

Megan Snow, M.S., CCC-SLP, Sensory KIDS, Portland, OR

"Marge beautifully demonstrates how children develop language and how natural language development can be!

"This is a 'must read book' for every parent who wants to understand how language development can be built into speech and language therapy. And it is the perfect book to help you decide the balance of approaches (play/ABA) you want for your child.

"While the author intended this book primarily for families of kids on the autism spectrum, the concepts equally apply to language-delayed children who are gestalt learners, but who are not on the autism spectrum! As the mother of such a boy, I understand that echolalia is part of the learning style of very typically-developing children. I found that most people don't know that, and think that echolalia equals autism—just like that!

"This book helped me think through the stages of language development for my son, and I realized that the book was written for my son, too, and to help my family with its own journey!

"Thank you, Marge, for your wonderful work!"

Satya Kusumanchi, Parent, Seattle, WA

Natural Language Acquisition on the Autism Spectrum

The Journey from Echolalia to Self-Generated Language

by Marge Blanc, M.A., CCC-SLP
Speech-Language Pathologist
Illustrated by Jon G. Lyon

Communication Development Center
www.communicationdevelopmentcenter.com

Illustrations courtesy of Jon G. Lyon

ISBN 978-0-615-69610-2

Communication Development Center, Inc.
700 Rayovac Dr., Suite 200
Madison, WI 53711
(608) 278-9161

www.communicationdevelopmentcenter.com

Contents

About the Author

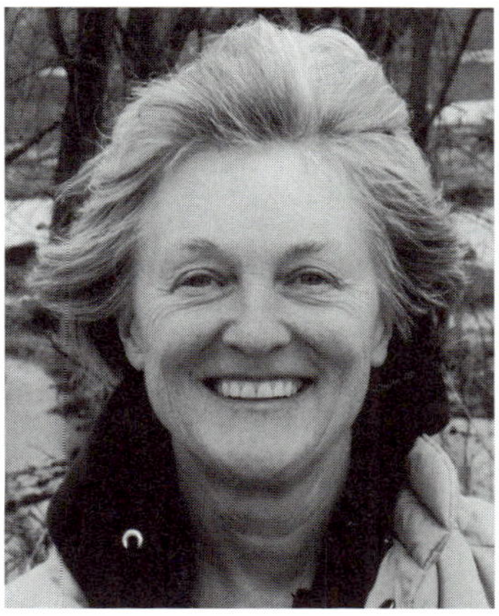

Marge Blanc has been a clinical Speech-Language Pathologist for 35 years and founded the Communication Development Center in Madison, WI, in 1997. Specializing in physically-supported speech and language services for children with ASD diagnoses and others who benefit from physical support and movement, CDC is devoted to helping children become communicators as they move through the stages of speech development and language acquisition outlined in this book.

Marge and her colleagues have presented workshops on Natural Language Acquisition to Speech-Language Pathologists, educators, and families of children with speech and language delays and challenges. She has also written numerous articles and columns for the *Autism Asperger's Digest* since 2004. Topics have included augmentative communication, self-regulation, speech supports with dyspraxia, language retrieval, and, of course, natural language acquisition. Articles can be downloaded from the CDC website at: www.communicationdevelopmentcenter.com

The illustrator, Jon G. Lyon, Ph.D., CCC-SLP, is the author of *Coping with Aphasia* (1998). Combining his love for his wife with his love of drawing, Jon became well-versed in the words and wisdom of the kids at CDC through filming them for a CDC workshop. One of his earlier gifts to the clinic was the logo seen on this page, one rendition of which appears throughout the book.

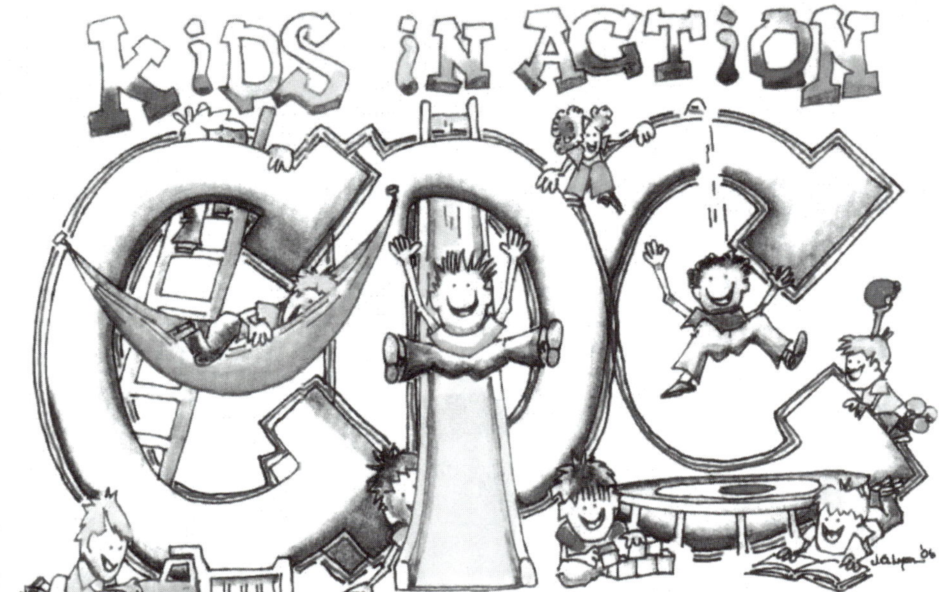

Acknowledgements

This book is dedicated to my mother, Florence Code Blanc, who has inspired me daily and once said to me, "If there was ever a reason you were born, it was to write this book." And she lived to the age of 100, to make sure the book made it to print. From the bottom of my heart, I thank you for your constant love and encouragement, and for the example of your life.

A sincere thank you goes to all the families who have requested this book and to the kids who have lived it.

Thank you also goes to my husband, Jon Lyon, who illustrated the book, and encouraged me, every day, to finish it: with his reminders, his love, and, not incidentally, his promise to do the illustrations.

And to my brother, Paul, who supported me through the last chapters, not to mention the printing; to my sister, Christine; my father, Milton; my mother-in-law, Barbara; and Jill Trick, John Anderson, and Vilje, who have supported me every day of my life.

To my friends, Nicko, Benjamin, and Cyrus, who have taught me through their poetry and metaphors that not all language is created equal! Nicko kept me laughing until the "stupid book" was done; Cyrus kept me well-fed; and Ben is my spiritual advisor and muse. These three have delighted my heart for the last decade with their love and wisdom.

To Kjersten Sandin, who lovingly referred to "the book" for ten years, and constantly inspired me with her brilliance and the new topics and stories she kept putting on the piece of butcher paper above my desk.

To Megan Snow, who helped develop NLA with her creativity and her incredible therapeutic support of her clients over the years.

To Leslie Wellauer, Kristen Powell Lee, Jessi Schmidt, and Meghan Matthews, who expanded our world with their amazing therapy and who, along with Megan Pierce, Zadock Cropper, Kayla Wiedenbeck, Shannon Lisowe, Renee Reszel, and Sarah Levinsky, applied the principles in this book and helped so many children become the "real kids" they already were.

To Jane and Randy Lambert and Linda and Wallace Carter, who tell stories far better than I ever will.

To Jessika Rumbaugh, and other educators, who see their students as "real boys" and "real girls" every day.

To Sheila Frick, OT, for her pioneering work in listening therapy, and Laura Quast, OT, Tracy Bjorling, OT, Dave Bogenrief, PT, and Todd Nierman, PT, who came to my rescue and provided our kids and countless others the tools for self-regulation that allowed them to continue their language journeys through the hard places.

To Jo Sandin, Peg Lemme, Katharine Odell, Jim Statz, Jr., and Jim Statz, Sr., who helped through their support of our clinic, and to Renee Wilson, who supported me through the last chapters.

To Michael Proctor, who saved a whole species during the time it took me to write this book.

To Veronica Zysk, who, through the *Autism Asperger's Digest*, gave me the opportunity to first tell these stories, and encouraged me to put them together in a book.

To Kayen Cheung, who made the book come alive with her visual genius, Bonnie Brinton, who helped with her suggestions, and Anna Keaney for her fine-toothed comb.

To Sandra Levin, my former colleague at the University of Wisconsin, who showed me the first roadmap for this journey, and to Barry Prizant, Amy Wetherby, Patrick Rydell, and all the other pioneers who lit the way for a sourcebook like this.

And, finally, to Annaliese, who lives a brilliant, gestalt life and reminds me every day how loving and beautiful the world is. Annaliese, Madeline, Marin, Nathan, Miles, Isaac, Lizzy, Charlie, Georgiana, Maya, Tara, Gwendolyn, Gibson, and their age-mates are the soul of the next generation.

Foreward

"Mrs. Carter, I know of a woman who is quite different in her approach to kids like your son. You may want to just visit her clinic and see how it feels as a next step in caring for Ben." I walked into Marge's clinic and the sun came out. The place was covered in color: layers and layers of lycra hang from the ceiling, swings and platforms, slides and huge pillows everywhere. Mirrors and TV monitors, rooms of toys and kids running all around with smiling adults who appear to be having such fun.

As a family, we had exhausted every mode of therapy for our boy with autism and in the process, had exhausted him, our resources, and ourselves. Ben was frustrated, angry and bottled up tight as a drum. I scheduled a visit with Marge for Ben. He walked into "Marge's" and the magic began to bloom from his insides out.

I asked Marge early on, "Is there any way you can make him stop that blasted movie talk? He is making me nuts!" Marge grinned and, with a twinkle in her eye, said, "That boy is brilliant and he is talking to **you**!" From the depths of my heart, I had no idea what she was talking about—and did I just hear a professional say my son was brilliant? I have heard them say retarded, stunted, slow like molasses, autistic, speech delayed and disabled, but this woman is grinning at me, winking at Ben, and calling him brilliant.

A few sessions pass with Marge and Brilliant Ben. I truly had no clue what they were doing together, but I do know that Ben ran down the hall, up the steps and down another hall as fast as he could to get to "Marge's," and he did not want anyone to interrupt them when they were together.

In a few short sessions, a change comes over Benjamin the Brilliant: for the very first time in his young life, he made a human connection! Marge owned a knowledge of Ben that captivated him, propelled him to therapy, settled him, and inspired him. Marge was magical with Ben and he could not get enough of her. As the mama, I ask myself, "What on earth are they doing in there?" It was loud, it was messy, a lot of banging and singing and bouncing and most of all, it was a whole lot of fun for that kid. Marge was laughing and my Ben was shining and grinning and changing.

We found a very mysterious help in this woman when brilliant Ben met his friend and teacher, "Marge's." Our life as a family was about to improve drastically. If I had known that we would find Marge, I would not have cried so long and so hard and so often all those previous years! Brilliant Ben—she called my Ben 'brilliant'—imagine: brilliant.

Read on. You will discover the mystery.

Linda Carter, R.N.
University of Wisconsin Medical Foundation
Madison, Wisconsin

Preface

This book is written for you, the family member of a child diagnosed with an Autism Spectrum Disorder (ASD). Whether the child you love is considered verbal or not, whether your child's speech is considered communicative or not, it is you who will find the hidden gems of meaning inside your child. It is you who will see the uncut diamonds that exist there. Even though you may not feel qualified to be the one who analyzes your child's language or discovers it in the first place, you will find things no one else has the depth of understanding to see. And, just as importantly, you will become your child's best partner in language development. So, this book is for you.

This book is also written for others like me, who have been entrusted with helping parents and family members with their precious children and their children's language. It is a privilege to be here with you; please join me in the journey we will take here together.

You will find the hidden gems of meaning inside your child. You will see the 'uncut diamonds' there.

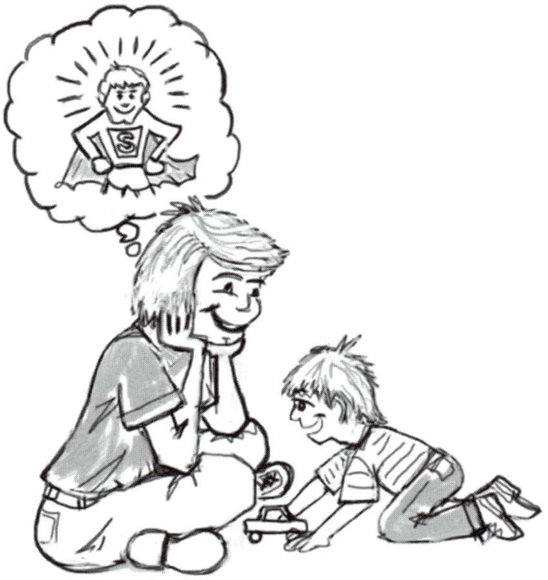

For me, the journey began eighteen years ago with a wonderful experience. I was working as a Clinical Instructor in the Department of Communicative Disorders at the University of Wisconsin and was introduced to my first group of children with ASD diagnoses. I had worked as a Speech-Language Pathologist (SLP) for 20 years, but only with a handful of children with labels on the autism spectrum. So, working with my new charges might have seemed daunting. But, it was not. They were wonderful children, and I quickly got to know them as 'children, first,' and helped my university students do the same.

Echolalic language systematically develops towards self-generated language.

At about the same time, a clinical colleague introduced me to the work of Barry Prizant, Amy Wetherby, Judith Duchan, and Ann Peters: communication research and linguistic theory that supported the idea that kids who started out echolalic could move towards becoming competent generative language users.

Language emerges naturally in our kids with ASD.

I never questioned that language could develop naturally in the ways these Speech-Language Pathologists and linguists predicted. Somehow, it rang true with what I knew about another group of children, a group of children we often see in speech and language clinics. They are the story-tellers, often boys, who use long streams of well-intoned but unintelligible speech and seem to lag behind their peers on language milestones. That our kids on the Autism Spectrum could be like this, but more so, made intuitive sense to me. It also would help explain what I was seeing and hearing.

So, I went to work with these kids, using the material Prizant and others had added to our clinical knowledge, and we began to systematically facilitate it with the ASD children at the UW Speech and Hearing Clinic. It worked beautifully.

Echolalic language can be analyzed and a progression outlined to move it towards self-generated language.

Eighteen years, a specialized clinic, and scores of ASD children later, I am now firmly ensconced in our local autism community. In our own physically-supportive clinic, we have seen and documented this process of language development unfolding time and time again with considerable individual variation, but always in the direction of more flexible, creative language. It is still wonderful to be a part of this process, but it no longer seems remarkable. It seems only natural, while needing support and facilitation along the way. We diligently recorded language samples of all our kids, wrote innumerable progress reports, and, in this way, the regular process of natural language acquisition in ASD became better documented.

Finally, in the year 2000, we gave it a name. We devised an assessment protocol and began inviting others to look at their kids the same way. More documentation was accomplished, and it was time to write about Natural Language Acquisition (NLA) for the autism community.

What motivated me was the fact that this progression of language emergence in our ASD kids was not more widely understood and targeted in the larger autism community. Largely remaining in the realm of language research circles, it seemed to be silently usurped by innumerable language programs which focus on teaching language rather than supporting natural development. Well-meaning though they are, these programs have made the natural process almost impossible for our kids to access.

Over the years, I have felt determined to reduce this widening gap and to get this life-changing information out there to you, the families and professionals who can use it best. I devoted a column series in the *Autism Asperger's Digest* to this endeavor, and this book is sprinkled with material from "Finding the Words ... To Tell the Whole Story" (July–Aug 2005 through Jan–Feb 2006). My colleagues and I have also conducted workshops on the subject, introducing parents to NLA and showing SLPs how to analyze language samples using the principles you will learn here. In this practical way, Natural Language Acquisition became a tool for others to use and, with this book, has come to fruition.

And while this book teaches the 'how to's, it is mostly a collection of children's stories, each one illustrating something important about the development process. Taken together, these stories trace the acquisition of language in children with ASD. Through these stories, you will find parts that speak to you, that remind you of your child. During the course of this journey, you will learn that your child is engaging in a common, natural process: one that is shared with roughly half of all kids, including typically-developing kids. It is that natural and that common.

Yes, most of our kids need some support to get there (sensorimotor supports and an abundance of language models), but the process is just as natural. The biggest help you can give your child is to recognize that this process is one that will unfold over time. And in this book, you will learn everything you need to know to help your child move in the direction of more flexible, creative language use.

The process of witnessing language develop and flourish continues to be an exciting one for my colleagues and families, but it is especially exciting for the children who have benefitted from our faith in them. You are invited to come along and to help your child progress along this path toward intentional, interactive communication.

Echolalia is hard to hear in a child with little speech and impossible to hear in a silent child.

This book was designed with parents, teachers, and SLPs in mind. It is meant to be primarily reader-friendly and usable, so the theoretical principles involved have been relegated to their own section (Section 2), the assessment and intervention principles have been put into another (Section 6), and the rest of the book is filled with relevant stories you are sure to relate to. All of them are real, about real kids with ASD whom we, in our clinic, have known and worked with. These are kids, some just like yours, who found an understanding ear, just like yours, to help them develop useful, flexible language in this natural way.

Many of the children I have met along the way were already vocal. Some were very vocal. But some were not. There were many who were called dyspraxic, some severely dyspraxic. Some children, in fact, were nearly silent. Here is something important to consider with those children: the echolalia that is a hallmark of autistic language is hard to hear in a child with little speech and impossible to hear in a silent child. We all understand and formulate language in our heads, not with our lips. So even a complete lack of speech doesn't mean a lack of language or a lack of language development. The language process described in this book is still relevant. If you are one of the many parents who is thinking, "But my child isn't talking—at all!" please do not despair. We have a chapter especially for you and your child: one that addresses the development of motor speech and which will help you discover the 'gems' that are sure to be found inside the heart and mind of your silent child!

Lack of speech doesn't mean a lack of language or a lack of language development.

So, please join me in this journey. I think you will find something familiar in many of these stories and find yourself identifying with the families featured. Then, as you see where your child fits compared with the children in this book, you will begin to see how you, too, can apply the principles of Natural Language Acquisition for your child.

section 1

Getting Started with Natural Language Acquisition

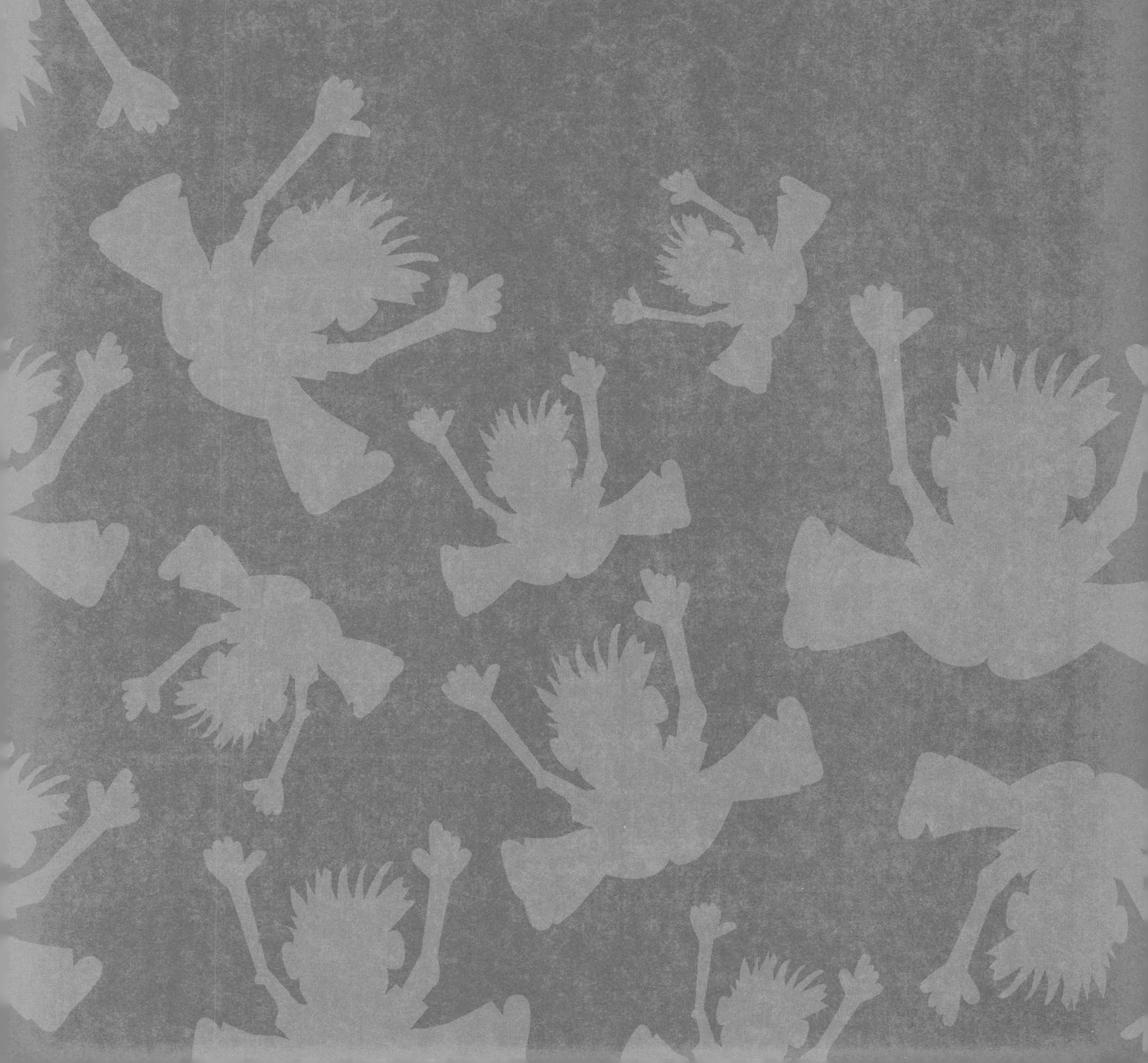

Introduction

"Help! He's using 'movie talk' all day, every day!"

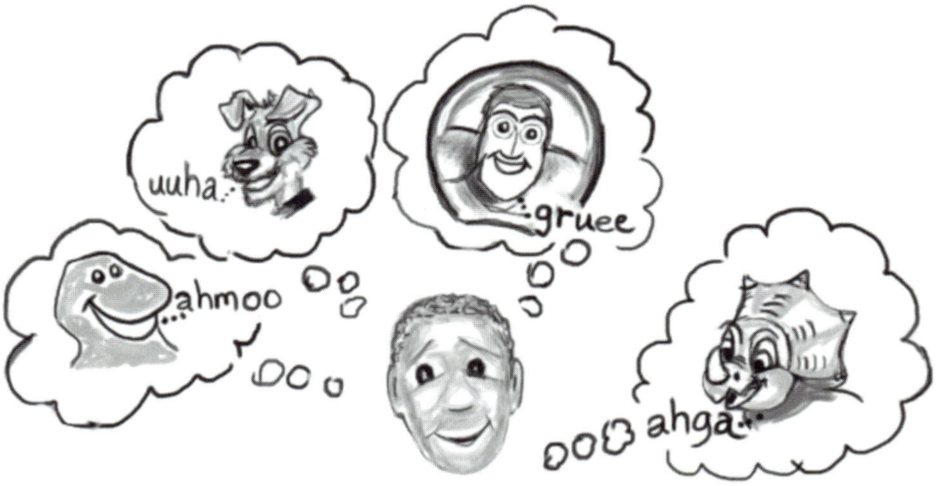

Bevin's mother was exhausted—and desperate. When she first called me about her ten-year old son, she admitted that the only reason she was doing so was that a friend, a well-regarded person in our local autism community, made her do it! "Kathy told me I had to call you. She told me to trust you and to do whatever you said. She told me that I wouldn't necessarily understand what you were doing but that I had to do it anyway!"

Our kids' language is not categorically different from that of other gestalt language processors—just more pronounced.

I laughed at the veiled compliment but understood what she was saying. Our clinic looks a little different, and this makes it harder for some people to 'get.' First of all, it looks more like an Occupational Therapy clinic than a typical Speech and Language clinic. It's filled with colorful lycra swings, slides, pillows, and trampolines. We actually don't even have a table, except in our waiting room. And we play a lot—all the time.

The most unique thing about our clinic, however, might be our philosophy of language development. We don't despair over kids' echolalic language or talk about the challenges it seems to suggest to many people. Instead, we look at language development on the spectrum as a common, natural process. Yes, it usually needs more direct intervention than does the language development of kids off the spectrum, but it is not categorically different, or at least not categorically different from that of the other kids out there who tend to develop language in big chunks, or 'gestalts.' Our ASD kids are actually in good company, but they tend to be the extreme of those 'gestalt language processors,' and this makes them stand out.

Yes, I know it will take you some time to digest this news. But you will, I promise, as you undertake the journey that is this book. As you travel along, some of your assumptions about echolalia will be challenged. But that's a good thing: thinking of it as gestalt language processing will be much more helpful and hopeful.

But, I digress—more about language development in due time. For now, suffice it to say that our clinic is unique, and our approach takes some rethinking of the common assumptions made about how different our kids' language is. But, believe me, the rethinking will be helpful. It will turn the tedium we often associate with 'teaching language' to our ASD kids into limitless, creative language development. In turn, it will be hopeful, fun, and productive.

Natural language development is hopeful, fun, and productive.

Let's start our journey with a story, the story about Bevin, who, beyond a doubt, was echolalic. According to his family, he was echolalic about 24/7. His mother was more than justified in her fatigue, and I sympathized when she told me that Bevin's "movie talk" was making her entire family tired all day, every day. It was no wonder that his parents pleaded with Bevin to "turn off the movie."

His mother told me that Bevin could recite many things and did, pretty much non-stop. He knew all the words of the Barney songs—at least she was pretty sure he did, because the tunes were familiar even if the words were slurred together. He recited his favorite scenes and would spend hours saying the dialogues, with his sister taking one of the roles until she tired of it.

Bevin's favorites at the time I met him were every Barney movie ever made. He would play one of them over and over, literally hundreds of times, saying all the lines along with the movie. When even his family was beginning to know one by heart, they tried to hide it just to give them all a break.

When his family asked, Bevin could "turn off the movie" verbally. But his family wondered if he was still playing it in his mind. They suspected he was, because the words would erupt again and again throughout the day.

I couldn't wait to meet Bevin!

Chapter 1
Echolalia Revisited: Gestalt Language Development

"The wonderful thing about Tiggers"

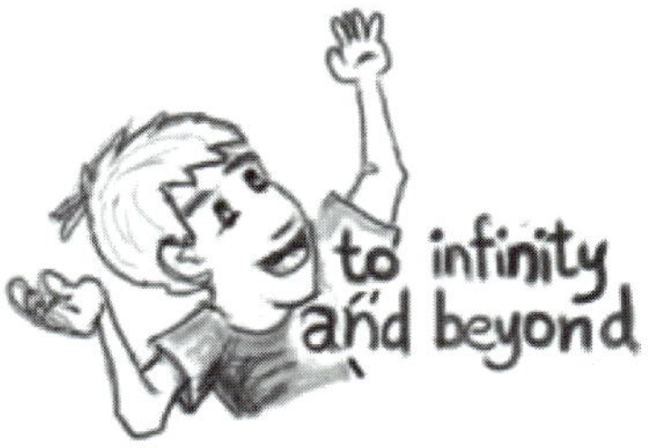

Some of the lines our kids say are common; others are more elusive. But family members usually know just where they came from, because our kids sound just like their source. **"To infinity and beyond"** is classic, of course. But other lines are known only to the true aficionados, like these from *Blue's Clues*: **"Blue skidoos; you can too!"** And we hear our kids say some of Pooh's lines at vaguely appropriate times: **"You never can tell about bees," "And I'm the only one!"** Even words like 'cheeky' find their way into our kids' speech because of *Thomas the Tank Engine.*

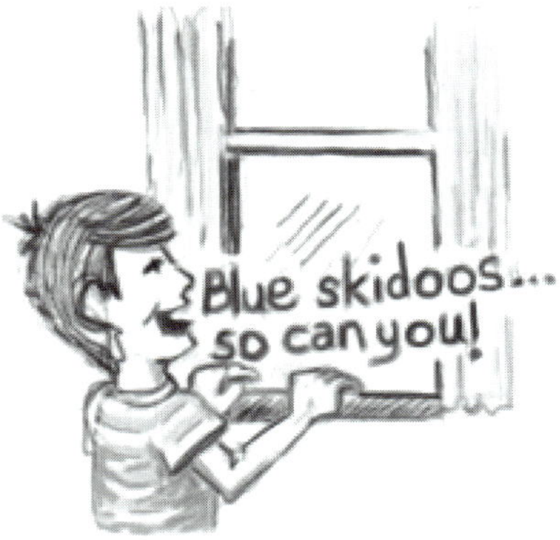

Consider this: when any one of us uses one of these lines, it's a quote. But when these colorful expressions make up almost the entirety of a child's language, we refer to it as echolalia. It's not strange at all, just pervasive. It used to be called 'delayed echolalia,' meaning that kids echo the words not right after they hear them ('immediate echolalia'), but later, or 'delayed.' Of course, sometimes our kids do say the lines right after Christopher Robin or Steve, and sometimes right along with them. We even hear our kids anticipating the next line and saying it before the movie even gets there. It's all echolalia, but it's the delayed kind we notice. And it's often when our kids surprise us with a line they got from somewhere else, but somehow pulled out of their heads at this particular moment.

No matter the source or the timing of it, all of this echoed language is what our kids repeat verbatim from other sources: movies, books, things people have said to them, and things they have overheard. Granted, a lot of the time it seems pretty meaningless to us. We think it must just be interesting to our child to hear or interesting to him to say or just **interesting**. We think it keeps our kids "awake" or "alert" or "stimulated." We even call it a "stim" of sorts; a "verbal stim." And, truth be told, we worry about it. We try to tune it out. And we ask kids to "turn it off."

When any one of us uses a movie line, it's a quote. But when a child quotes extensively, we call it echolalia.

But sometimes it surprises us—in a good way. Sometimes our child might say an echoed phrase at just the right time so that it seems to have real meaning. I remember one of the first parent stories I ever heard about a particularly well-timed delayed echo. Cam and his mom were in an ice cream store when Cam piped up and proclaimed, **"I love chocolate!"** This wouldn't have been so surprising except that Cam rarely talked and certainly didn't have the grammar to say sentences. That Cam's mother recognized this line from an *Arthur* story solved the mystery. But what this mom also learned at that moment was that echolalia can communicate, and that for her child at that moment it can communicate just what he intended it to. Cam did love chocolate!

Now let's look more closely at the gamut of common echolalia among kids in general. First are the transparent phrases we tend to hear at appropriate moments in kids' lives. We all recognize them as "kid talk" and rarely think twice about their origin. But chances are, they are echoed:

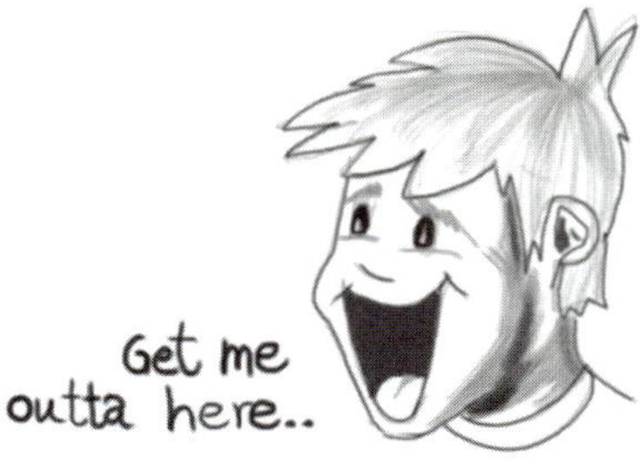

"Get me outta here!"
"Game over!"
"It's a match!"
"Are you OK?"
"That is not OK."
"Come on, guys!"

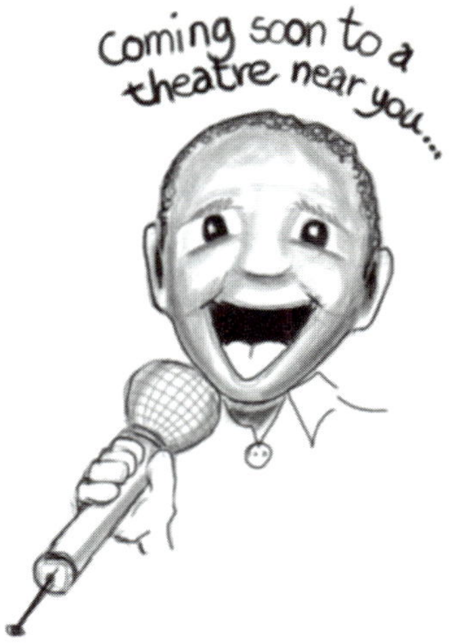

The next set sounds a little too theatrical to dismiss quite as easily as the first group. They might sound familiar, particularly the drumroll quality delivered with dramatic intonation:

"It's showtime!"
"Coming soon to a theater near you."
"And now, our feature presentation!"

Echolalia consists of the commonplace and the theatrical, whatever catches the ear and the heart of a child who processes them. That these same lines resurface later, under real-life conditions, is what makes them important to gestalt processors, and to us.

It's time to delve further.

Echolalila revisted: in the research

Until about twenty five years ago, we thought of delayed echolalia in ASD as deviant behavior, meaningless at best and a "self-stim" at worst. People tried to ignore it or extinguish it, and thought that kids could be taught "appropriate language" to take its place. Lovaas programs literally beseeched kids, "Don't echo," and tried to replace echolalia with rote statements like "I don't know" (Prizant, 1982).

Echolalia communicates.

But during the decade between 1980 and 1990, language researchers discovered the same thing that Cam's mother had discovered: echolalia can communicate. In 1984, Prizant and Rydell reported on their analysis of hundreds of delayed echolalic remarks and found that many of them serve the same communicative functions we associate with generative language. Rydell and Prizant found that most of ASD kids' echolalia fell into "fourteen functional categories," seven of which showed evidence of both interactiveness and comprehension. Those seven functions were labeling, providing information, calling, affirming, requesting, protesting, and directing. The researchers noted that in the case of these seven functions "there was clear evidence of communicative intent." Additionally, kids were seen as using echolalia to take a turn in conversation.

Rydell and Prizant outlined a process for helping kids move from echolalia to generative language.

With the evidence that echolalia serves the same communicative functions as other kids' language, many of us began to treat echolalia more respectfully. And because language researchers have reported that echolalia is used by "at least 85% of the children with autism who acquire speech," that was a good thing (Rydell and Prizant, 1995).

In 1993, Rydell and Prizant reported that their research subjects "frequently recombined and conjoined language chunks." Noting that "children with autism who acquire spoken language may be limited to an extreme form of a gestalt processing style," they outlined a process for helping kids move from echolalia to generative language. Their first step was to acknowledge the echoic utterances as communicative and promote their increased use for a variety of purposes.

Prizant et al. (1997) further commented on the usefulness of echolalia. "The majority of verbal children with autism use echolalia, the imitation of another person's speech, as a language-learning strategy." They stated that "echolalia of children with autism usually consists of longer and more rigidly repeated utterances, but appears to serve important communicative and cognitive functions for these children" (Prizant, Schuler, Wetherby, and Rydell, 1997). Finally, these researches noted that verbal ASD children "have been found to acquire grammatical and lexical aspects of language in the same general progression as typically developing children."

Research shows that ASD kids develop vocabulary and grammar and in the same order as typically-developing kids.

In 1999, Wetherby and Prizant presented assessment and intervention guidelines for "enhancing language and communication development in autism." As they noted, "many children learn to use these 'gestalt forms' purposefully in communicative interactions, and eventually are able to break down the echolalic chunks into smaller meaningful units as part of the process of transitioning to a rule-governed, generative language system." At the same time, research emphases expanded in the area of social aspects of communication in ASD, with increased focus on 'joint referencing' with gestures and language. Wetherby and Prizant stated that "children with autism in the early stages of communication and language development have been found to show limitations in the range of communicative functions espressed." Noting that in 1986 Wetherby had suggested that "the easiest and first emerging category of functions for these children is regulating others' behavior, whereas the most difficult is referencing joint attention," these authors recommended that "assessment should determine the sociability of communicative functions expressed."

But the autism community forgot, and replaced language development with teaching a little functional language.

At the same time, the number of children diagnosed with autism was growing at an unprecedented rate. While echolalia was well recognized as a diagnostic marker, the process of language development from echolalia to generative language seemed to have dropped out of sight. As behavioral therapy quickly expanded to address a growing need, the term "language learning" was used more commonly than "language development," and programs that taught specific pieces of functional language proliferated (Lovaas, 1981).

We all recognize echolalia—but what do we do about it?

The last decade feels like a kind of fast-forward in autism. The sheer number of kids with new diagnoses has challenged our educational systems, and we read in their IEPs our desperate attempts to help kids become communicatively connected with their environments. We also see our watered-down attempts at providing the growing population of ASD kids with at least a modicum of functional communication tools.

Program decisions often seem to reflect the challenges providers feel. Systems of choice-making have been devised to emphasize functional communication, either with or without language. Even when spoken or written language is addressed, the trend has still been towards ease of communication. Thus, functional language programs for kids with ASD have proliferated. And because behavioral therapy is so often used with children with autism, and it regards language is a behavior, a child is often taught to produce (or choose) something like "I want chips" soon after he can produce (or choose) "chips," without regard for the developmental appropriateness of the decision.

Those of us who believe that our kids with ASD can achieve much more have felt outnumbered as the term "functional speech" has proliferated in the autism community. Indirectly suggesting that our kids lack the capacity for normal language development, a set of learned survival phrases are selected as practical targets. Sadly, in the name of "function" our kids are short-changed, with little regard for their intellectual or linguistic potential.

In the name of "function" our kids are short-changed, with little regard for theirintellectual or linguistic potential.

In the midst of this trend, too few of us realize or remember that echolalia communicates, and even fewer of us know what to do about it. Since 2004, this author has written articles and given workshops to try to fill this gap. But until now we were lacking a complete source material for Speech-Language Pathologists and families to support their students step-by-step from echolalia to self-generated language.

This progression is embraced by Prizant et al. in *The SCERTS Model* (2006), however. Developed by Prizant and colleagues, SCERTS approaches social communication and emotional regulation in ASD children by targeting shared attention, affect, and intention. As children develop joint attention, SCERTS describes language as developing "from using primarily chunks of language to using more frequent mitigated echolalia ... and ... making novel combinations" (p. 41). The SCERTS assessment notes non-communicative echolalia giving way to communicative echolalia as a child develops from a "social partner" to a "language partner," and language becomes symbolic. Communicative gestalts become mitigated as joint attention develops.

But in the larger education and autism community this connection appears vague, and echolalia seems to represent an on going conundrum. For example, the *Practical Guide to Autism* (Volkmar and Wiesner, 2009) offered this: "Often, as language increases, unusual aspects of language also become more apparent. These can include echolalia ... Some children use idiosyncratic language ... some word or phrases whose meaning is unique to them" (p. 173). More often than not, echolalia seems to represent a conundrum.

Moving our kids forward

Echolalia often represents far more than a conundrum. Frequently seen as simply "self-stim" or "movie talk," its communicative value is rarely lauded: "Oh, Johnny is so communicative. When he's about to have a meltdown, he warns us by saying, 'Sharptooth attack!'" Think how foreign this sounds: "Johnny communicates effectively by saying, 'Back off!' when kids brush against him when they line up at the door."

And we rarely see gestalt language legitimized in an IEP goal: "The student will use his gestalt ("Back off!") with his peers 75% of the time when they are getting too close to him." Nor do we read a goal statement that encourages the pragmatic use of a child's echolalia: "The student will expand his pragmatic uses of gestalts to include 'Let's get out of here!' when he needs a sensory break, 'Hey, what's going on here?' when he has a question, and 'Game over' when he's done with his work."

We don't honor echolalia because we really don't like it.

The reason we don't encourage echolalia or want it to generalize, I think, is because we really don't like it. We have real trouble recognizing that echolalia has value. If we did, we would have to accept it, and we really don't want to. We don't think, "I'm excited about helping him use some other movie lines he seems to like." We wouldn't think that way because we don't really like echolalia at all.

Yes, we recognize it, and we might be entertained by it, but, quite honestly, we worry about it—and this determines our strategies for dealing with it. Our strategies, in fact, are almost exclusively limited to one of these alternatives: we try to ignore it or we actively try to make it stop. All too often we still call it "verbal stim" and assume that it can't be good. We just want it to go away and be magically replaced with "real" language.

If we recognized echolalia as valuable, we would have to acknowledge it when our kids used it.

Our children's birthright to develop language

Sadly, we've misplaced our past. As we valiantly try to replace our kids' echolalia, their natural language, we feel validated when they learn to say new things. We teach our kids a dozen functional phrases and sentences and feel satisfied that we have taught "functional speech." The tragedy is that while IEP goals are met, children's linguistic potential has been ignored—and undermined. We have forgotten how to assess a child's developmental language level and his capacity to develop generative language. And we have also failed to consider that the functional phrases we've taught might actually interfere with his potential to develop language competence. And in the process, the echolalia doesn't go away.

Teaching language can interfere with language development.

Bevin provides a good example. His IEP contained well-meaning goals which addressed teaching him more typical-sounding language, deemed the functional phrases that would help him communicate his needs. And he did learn some of this language. He could request, "Help me" when he got stuck. He could ask, "Where's Papa?" appropriately. Amidst his pervasive echolalia, Bevin had a good dozen sentences he'd been taught to say, and he was successful using them.

On further analysis, we can also see that Bevin learned these phrases—as gestalts. People had hoped they would represent "real language" that was different from the movie gestalts, but, to Bevin, they weren't. Each was learned and used as a whole phrase, just like "Back off!" or any other of the dozen movie phrases Bevin used at school. Bevin had learned a few new phrases that sounded more acceptable, but from a linguistic perspective they were still gestalts rather than building blocks of unique language.

All of us have probably put in our time teaching kids to say phrases like "Help me" or "I need help, please," that certainly do sound more like typical language. And some of them have great survival value and need to be a part of every child's repertoire. But think about what's wrong with this picture. Do kids who have been taught "Help me" ever say, "I need help, please" or vice versa? No, because each one is a different learned gestalt. Kids don't cross over between them grammatically because neither of them was acquired by the child via grammar. To carry this example a little further: does either group ever vary their request with, "I could use a little help now" or "Could you help me with this one?" Absolutely not, since again, their original phrase wasn't acquired grammatically, so kids have no way to use grammar to build a new phrase.

Since our friend, Bevin, was dutifully taught language that had nothing to do with grammar, it should be no surprise that none of the language he learned in his in-home intervention lead to developing, or even learning, more language. Each phrase he learned was an entity of its own and had nothing to do with developing a useful, flexible language system. Why? Because Bevin wasn't ready for anything but acquiring more gestalts. He wasn't ready for developing useful, flexible language, because that's actually a later step for a child who is a gestalt language processor. He was only ready for the first step, which is acquiring language gestalts. So, whether these gestalts were supplied by Walt Disney, his family, or his teachers, that's what he would learn.

Teaching language outside of a developmental progression fails to lead to developing more language.

It's time to reframe the misconceptions we have had about kids like Bevin who use echolalia. Being echolalic isn't what makes our kids different; it's being echolalic so late in their lives. Typical echolalic kids move on to the next stages by the time they're five years old. By the time they start school, they've been able to break down gestalts, use mix-and-match mitigations, and even isolate single words and start to build phrases and sentences. They might sound delayed, but not deviant. Kids like Bevin are delayed too—just by more years. That's what makes them different and stand out. They still need to go through the steps that other echolalic kids already have, and we need to recognize that and help them. Because their echolalia sounds so aberrant, we often don't think they have the capacity to develop language, that they are too "concrete," that they can't "generalize," or that they really don't want to. We surmise that if they are going to learn "functional speech," we need to teach it to them.

But now is the time to recognize what has really been going on with our kids. They picked up movie phrases because they could "see" the movie in their heads, internally "hear" the sound tracks, and use their speech skills to reproduce them. Maybe not all our kids could process language in real time, but with enough rewinds they learned plenty of language. In this light, we can now see how competent our kids actually are.

Gestalts are a powerful form of language—to gestalt language processors.

The irony is that using this same competence, our kids learn other gestalts: the ones taught through countless hours with well-meaning adults. So, in addition to their "movie talk" phrases, they now have another set of phrases we taught them. Indeed, once they've heard, "Can I have a turn?" a bazillion times, kids learn it—and use it. I'm sure you know the kind of gestalt I mean. "Ready, set, go" becomes so well-learned that kids never seem to be free of it.

Gestalts are a powerful form of language—at least to gestalt language processors!

Half of all young children are gestalt processors, often unrecognized because they cannot produce their long gestalts clearly.

So, what did we do when we tried to replace "movie talk" with other language? Inadvertently, we acknowledged our kids' ability to use gestalt language by teaching it to them. And, without realizing it, we proved that our kids are part of a large population of kids who are natural, normal gestalt language processors. We weren't actually aware that a huge group of neurotypical children are gestalt processors, but it's true. In fact, half of all young children are gestalt language processors, hard to recognize because their early lack of speech clarity renders their long gestalts impossible to understand. They sound more like jargon. But the legions of children, mostly boys, who eventually "catch up" with their peers, mostly girls, once processed and developed language from a gestalt perspective too.

There is an important segue here: our kids are not alone. A few people once knew this, but their knowledge appears long-buried. It is time to resurrect it, and make it relevant and useful to our current generation of kids. So, let's begin.

Life after echolalia

Barry Prizant, Amy Wetherby, Patrick Rydell, and others have long reported that kids on the spectrum are capable of moving beyond gestalts. With some understanding among the people around them, kids discover how to change those language wholes or gestalts, to mitigate them, and to recombine them more creatively.

Cases of individuals using mitigated echolalia as they develop language have been reported in our literature for over a century. And 40 years ago, young children who used echolalia were reported to mitigate it, or break it down, and recombine the parts to make the language their own. For too many decades, however, these reports seem to have remained within language research circles, buried under the plethora of information in the larger autism community. Today, too few people remember or understand it. That the SCERTS model acknowledges echolalia helps; now our kids need people around them who can directly help them with natural language development.

The mitigation process involves identifying shorter phrases and, eventually, words within sentences and mixing them in personal ways.

So, if we could help give our kids' language systems new life again, where should we start? We could start with this question: what is this process of mitigation and why is it important? Mitigation means changing the language that the child first heard, not just repeating it in its entirety, or gestalt, but changing it in some way. If the original song phrase was, "It's a whole new world," and the child says, "It's a whole new pizza," that's a mitigation. Or if the original jingle was, "Have it your way!" and the child says, "Have it my way!" that is a mitigation. Likewise, if the question was, "What do you want to do?" and the child counters, "You want to do—counting," that's a mitigation, too.

The mitigation process is natural but complex, and there is cause for celebration when kids accomplish it. It involves identifying shorter phrases and, eventually, words within sentences they've heard many times, and mixing them in personal ways. Kids who are gestalt processors eventually do this with all their language, and it is truly an awesome process. Neurotypical kids do it regularly, and our kids can do it too. We may need to support them, or at least not make the process more difficult. When we know what they're doing and why, that's all the help some of our kids need.

So, the next time your child rewinds and replays a short segment of a movie, consider that he's not just "stimming" on it (or trying to drive you crazy). He is actually trying to work on language development and communicating. He is isolating it from the whole story: isolating a bit of language so he can study it and use it. He's heard it so many times that he's found it in other places. He recognizes its commonality with other sources, and he's about to mitigate it.

And here's the proof: when you begin to hear not only "Let's get out of here! but "Let's get out of **there**!" your child has mitigated successfully. This example might not sound too sophisticated, but it will when you hear your child say, "Let's get **it** out of there!"

This amazing process just continues as long as people acknowledge it as meaningful, and no one interrupts it. Eventually, when a child can use many, many of these snippets of language in a mix-and-match fashion, he or she will be able to communicate with some flexibility.

Temple Grandin is one such person. She is a self-described "mitigator" who can describe the process of language recombination she has used. During a radio interview in 2005, Grandin was asked about her considerable success as a communicator. The interviewer began, "Tell me about the process that you went through to become as remarkably verbal as you are. You write early on that people said that you were a tape recorder. You had certain phrases that you said over and over again. And listen to you now!" (Conversations with Kathleen Dunn, Wisconsin Public Radio, 2005).

Grandin then described how mitigation worked in her own life: "Well, what happens is, as I put more and more and more information on the hard drive—and I do have a big hard drive; tiny processor, big hard drive—as I get more and more phrases on the hard drive, I can recombine them into different ways, and then it's less tape recorder-like …"

Grandin continued: "The thing is, it's a gradual learning. You know, you gradually just keep getting better and better and better, and … gradually get more and more insights. And more and more details are loaded onto the hard drive." It's hard for us to even imagine the complexity of the recombinations Grandin achieves, given the formidable size of her "hard drive."

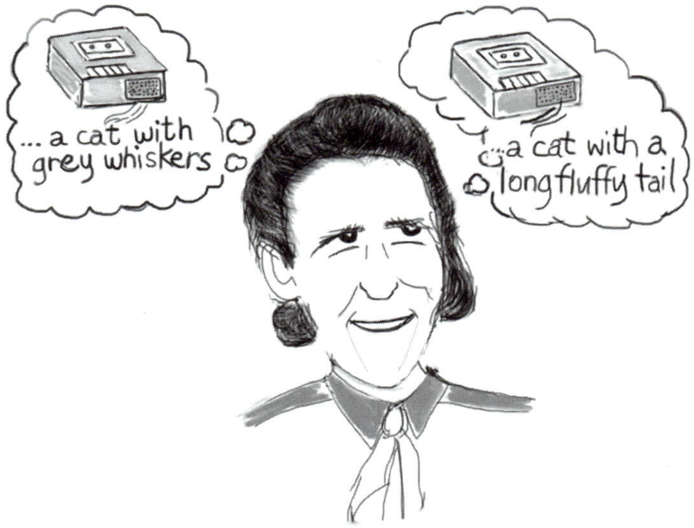

We are not all as gifted as Grandin, pictured above. So, fortunately, the process provides a short cut, which we'll describe as we return to the work of Prizant, Wetherby, and Rydell. As more and more phrases become separated out, a word itself can become isolated. Imagine the "recombinations" then. Well, that's exactly what we accomplish every day when we string words together in their infinite combinations. It's what grammar and vocabulary combine to do every minute of every day. We can actually "recombine" all the single words of our language—as long as the rules of grammar allow it—in an infinite number of ways. It is this infinite possibility that makes our language so rich and individual.

So, can our kids do this? And if they can, how can we help them?

Yes, our kids can do this too. It's a process of mental rewinding and hearing the commonalities of language. It's about mitigating out the parts and recombining them to be a bit more original. Next, it's about whittling it all down to the lowest common denominator of language: the word. At this point, these words become the building blocks of self-generated, grammatically-constructed sentences. Our kids' language begins to sound like what we'd hoped for all long: original, but very delayed.

If a child is echolalic, he will echo single words but not be able to build language with them.

But, no, they can't start with single words like analytical processors. That's not how their brains work, and if we try to teach them language that way, they will learn those single words as single gestalts, impossible to mitigate and impossible to build with. It doesn't speed up their process; it slows it down and lengthens it.

But now we need to hear it from the kids who have been there.

Putting the theory into practice

Eighteen years ago, when I was a Clinical Instructor at the University of Wisconsin Speech and Hearing Clinic, I read the information from Prizant et al. cited in the last section. As graduate students and I began working with Cam ("I love chocolate!") and other children like him, we applied these principles, realized how well the blueprint applied to them, and, best of all, how well it worked.

One of the children back in those days provided us with a beautiful case study, because we video-taped and transcribed almost all of his weekly therapy sessions. Dylan was nearly four years old, and he seemed to move through the stages of mitigation and self-generation in near-textbook fashion. At the time, however, I didn't realize there was no textbook. Nor did I realize that not everyone was treating ASD language this way. Limited longitudinal data existed, even though it had been a decade since Prizant had challenged SLPs to collect it. Dylan's story was more valuable than I realized.

A few years later, our clinic, the Communication Development Center (CDC), was born. There, Cam, Dylan, and others continued to grow, and the description of gestalt language development over time continued. It was time to do something with it.

In 2005, the stories of Dylan and his peers were presented in the *Autism Asperger's Digest* in a series of four articles, and the process of Natural Language Acquisition was explained. Since the time the articles were published, our Center has provided them for download to interested family members, SLPs, and others who work with ASD kids. Since that time, too, my colleagues and I have presented this material at various Autism Society conferences and other workshops. We have fine-tuned our assessment measure and have a protocol for its use that is clinically useful and user-friendly. And now, you will have the benefit of what we have learned in the process.

The stages of Natural Language Acquisition

There are six developmental stages in the Natural Language Acquisition process. Based directly on the pioneering research of Prizant et al., the steps have been demonstrated through longitudinal language sampling with children in our clinic between 1997 and the present.

An overview of the process is presented here, with a variety of illustrative examples taken directly from the stories of kids we have known over the years. We will then return to Dylan, whose process and progress is easy to see. Tables 1 and 2 display his evolving language as he moved through the stages, making the principles of the process clear.

To set the frame for what is to come, here are the six stages of Natural Language Acquisition. You will note that the process begins with the gestalts our kids pick up from their language sources—which, by the way, include us. Those gestalts are broken down in Stage 2 and further broken down in Stage 3. Single words begin to be recombined in Stage 3, and in Stages 4–6 those recombinations occur with the benefit of grammatical rules.

Stage 1: Use of gestalt language wholes
Stage 2: Mitigation of wholes into phrases; recombinations of phrases
Stage 3: Isolation of single words; recombinations of single words

Stage 4: Beginning grammar
Stage 5: More advanced grammar
Stage 6: More complex grammar

Stage 1: Use of gestalt language wholes

Stage 1 is when our kids use multi-word language gestalts lifted in their entirety from elsewhere.

Stage 1 is when kids use multi-word language gestalts lifted from elsewhere in their entirety. It's all or nothing at Stage 1, and kids can't use these gestalts any other way. The language wholes can be phrases, sentences, paragraphs, songs, or entire movie scenes. They can be so monsterously long that young children can't say them with any clarity, and they often go unrecognized as language at all.

Unfortunately, these often-unintelligible sound bytes seem like nothing more than "jargon" or "stims," but, once kids can say them better, we start to recognize them as jingles, slogans, or other language we've heard before. As they become easier for kids to say, parents begin to recognize where some of these often-repeated lines came from.

I can remember one of the first retrospective stories I heard from a parent, a meticulous mom who kept a journal of everything that happened in her young child's life. When Cam was two years old, he said something that sounded like **"Uh poo"** and other things Kay disregarded as babble or jargon. Because she was so meticulous, though, Kay wrote them down. And, two years later, Cam was regularly naming the characters from *Winnie the Pooh*, until, you guessed it, Kay realized "uh poo" was "the Pooh."

So, the next question is about this language kids lift from their media or from other people: is it meaningful to them?

Our kids' first gestalts often come from the sound tracks that run through their minds as they mentally watch movies.

Yes, it turns out, even if it was two years later that Kay discovered that Cam loved Winnie the Pooh and wanted desperately to refer to this little bear and his friends. Prizant et al. had also figured this out, and from them we know that kids use gestalt language for a great variety of reasons. At first, though, the language seems to just course through the minds of our visual children as they replay movies in their minds. The sound is something like the "fast forwarding" you might recognize as you listen to your children. A string of sound of this type is more like a sound track, until a child finds what he wants and pulls out some chosen language. At this point, a child might be trying to understand something about the movie or something about the sound—or he might be practicing saying it—or he might be communicating.

Cam's mom eventually learned that when he said "Uh Poo," Cam was communicating, but exactly what he meant was unclear. His mitigated phrase seemed to her to be a declaration of love somehow, but, like all early words, the exact meaning to the child who says them is unclear. And, communicating with gestalts can be even more fuzzy, since the phraseology comes lifted straight from the movie, the book, or the song. What the original song meant to Cam is hard to know.

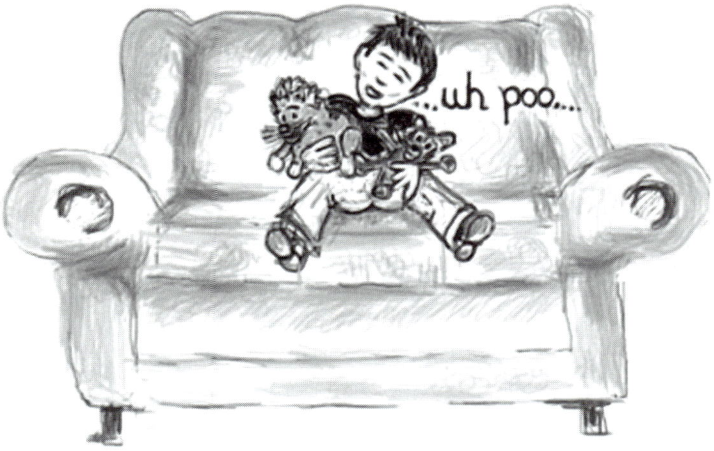

So, language gestalts can communicate. This is wonderful, of course, but doesn't necessarily help the deciphering process. Understanding the meaning behind these sometimes-odd expressions takes some detective work and translation.

Here's one hint: nothing at Stage 1 can be taken literally. The following examples will show you what we mean. Because each has been lifted in its entirety from one context to another, they're not an exact fit for a child's specific circumstances. All but one are real examples from children we know. See if you can guess at the translations.

Nothing at Stage 1 can be taken literally.

Examples of Stage 1 communicative gestalts

The first example, used by many children we know, is **"And now for our feature presentation."** Once you have heard this line numerous time after watching previews of your child's movies with him, you get the gist of the meaning to an eager child: "Here it comes; this is what we've been waiting for; here's the main event." The kids we know who used this language gestalt communicated the arrival of an important event or topic this way.

"You gotta love it!" says another young friend of ours, and this, too, is fairly easy to interpret when it is applied to a particular referent.

"Let's get outta here!" is another common expression used more or less specifically, depending on the sophistication of the child using it. A little "rough around the edges," maybe, but this one effectively communicates that a child needs to be taken seriously about the conditions at hand.

"This can't be good," says another child. A fairly transparent comment, it's true, but certainly stronger than this child probably meant when he said it. Of other expressions kids say that sound a little more extreme than they actually meant, **"What a nightmare!" "That's stupid!"** and **"Never!"** quickly come to mind.

"Welcome to my world" is certainly a transparent greeting, if more grand than probably intended. **"Welcome. You've got mail!"** is a little less "welcoming" and causes the listener to come away with a question mark more than a feeling of being greeted.

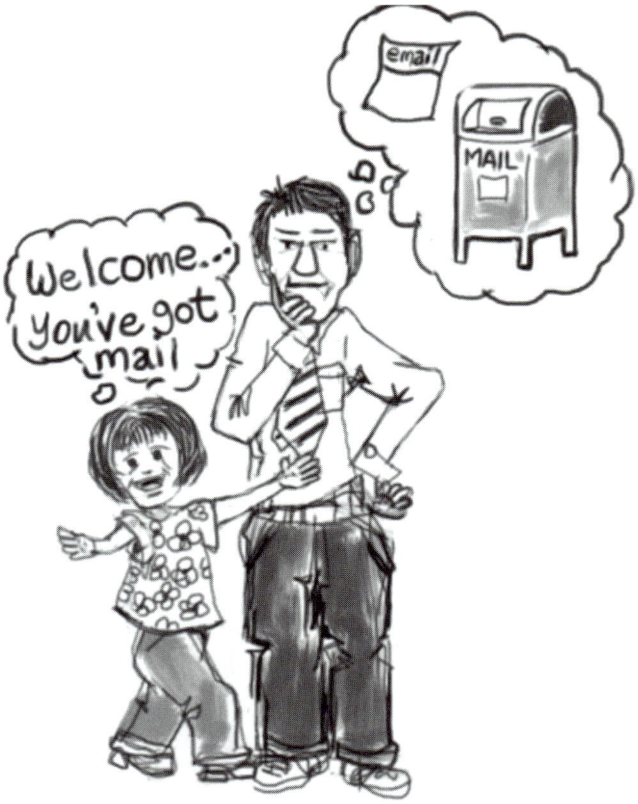

"Back off!" is a gestalt I have heard many times, and it still induces a little recoiling. I know not to take it literally, but it's hard not to feel offended if you are the one who was trying to help. I try to remind myself before my reaction shows that it's not about me; that the child in front of me is communicating something important; that it is my job as the adult to listen and to read between the lines.

"Available December 9th, wherever videos are sold" might not be used by a child who wants a video, especially in this post-video era, but rather by a child who wants to procure something else he hopes will become available regardless of the date. Remember not to take any gestalt literally!

There is no grey; there are no shades of meaning at Stage 1.

"I don't think so!" is common in adult conversation, and coming from a child sounds pretty cute. That it means 'no' is apparent, but what is not apparent is that your child probably means it to be more adamant than the words, taken literally, suggest. This is a good example of the 'all or nothing' principle of gestalts. You get it full barrel, as in **"Shut up!"** or so polite as to mask the meaning completely. There is no grey; there are no shades of meaning at Stage 1. We have that to look forward to at Stage 2, but it is all raw footage at Stage 1.

Another example is **"Well??"** used to seek more information. It's also pretty cute, but its use by a child might belie how desperately he wants to find out more! To reiterate, it's communicative but not to be taken literally!

As these examples show, once kids spend enough time at Stage 1 and have amassed enough language gestalts in their minds for them to live there, it's no longer just about the material they came from. The language starts to develop a life and a legitimacy of its own. Yes, listeners might need to know the source in order to understand the feeling behind the words, but as the language is used in multiple situations it takes on more shades of meaning in various life situations.

Now let's see what our textbook friend, Dylan, was producing at Stage 1. Dylan had many Disney-style gestalts, some too long to understand, but other short ones we could. **"Sh, there's Aladdin. Quick!"** and **"Take that!"** peppered his play, giving it a dramatic quality. In the clinic, we were careful to surround him with language gestalts that were easy to break down and, eventually, recombine. Since we supplied the right language at just the right moment in play, Dylan picked up several of our language models in the first month of therapy. And since we wanted them to be useful to him when he was ready to move from Stage 1 to Stage 2, we picked language that could be mitigated when the time was right, e.g., **"Let's get out of here!"** and **"Want some more?"**

In our sessions, we made sure Dylan had meaningful play opportunities to hear and use these social sentences and others like them. We wanted to make sure Dylan liked our gestalts and that they matched his communicative intentions. We wanted to make sure he would use them often so he could discover the component parts they shared with other gestalts. In this way, he'd be able to engage play partners with these social sentences, and, once he recombined parts of them at Stage 2, have lots of language material to move more flexibly into the future.

Stage 2: Mitigation of phrases and recombinations

When language becomes separate from its original contexts at Stage 1, kids start to hear it and use it as their own language. It's not just language the character in the movie or the therapist in the clinic uses. As a child gets used to saying it himself, it becomes his own language.

Once a child has amassed enough similar language in his mind, he starts to hear the embedded pieces that are shared from one gestalt to another.

And, once a child has amassed enough similar language in his mind, he starts to hear the embedded pieces that are shared from one gestalt to another. Kids who once could hear only the larger gestalt start to hear smaller chunks within larger wholes. This is the process of mitigation.

For Dylan, one example is **"Let's get"** as heard in "Let's get out of here," "Let's get something to eat," and "Let's get going," all invitations to action that the child finds important. "Let's get" becomes sifted out and the original sentences become mitigated or "softened" from their rigid meanings, so at least a part of each can be used in different ways.

Let's look more closely at how Dylan accomplished this task through the threads of language in the following table:

Stage	Example
1 – Communicative use of whole language gestalts	"Let's get out of here." "Want some more?"
2 – A. Mitigation into chunks	(1) "Let's get" + "out of here" (2) "Want" + "some more?"
2 – B. Recombining these chunks	(3) "Let's get + some more?" (4) "Want + out of here."
3 – A. Further mitigation: isolation of single words	"get", "more", "want", "out"
3 – B. Recombination of single words as two-word phrases	(1) "Get—more." (2) "Want—out?"
4 – Generation of first sentences	"Hey, I got some more." "You wanna go outside?" "Come on—we gotta play inside."

Table 1: The First Four Stages of Natural Language Acquisition

This table shows how tidy Dylan's progress looked once we analyzed it, and how it could be predicted because of the easy-to-mitigate gestalts we surrounded him with. Outside of planned intervention, however, it can be quite individual which phrases become kids' first mitigations. We hope that first experiences with language contain enough commonalities and enough positive connotation that there will be many such phrases that get parsed out. We can plan this for kids, of course, and certainly do so once we realize how important it is and how much it matters to our kids' language development. Now that we begin to understand how Stage 2 is the platform to flexible language, we would prefer not to leave it to Walt Disney to give our children the bulk of the language commonalities they can find.

Imagine the power at this stage of development. Kids are no longer stuck with unmodifiable language and able to say only things like, "Let's get out of here!" as a way to suggest another idea. They no longer risk being misunderstood when all they really meant was "Let's do something else now." At Stage 2, they can take the softer "Let's get" and maybe even use it to invite others to join them in different pursuits. Imagine, in our example, that they have also been saying, "Ready, set, go!" with enough understanding to mitigate it, too, and take the words "set, go" out of the whole. If they have "Let's get" from one gestalt and "set, go" from another, then they might be able to say, "Let's get—set, go!" The grammar is a little rough, to be sure, but you can see what I mean about power.

Stage 2 is the mix and match stage.

Stage 2 is the mix and match stage. The results are softer, less rigid, more original, and a pure delight for you and for your child.

But, a caveat is in order here. Looking at the list of gestalts cited above, consider how many, many movies our kids would have to watch to realize that there are commonalities among gestalts, much less to figure out what they are. The thought is overwhelming. Most movie songs and dialogues don't mitigate very readily, and that's a big problem for our kids. Movies can be great, of course, when real life goes by too fast for our kids to hear. And rewind can be a blessing when our kids don't have the motor control to engage in many real-life interactive conversations. Think of all the other little boys you have known and consider the many hours of play they naturally engage in. It takes that kind of language immersion to hear and learn from the gestalt language of real life.

As you tune into your own family's mealtime conversation, you hear multi-generational chatter that might sound like this: "Can I have some more bread, Mom?" "After you finish your peas." "But I don't like peas this way, Mom!" "I just found that out, darling. But more bread isn't going to change that." "Oh, Mom …" "Oh, darling …"

Imagine that if you were able to process this language in real time, you would learn that "oh" was common in this family's language repertoire, that "Mom" and "darling" were too, and that "but" was a word people used in animated exchanges. "Peas" was associated with unpleasantness, and "bread" was a mystery.

And as you tune into sandbox play between a neurotypical boy and his friend next door, you hear animated exchanges filled with sound effects, long strings of intonation mixed with a modicum of recognizable words: "Heeeeey—Woody, you wanna fly?" "Nooooooo!" "Whaaaaaat?" "OK, Buzz, geeeeet your rocket!" "Whoooo. Whooo!" "Whoa, aaaa, get out of here, you toys!" "Whoooooaaaa!" "Heeeey, this is my house, you got it?" "Nooooo, that's mine!" "Nooooo; I had it first." "It's miiiiiine! Waaaaaa! Get your oooooown Woody."

And as you listened to the language these children use, you would also learn that Buzz and Woody spoke in ways off screen that were completely different from how they spoke on screen, and that when they shared sandbox time, the former language style predominated. It's easier for little kids to say, of course, and much more flexible. But even neurotypical boys attempt to articulate "To infinity and beyond!" with more or less success; and yes, even typical boys have no idea what it means outside of the limited movie context. They just know, like our ASD kids do, that it is grand and glorious, and a wonderful thing for two friends to yell when they are as close as Buzz and Woody.

While typical boys play from sun-up until sun-down, our kids tend to lack the motor coordination to play at all and rarely stay focused on conversations long enough to hear the commonalities.

But the language similarities from the sandbox to our kids' worlds stop there. While typical boys play from sun-up until sun-down, our kids tend to lack the motor coordination to play at all and rarely stay focused on either family conversations or kid conversations long enough to hear the commonalities. Most of them miss the opportunities to learn to mitigate in real time and need the many, many rewinds of *Toy Story* to hear the same phrase in more than one context. When they learn that "Hey, guys!" is spoken by many characters in many situations, it can become a nice mitigation from the longer dialogue. But movie language isn't the language of real life, so the gestalts and mitigations our kids use have a theatrical quality to them and often sound more rough-and-tumble than the kids intend. I remember going back and counting how many times "Shut up!" was used in a popular kids' movie, trying to figure out why so many ASD kids said it. Amazingly, I heard it in "friendly" dialogue more than a dozen times, and I understood how our kids found it so "socially acceptable" and just as viable an expression as "Hey, guys!!"

But not all language is created equal, and movie extractions make our kids stand out—and often get them in trouble. Certainly they have enough challenges without "innocent" phrases like "Back off, bozo!" and "Take that, sucker!" causing undo calamity.

You will become the human rewind as you pepper sentences with common phrases like "Let's get ..." and "Hey, we can ..." throughout your day.

That's where you fit in. You now know what kind of language matters to your child's language development process and how you can help. You know you can, and should, present everyday language in exciting ways and set up a language-rich household your child can learn from. When you do that, your child will not have to depend on movies for his language enrichment. You will become the human rewind as you pepper sentences with common phrases in them like "Let's get ..." and "Hey, we can ..." and "How about ..." and "I wanna see ..." throughout your day. You will be able to set up language experiences that are tailored to the gestalt processor in your midst and give him the head start he needs to get from Stage 1 to Stage 2—and then Stage 3.

A wonderful mother-author writing at her blog, MOM-Not Otherwise Specified, has added to our common experience through ongoing stories of her son, Bud. On March 20, 2006, she posted that the "Finding the Words" series had been recommended to her:

> "It was in the midst of this transformation that I attended a workshop led by SLP Barry Prizant, and during one of the breaks I told him about Bud's increasingly complex modification of movie scripts. Dr. Prizant told me that Bud was using 'mitigated echolalia,' and that it was an excellent prognostic indicator for future language development.
>
> "'I'll bet you'll start seeing spontaneous language soon,' he said. 'We already are,' I said. Dr. Prizant smiled and said, 'And I think you'll probably see a lot more.' He pointed me in the direction of some great articles on echolalia. One of them was "Finding the Words" by Marge Blanc in the May–June 2005 issue of *Autism Asperger's Digest* magazine. The article talked about 'gestalt language acquisition,' or exhibiting delayed echolalia with whole sentences repeated verbatim. I read the article with fascination: it seemed that she was writing about Bud."

In fact, Bud's Stages 1–4 sounded much like Dylan's. Here are examples from the blog:

Stage 1: **"Quick, Dipsy. Help Laa Laa catch the ball!"**

Stage 2: (a) **"Quick + Daddy. Help Mama + catch the ball!"**
(b) **"Daddy catch the ball!"**
Stage 3: **"Daddy ball?"**
Stage 4: **"I playing ball with you, Daddy!"**

Yes, Bud's language development process looked pretty neat and tidy, like Dylan's, once it was analyzed and written down. Of course, real life feels much fuzzier and messier, but that's because our kids are working on many, many mitigations at once. Please remember, though: that's what makes this a developmental process, and not just learning a phrase or a script. The beautiful thing is that the process is a natural one. When we support it in our kids, we give them the benefit of tapping into what is right for them!

Stage 3: Isolation of single words and recombinations

With Bud's progression in our minds, let's now revisit Table 1 and recall Dylan's Stage 1 gestalts and Stage 2 mitigations so we can put Stage 3 in context. This stage is really a refinement of the mitigation process. It is the stage where phrases are further broken down, this time into single words. Notice that the Stage 2 mitigation "Let's get ..." was further mitigated into single words "let's" and "get." Just like his jump to Stage 2, Dylan's jump to Stage 3 occurred once he had spent lots of time at Stage 2 and heard lots of examples with each of these kinds of phrases: "Let's go," "Let's not," "Let's try it," "Let's cut that," and "Get it," "Get me," "Get some more," "Get it out."

At the same time, Dylan was separating out "more" from "some more," because he had heard enough phrases such as "one more," "no more," and "lots more" so that "more" was becoming a meaningful language component to him. This was the bridge to Stage 3.

Stage 3 is about combining concepts: about thinking and mental gymnastics.

Stage 3 language is mostly single words, but remember these single words came from gestalt sources and derive their richness and meaning from the ways they were used in context. Our kids are context kids, and we sell them short when we try to make them be something else. With well-meaning hearts, we'd love to bypass Stage 1 and 2 mitigation and "just teach them how to talk." And even when our efforts seem to have some initial success, they don't promote language development. We are excited when our kids learn "more" and can sign and say it to get more swinging, more chips, and more tickles, but then we are dismayed when it doesn't lead to more language. Now you know why. When our kids are yearning for Stage 1 gestalts, "more" is just one more. It doesn't become part of a new sentence any more than "To infinity and beyond" does. Gestalts are supposed to be broken down, not added to.

But, when we do it right and support our kids in the natural way their brains were intended, Stage 3 single words are true building blocks for self-generated simple phrases built from scratch. At Stage 3, our kids are able to form original recombinations of single words like their analytical sisters did. When our kids can combine "get" + "more," they can form two-word combinations which sound like those of other, albeit younger, children. And they are fully original. While "Get more" may not sound like much, especially when we're used to our

The more kids experiment with creatively combining words, the more they creatively combine concepts.

kids saying, "To infinity and beyond," it's original. And, although it sounds far less grammatical than Stage 1 or Stage 2 language, it demonstrates progress.

When kids get to this stage, parents often relax. It just sounds so "normal." Granted, it's late in coming, and, depending on how old he is when he gets there, a child may sound misplaced among his peers. But he's not using just gestalts any more, and that is music to our ears.

Part of the communicative flexibility at Stage 3 comes from the sheer variety of word combinations possible in our language. The sky is the limit. No, that's not true: the possibilities are limitless. And before the specificity of grammar rules ties our kids into patterns at Stage 4, we want them to spend lots and lots of time in this mix and match of words. The more kids experiment with creatively combining two and three words, the more they creatively combine concepts. This kind of mental gymnastics provides a way of looking at the world conceptually and linguistically, and Stage 3 nicely sets the foundation for further spontaneous language development.

The more varied these two-word combinations are, the easier it will be for Stage 4 grammar to express real meaning.

We will talk much more about Stage 3 later in this book, but for now it is enough to know that a rich environment provides the material for a rich experience with the mix and match of concepts and words. These combinations are grammar-free, and the more varied these two-word combinations are, the easier it will be for Stage 4 grammar to express real meaning and keep kids from falling into the scripting trap of canned phrases and sentences

Stages 4, 5, and 6: Use of grammar

Experience with two-word combinations is rich and rewarding, and once kids develop competence and variety at Stage 3, they have the whole world of grammar ahead of them. Grammar includes a few layers early on at Stage 4, but continues to develop complexity at Stages 5 and 6. As they develop grammatical competence, our ASD kids look very much like every other language learner, albeit older.

Depending on their age and the sources of language—particularly vocabulary—they have to work with, there are some differences for a while. But at Stage 4, our kids can start to develop grammatical sentences and can begin to sound like we thought kids ought to sound.

We will go into great depth about Stages 3–6 in Chapter 5. For now, a brief illustration will show you the path language takes through all six stages. Table 2 follows a thread common to Dylan's utterances. While I was not privileged to work with Dylan after Stage 4, I know he did well in public school Speech and Language, and so the threads of his sentences will be continued here as they would have in Stage 5 and Stage 6.

Yes, there's much more to the story, but the outline is now complete. And, yes, there's plenty more to learn about it, but please remember this natural process is what neurotypical gestalt processors do all by themselves. No, your child isn't Dylan, nor does he necessarily have the same kind of support. But I can tell you from eighteen years of experience that our kids can do it, if we know when to help and how. I promise that we will show you how. As you pick and choose among the chapters of this book, you will find ample illustrations that will remind you of your own child and give you a sense of camaraderie with others who are in the same boat with you.

Stage	Example
1 – Communicative use of whole language gestalts	"Let's get out of here." "Want some more?"
2 – A. Mitigation into chunks	(1) "Let's get" + "out of here" (2) "Want" + "some more?"
2 – B. Recombining these chunks	(3) "Let's get + some more?" (4) "Want + out of here."
3 – Further mitigation: isolation of single words; recombination of words, and generation of original two-word phrases	"Get—more." "Want—out?"
4 – Generation of first sentences	"Let's get some more toys!" "You wanna go out?" "Hey, we gotta go back in!"
5 – Generation of more complex sentences	"I don't want any more, but you can have mine." "How long do you wanna play outside?" "I know what to do: play inside!"
6 – Generation of the most complex sentences	"Do I really have to go out to play today?" "How 'bout if you go out and play instead?" "When do you wanna come in, 'cuz that's what I want to do."

Table 2: The Six Stages of Natural Language Acquisition

Dylan compared with your child

First of all, I will grant you that the examples above may seem a little too neat and tidy to remind you of any of our older kids. And perhaps Dylan's Stage 1 gestalts sound like a dream compared with your child's. But remember that Dylan was a preschooler and hadn't learned many mega-gestalts. Besides that, he had the best of all worlds. He got to play with eager graduate students at a University clinic, students who could provide great language models, listen to him, and see how their intervention was working. We carefully chose the language Dylan was exposed to in our clinic, presented it from his perspective, and, as best we could, matched it to his intentions. We wanted Dylan to be motivated to use our language models and use them a lot so he could hear their commonalities and eventually mitigate them.

So, knowing Dylan, we picked sentences like "Let's go outside," "Let's get the toys," "Let's find the big ball," and "Let's see what's in here." In this way, we were surrounding him with language that satisfied all our criteria: it would serve his needs, it would be easy to mitigate, and, not coincidentally, it would sound good to people, so he would get some nice feedback from family and friends early on. The process with Dylan worked in textbook fashion. But of course, the "textbook" hadn't been written back then; it's the one you are reading right now, and it is Dylan's example that is at its core.

But back to your concern. You might be thinking, "Dylan's echolalia barely sounds wrong at all and certainly doesn't sound like my child's. My child sounds like the examples you gave earlier; you know, the kind that are hard to mitigate. Besides, you could understand Dylan. No one can understand my child! If his sister didn't know *The Lion King* forwards and backwards, we wouldn't even know where our child's 'gestalts,' as you call them, came from!"

Yes, you are absolutely right, but not to worry. True, only the younger children can move through the stages as neatly and as predictably as Dylan. Rest assured, however, that we know lots of kids who are very much like your child, and they make good progress, too. And, yes, you will learn how to help your child make his own progress! You will learn how to introduce appropriate language models to your child from his perspective. You will learn what to do with the gestalts your child has already learned from his environment. And, yes, your child will be able to mitigate: not like Dylan, or Bud, but mitigate nonetheless—like your child!

And your child, too, will be able to continue language development, moving through the stages of Natural Language Acquisition. It's natural, and that's part of the reason it will happen. You will help, and that's the other part of the reason.

How you will help: assessing and modeling language

Sections 3 and 6 will cover how you can help, but here's a sneak preview.

Even at this early stage of the game, you might feel comforted to know something about how you will be assessing and supporting natural language development: the methods, materials, and, especially, what you will look for that will tell you are doing the right thing and your child is making progress. We will cover this in more detail in Sections 3 and 6, but I can imagine you will feel more relaxed if you knew something about this now.

If your child is vocal and you can hear some jargon or maybe even the hint of words, there is a sequence you can follow to get started. If, however, you cannot tell that there is anything resembling the sounds of singing or talking, you might want to skip to Chapter 9, which is intended to help you get started with silent kids.

But for those of you who can detect that your child is singing or speaking something that sounds like jargon, you will want to try this:

Listen intently to your child.

- First, listen intently to your child for a few half-hour periods of time. You may need to have another person there with your child so you can simply spend your time listening. If you can make a sound recording of your child, all the better. The first time you do this, you will just listen without expecting that you will understand anything. You will notice your child's environment and watch for clues to meaning: What movie is he watching? What are the melodies and songs that go with that movie? What is the sound track like? Which book is he looking at? Which part is he looking at while he's talking? Do you hear any song melodies or signature phrases, or any intonation that identifies the original character who said the lines. Can you find any matches in his environment?

- While you are listening, or later on with your notes or sound recording, learn to 'sound like your child.' Say or sing your child's melodies with your lips and in your mind. Hear your child in your head. Hear him well enough that, with some practice time in the shower, you can sound like him. Whenever you have something to write down, do so. Take notes with squiggles and lines to remind yourself what his melodies sound like. A trick I taught myself over the years is to quietly play a child's sound on a toy piano. After a while you will recognize recurring themes and, even if you are as tone-deaf as I am, hear 'middle C' again and again.

Learn to 'sound like your child.'

- Next, sit down with your notes and see if you can make any sense of them. If you have a sound recording, listen again. Or watch his favorite movie again. Or read the book again. Does anything ring a bell or sound like a match? If not, go back to the original excercise and spend another half hour with your child, but this time make sure you record everything with an audio recorder or movie camera. This will give you something to listen to later on and jog your memory about what you heard. Did this help, as you listened to it later?

Find a match in your child's environment.

- If you came away with something, great; you can move on. If not, you will want to continue the first exercise. Don't worry if you don't have any clues yet: this process will eventually pay dividends, because you will learn the source of your child's language.
- Once you have found a match, try for some others. Once you have 3–5, report them to someone else. You will solidify your thinking by talking about it out loud. Be sure to keep your notes so you can begin to put together a journal of your child's language.
- Now that your ears are starting to become well-tuned, you are ready to try a language activity with your child. You're going to remain a listener, a quiet one at first, but you will be engaging with your child. Just quietly be with your child; this will let him know you are listening and interested. Does he continue vocalizing, knowing he's being listened to? Does he sound the same? If so, you can move on to the next step: adding some vocalization. If he seems different once you've joined him, however, you might need to move back so he doesn't perceive that you are "expecting" something of him.
- After some minutes go by, join your child vocally. Try out quietly repeating your child's sounds or language here and there. Even if you don't get it at all, you will be amply rewarded the first time he looks you straight in the eye as if to say, "What? You're listening?" This is a heavenly feeling for both the child and the adult.

You will be amply rewarded the first time your child looks you straight in the eye as if to say, "What? You're listening?"

- If you get that much reward from your child, keep going as long as you and your child are enjoying the process. The more you stay in the

It takes two to communicate, and when you became a gestalt translator, you became that second person.

conversation with your child, the easier it will become. As it becomes easier, you will relax, and your child will feel that relaxation.

- Before too long, your child may give you eye contact of an even deeper variety. More than just a startled reaction, your child may actually look at you with a surprised, delighted look, one that I have dubbed the "Bingo!" expression. It says, in essence, "Bingo, Mom. You got it!" What pleasure that is for both parties.
- Now you are on the road, and your child will look forward to sharing "conversation" with you, because it really is conversation. It is two-person sharing: the dance of reciprocity. And as your confidence in yourself grows, you will get better and better at it until you may find yourself understanding some things your child says.
- The next step is equally exciting: you realize what your child meant by something he said! You will suddenly realize that "wone chew say" is actually "won't you say," which is part of Barney's song: "Won't you say you love me too." Translated, that says, "I love you" and is an invitation to you to tell your child you love him. Congratulations! You have now become a gestalt translator.
- As your repertoire of translations grows, you will find that you and your child are truly communicating, and you will have discovered with surprise that it wasn't your child who changed anything. It was you! Yes, it takes two to communicate, and you became the second person.

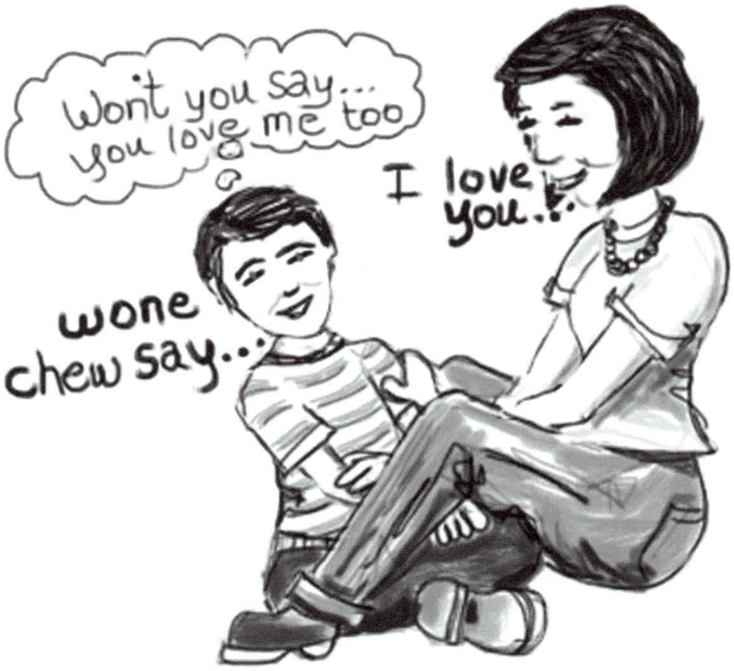

A story from MOM-Not Otherwise Specified illustrates the process this mom used with her son, Bud:

> "So I learned the scripts, and climbed into his fantasy world with him. I tried to engage him in dual-scripting—you say one line, I'll say the other—to approximate the reciprocal flow and give-and-take of conversation. I worked with him to develop scripts of our own—private jokes that we shared with each other. And whenever I could, I looked for the moments when he was well regulated and I tossed a little chaos into the creation, hoping to provide just enough dissonance to move him forward a bit, to expand the possibilities of language, to help him consider that there could be more to talking than scripting alone."
>
> The story continues: "Bud continued to script, but as time passed I noticed a clear evolution in his scripting. It became less random. He began to assess his surroundings and select the script he had that best fit the circumstance. So if he wanted to play ball, he would approach us with ball in hand and say 'Quick, Dipsy. Help Laa Laa catch the ball.' After more time passed, he began to modify his scripts … (and) swap out the pertinent details, so that 'Quick, Dipsy. Help Laa Laa catch the ball' would become 'Quick, Daddy. Help Mama catch the ball.'
>
> "As his talent to modify scripts became more sophisticated … Bud's confidence seemed bolstered by his ability to be understood …(which) allowed him to start taking risks with language and start putting words together on his own. Using creative, spontaneous language was much more difficult for Bud and took a great deal more time than it did for him to assess a situation, mentally thumb through hours of memorized scripts to find the most relevant script to the given situation, and modify the script by swapping out a few details. As a result, his creative speech was much slower and less polished than his modified scripts. But, in time, 'Quick, Daddy. Help Mama catch the ball" became 'Daddy ball?'."

Now, with Bud's story to remind us of the steps we took with Dylan, we are ready to return to Bevin. Even though he was quite a bit older than Dylan or Bud, I approached him in much the same way. Now let's continue our story to the first time I met Bevin.

Chapter 2
Back to Bevin: Out of the "Textbook" and into Real Life!

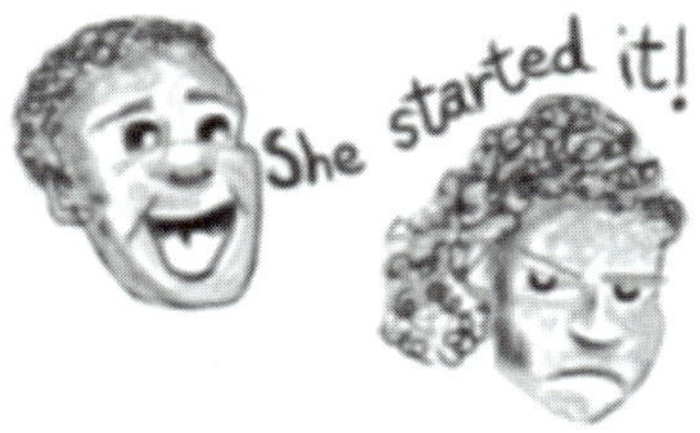

Just "turn off the movie!"

Back in the Introduction, we left Bevin (age 10) with his family, who wanted him to "turn off the movie." He actually did sometimes, to try to please his family. The trouble was, though, that when he did, he had precious little else to say.

I decided to spend the afternoon with Bevin and his family, and to see first-hand how Bevin communicated, what his echolalia sounded like, and what his interactions looked like. Bevin's family was wonderful. Their life together was a rich tapestry of talk, song, play, love, food, and good times. And Bevin did communicate many times, at least forty times in two hours. While these communiqués could easily be overlooked among the hundred of other lines, they were there. Sometimes Bevin communicated with movie lines, sometimes not. And his family was right, of course: he did use tons of "movie talk!" I could see how his family could get worn out. But he was a delight, and I couldn't wait to see him again. That would happen the next week.

I learned something important during my first two-hour home visit: if I waded through the echolalia and didn't give up listening, I could hear that Bevin really did have a small assortment of comments he could apply at the right time. He even had some jokes and dialogues he and his family had developed together. Bevin would tease his sister by calling to his mother, **"She started it!"** Tori would playfully retort that, no, she hadn't done a thing. Bevin would take another turn, and they would go on and on until one or the other was tired of the game.

In another game, Bevin would turn to someone and say, out of the blue, **"Shut up!"** The second person would laugh and say something in response, and Bevin would reply, "Shut up!" This game, too, could go on for as long as there were players.

Bevin knew some "survival" language, too. He knew how to ask for help and used at least a dozen learned sentences that served him fairly well. Some of these, like **"Will you help?"** had been taught directly by teachers or in-home therapists. Others, like **"Stop it!"** were whole lines, or gestalts, taken from movies, stories, or life.

During my first home visit, I got to hear, **"Let's get out of here!"** which served to ask permission to go outside. Other echoed lines used communicatively included:

Look at your watch.
Watch out!
Yikes!
Run, Simba—run away!
Ready, set, go!
Uh—what is this?

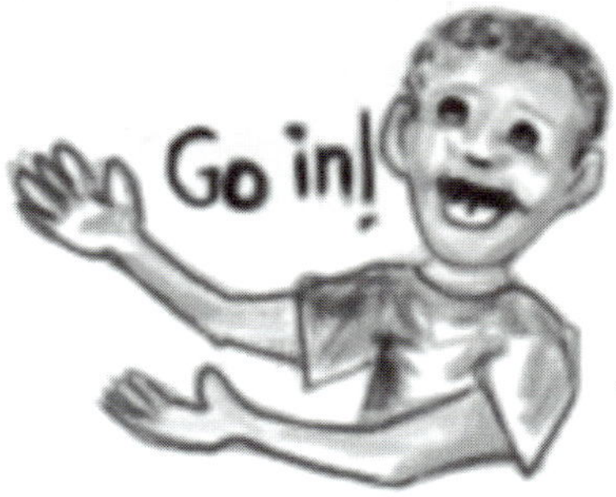

Echoed lines that Bevin used without clear communicative intent included:

What's all this?
Oh, thank you, man.
They're trying to take over.
That's what I heard.

Still other comments were Bevin's own reductions of lines, or mitigations, such as:

He burping.
I coming.
Go in!

There were also a few isolated single words used communicatively:

Terrible!
Banana.
Pizza.

But he's still echoing everything!

It was good that Bevin had a little variety but not surprising that his family saw him as simply echolalic. Because Bevin talked all the time, it was tedious to sift through everything to find the original kernels. And Bevin's family found it to be almost impossible to hear anything communicative.

Bevin's family had no idea what to do. Bevin loved to be with his family, and he obviously loved to talk. People had tried to teach him other things to say, but he wasn't using much of that language. And most frustrating of all was what Bevin did instead; he spent most of his waking hours reciting rapid-fire lines from *Aladdin*, *The Lion King*, *Hercules*, and whatever other movies and TV shows were his current favorites. His family felt left out of his world and lost as to what to do about it.

Bevin's mother was clearly exasperated with the extent of Bevin's echolalia. She saw it as a hindrance to what she considered "real" language growth. She really saw little hope and admitted that she wasn't even sure why she bothered to call me.

Echolalia is a stage of language development, and it has a doorway out!

On the other hand, however, I was quite excited. Yes, I had to agree about one thing: Bevin was echolalic, and he seemed to be operating primarily in Stage 1 of Natural Language Acquisition. A part of him did seem stuck there. He had a smattering of other language, Stage 2 and 3 at least, but it was as if he really lived in Stage 1 and had no idea how to move out. This made sense to me, knowing that this is a very natural process, and bit by bit, foot by foot, kids move through it. If Bevin wasn't ready for Stage 2, his own internal wisdom would not let him leave Stage 1 behind.

As I learned more about Bevin, I could begin to see why. The breadth of Bevin's repertoire of quotations made me realize what a gifted boy he was. Bevin had a veritable verbal "encyclopedia" in his head that included poetry (including long verses), songs of all kinds (from church, school, "PBS Kids," and "Disney Sing-Alongs"), and, yes, lines, lines, lines from Mufasa, Simba, Zeus—you name it. And even more astounding, these language sound bytes were often mixed together in what seemed like virtual paragraphs.

As astounding as Bevin was, I could see how tiring it would be to listen, or even to try **not** to listen, to his endless loop tape day in and day out.

Older kids have tried to open the door themselves.

Bevin's family had honored Bevin's echoed language in their own way, however. They themselves were encyclopedic in movie referents. Bevin's sister could name the origin of most of Bevin's lines. "Oh, I know what movie that's from," she would say, then proceed to recite the entirety of Rabbit's, Pooh's, or Piglet's speech. I began to realize that Tori was gifted, too. In fact, the whole family was gifted, but Bevin's gift was driving everyone to distraction.

Bevin starts language therapy

The next week, Bevin had his first session in our clinic. He couldn't believe his eyes. It was filled with lycra swings, a two-tiered loft, a trampoline, books galore, and pillows to nestle in. Bevin decided then and there to move in.

Once Bevin realized that he got to talk, too—really talk—and that I would not stop him, he completely relaxed. During our very first hour together, Bevin used literally hundreds of movie lines, but they were almost all spoken too quietly and rapidly for me to hear. But there were a very small number that were short, clear, and communicated nicely in the context of what Bevin and I were sharing. During this first session together, Bevin verified what I had seen at home: that he was a communicator. The mixture of short, communicative comments follows, some of them well-selected gestalts and others clearly mitigated or self-generated:

> **It's safe.** (hopefully, as he landed at the bottom of the slide)
> **Wait, wait!**
> **Let's play in here.** (seeing another room)
> **Stay all night.** (Bevin loved our clinic)
> **I'm faaaaalling.** (a dramatic moment)
> **Oh, this is great.**
> **It's too dark.**
> **Like a gym, like a home.** (commenting on the clinic)
> **Slow and steady wins the race.**

Bevin settled in, and we started to look at books together. Below is an example of a nice dialogue, mostly self-generated, concerning dinosaurs from one of the books:

B	**There's rooms there, and dinosaurs.**
M	(responding)
B	**And dinosaurs.** (a hopeful request for dinosaur toys)
M	(responding)
B	**Eat meats.**
M	Like—meat, like hot dogs.
B	**With blood.**

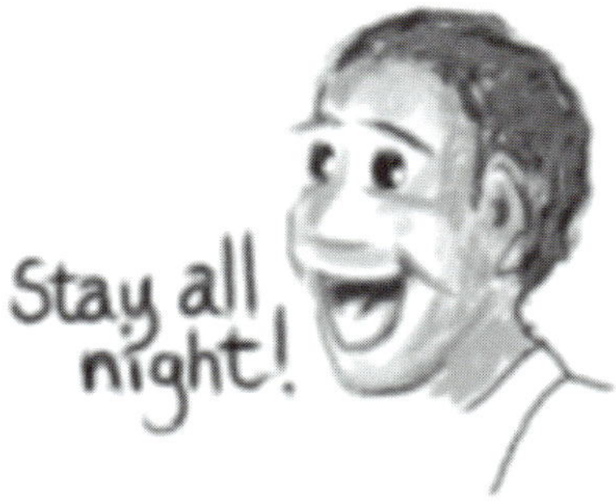

The first thing I could report to his family was how good these thirteen utterances looked on paper. But the other part of the story was that in an hour of non-stop talking, there were at least 200 utterances, with about 7% of them understandable enough to communicate. While a smattering was clearly mitigated or self-generated, it was also clear that Bevin lived in Stage 1, and that he had precious little to communicate outside of echolalia.

If I truly wanted to work with Bevin at Stage 1, which I knew I had to do, I needed to get to know him and his encyclopedia better.

Bevin's second therapy session

Our second session provided that opportunity. While I sat there, almost wordlessly, for an entire hour, Bevin talked and talked and talked. I tried to write down a word here and there just to document that I had been with him for an hour, but it wasn't easy. Most of it was an unintelligible blur of sound, with slight punctuation either when an echoed comment had a particularly well-stressed word or when Bevin really wanted me to understand.

When we listen to our kids, we prop the door open for them!

I wrote down whatever I could hear and tried to pay attention. I threw my "two cents" in very occasionally but only to repeat something Bevin said that seemed louder than the rest. I knew that the key to our fledgling relationship was for me to be quiet and just listen. I could tell that even the hint that I might stop him from talking could squelch the whole thing. Bevin's comfort with me was riding on my complete acceptance of everything about him, including all his echoed language. Frankly, I was just happy that Bevin's talk was often loud enough to hear and sometimes clear enough to understand. I knew I would learn a lot by just listening.

As Bevin and I sat together in the clinic's pillow room, we looked at animal books—not necessarily the same ones at the same time—and we certainly did not look at each other. Rather, we resembled little kids who are engaged in parallel play but not really interacting. I wanted Bevin to realize that he was safe there, that I was a completely accepting person, and that I was not going to stop him from talking. I wanted Bevin to be himself, so I could fully get to know who he was.

My notes from that second session were far from complete because Bevin talked non-stop, and I couldn't hear most of what he said. A small sample is included here, representing about ten minutes of talking. An **xxx** denotes speech that was not intelligible to me. This is close to what Bevin said: **"Hey, watch where you're going xxx. Xxx. Way up north in Canada.** [Bevin recited an entire poem, returning to it later and reciting it again.] **We're digging a hole they dug. Xxx, next week on Wisconsin Public Television. Xxx, Kogo—where's kogo? Come on xxx. Grasshoppers, scorpions,** [Bevin continued naming insects from a book]. **Uh oh, time for lunch xxx. Xxx don't play with your food. Wow, there you go. Xxx. Hang on. Mammals—looking for mammals. A life to begin—Why the book—read the book. Someday you will. Find any one. Bite. Oh, shut up. You idiot. You love—this story."**

I imagine the genre of this talk might sound vaguely familiar to many of you. If it doesn't, it may be because your child is too young to be able to talk this clearly. Remember that Bevin was 10 years old at the time I met him, and his speech, when it was loud enough and slow enough, was intelligible. This certainly helps us in our intervention for most older children: we can understand them.

On the one hand, extensive echolalia can be an auditory challenge for families. But from my standpoint, I am excited when kids' echolalia is clear enough that we know what they're saying. Children like Bevin are not hampered by the severe challenges of either auditory processing problems or motor planning; even though much of what they say is too complicated to be fully intelligible, their free-flowing echolalia is truly music to my ears.

So, just to make sure you're on the right page, this chapter is for those of you who know an older student like Bevin. It is not about little kids. In Section 3, we will be describing echolalia in preschoolers, so if your child is two, three, or even four and hasn't memorized whole movies yet, please feel free to skip ahead to that section. The theoretical premises involved in Natural Language Acquisition will be described most completely in the next section, Section 2. So, you might want to come back and read that section later.

But for the rest of you, whose child or student sounds like Bevin, let's contine with his story.

When his mother asked me about our second session together, I said that it went well, but, no, I didn't have any recommendations yet. I told her I thought it would be best for her family to not make any alterations in their daily life yet, but that within a month I would have plenty for them to do.

Bevin and his mom went home.

Bevin's third therapy session

The next week, Bevin returned for his third session, and I saw a qualitative difference in him. He sat closer to me and didn't look away from me the entire session. It seemed like he was more comfortable with me and was trying to figure out how I could possibly be "for real." In his in-home, intensive ABA program, new therapists were often low-key the first session, only to ask for compliance and performance the second session. I had made it past session number two and hadn't asked for a thing.

Our third session turned out to be pretty much like the one the week before, with Bevin dumping out boxes of animals and reciting lines from the movie, *Dinosaur*. This time, however, I began doing something more than repeat a few words here and there while frantically writing down as much as I could. This time, I took an active verbal role and began repeating back the parts of what Bevin said that seemed important. I was extremely judicious. I didn't want to look like I was judging him or criticizing him. And, most of all, I didn't want to interrupt him and risk stopping him if he perceived my comment as judgment. If he stopped, I would miss out on something more Bevin might want to say.

When we gloss our kids, they can move through the door.

Kids are trying to isolate the important words and communicate.

So, what did I repeat back to Bevin? I tried to listen for the parts of his monologue that were louder than the rest and just highlighted them, or 'glossed' them. Glossing kids is always a powerful therapeutic tool in communication therapy, because kids (like any of us) love to be listened to and acknowledged. And even though Bevin didn't demonstrate that he loved it, he did dare to look at me a few times, and I thought I caught the hint of a smile. That was enough for me.

So what, exactly, was going on between us? I was acknowledging just the parts of his recitation that were louder, not the parts that were blurred and muffled. I thought of the fuzzy parts like the fast forwarding in a movie. They were context, the parts that just didn't matter to what Bevin actually wanted to extract and say. I had come to realize years before that the unintelligible blur no one understood is not supposed to be understood. It is there because it is part of the original context, the original gestalt, and kids actively try to minimize it as they become more selective.

Let's put it another way. Fast forwarding is a step in the right direction: the direction of moving to Stage 2, complete mitigation. It is really 'almost-mitigation,' so no wonder it felt good to Bevin to have just the loud parts acknowledged. The words he mumbled were simply his place-holders that served to help him get to the words he wanted to use for communication. Bevin was not intending that the mumble be heard by anyone else; it was just for his own benefit in keeping the entire movie in mind. In this extremely labor-intensive way, Bevin was demonstrating to me just how much he wanted to communicate. He wasn't "talking to himself" or just replaying the sound track of the video in his head; he was talking to me!

Mitigation is hard work

Bevin was also demonstrating why mitigation is such hard work when kids are older. Smart kids like Bevin have a great memory, and the movies are so long! It's nice to have someone help you with the logic of your own personal take on *Hercules*, for instance, and whittle it down to a manageable size. To have to fast-forward in one's mind to find the sound bytes that make up a paragraph about heroism, for instance, takes considerable mental concentration. Mitigation at this level, at Bevin's level of sophistication, is about ideas as much as it is about language. At age 10, Bevin had a wealth of thought compared with a 4-year-old like Dylan, so mitigation was infinitely harder and more complicated.

And *Hercules* was just one movie Bevin had in his mind. To fast-forward through each of them, to pull out ideas, and to think about language mitigation would have been daunting if he had had to do it by himself. Clearly, if Bevin could have conquered mitigation by himself, he would have by then. No wonder he smiled to have someone take notes and help him. No wonder he was delighted that I could sift through his mumblings and find the kernels of meaning.

With so much language available at almost the same time, how could any child begin to analyze it for the grammatical commonalities?

But, of course, I wasn't really sifting at all. He was doing all the sifting by mumbling through the "filler" between gems of meaning. In his own way, Bevin was almost mitigating these giant gestalts himself.

So why hadn't Bevin conquered Stage 2 mitigation by himself? Here's the gist of it: Bevin was so good at appreciating and accessing the entire mega-gestalts that are full-length movies and books that he had to use his brainpower to sift among all those in his head if he were to organize them. This feat takes an intelligent child with a wealth of media experiences and an amazing archive system in his brain. His brain held not just a few movies, like Dylan's four-year-old brain did, but a hundred or more. What he accessed, I hypothesized, were movie clips, catalogued by themes: sometimes the same clip catalogued by several themes. With all that language available virtually simultaneously with the push of a mental button, how could any child begin to analyze it for the grammatical commonalities? When you're reciting poems about the frozen north and listing all the amphibians in the southern hemisphere—mentally jetting off here and there, all day, every day—grammar just isn't on the radar.

But, anyway, Bevin and I were off to a good start. Even though the process wasn't going to be easy or move along in "textbook" fashion like it did for Dylan, it was a worthy beginning, and Bevin and I were clearly on for the ride.

After a month: "Shut up and call me Frank"

Below is Bevin's language sample taken after a month of our being together. It is significant that the phrases and sentences that follow are the only ones I understood outside the context of all the dinosaur and animal names I could hear within the endless gestalts. We had been exploring dinosaur and animal books while Bevin talked in his familiar non-stop way. Most of Bevin's speech was far too fast and quiet to be intelligible, and it had the quality of talking to oneself. I could tell, however, that much of this process was weeding through dialogue from *The Land Before Time* and commentary from various nature videos.

The parts of Bevin's talk that were familiar and intelligible enough for me to gloss back to Bevin made up this language sample. In the course of an hour and a half, Bevin demonstrated that he had successfully mitigated some Stage 1 gestalts on his own and that his Stage 2 mitigations were useful to him. The theme of the session became apparent: Bevin wanted us to remain a team during the summer, to learn to deal with the **"bad guys"** through greater skill in **"speaking better,"** to have some **"incredible adventures,"** and to start **"making a room"** at home that would replicate our play room at the clinic.

As you read the following sample, remember that these were the only utterances I understood in an hour and a half. It looks pretty good on paper, but almost all of the fleeting blur of sound was unintelligible, with not much of it sounding like it was meant for me. As you read the following, note that the number before each of Bevin's utterances indicates which utterance it was in the entirety of the sample. Dialogues are indented, with B being Bevin and M being Marge. The first of the nineteen intelligible utterances was a nice compliment, I thought:

1	**B**	**Together, we're strong.** [gestalt, used selectively]
	M	Together, we're strong.
2	**B**	**Together, you're strong.** [mitigation]

In the next series, Bevin finally communicated that he did not want to go home.

73		**It's time to go home.** [gestalt]
74		**I said, "Come, Sara."** [same]
75		**x x No x x.** [isolated word]
	M	You wanna say, 'no.'
76		**I'm saying, "no."** [a supported, self-generated utterance]
77		**No, you're x x x.** [mitigation]
78		**Shut up and call me Frank.** [meaning unclear]
82		**I will x x x.** [Bevin seemed to be isolating "I …" phrases, as if trying to isolate "I" itself!]
85		**Together, we will make it.** [gestalt, used selectively]
86		**That's a great idea.** [gestalt, used selectively]
87		**Bad guys.** [mitigation]
88		**Bad guys—we're out of here.** [mitigation]
89		**Bad guys—we're out of here.** [repeated]
90		**I think.** [mitigation]
91		**It's time x x x on an adventure.** [fast-forwarded through the middle to create two mitigations]

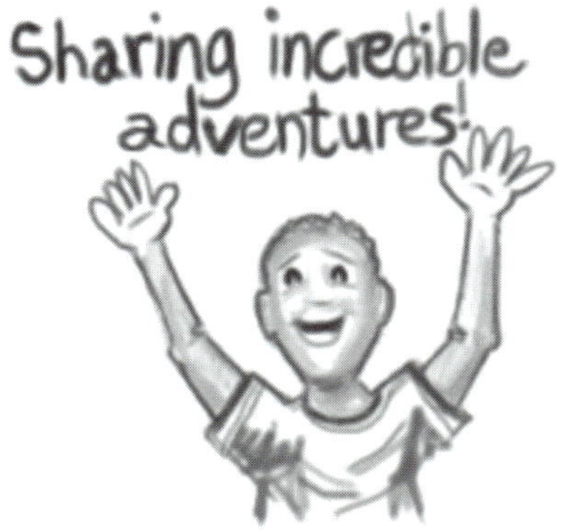

92		**Some incredible adventures.** [mitigation]
93		**x x incredible adventures.** [mitigation]
	M	(comments on sharing adventures together)
94		**Sharing incredible adventures.** [combination of mitigations]

Limited though it was, this sample of intelligible utterances was our beginning point. Other than dinosaur and animal names, however, all I could really discern from the plethora of recitations was that Bevin was happy to be there. Bevin had faith in my ability to listen throughout the hundreds of utterances it took to find these nineteen. I wanted to live up to his faith, so I guess we both had our jobs established for us.

The next year

Bevin was an amazing student of language. Our sessions were only once a week, but they were 90 minutes long; this allowed us to set things up, talk about them, and have plenty of time for sensory breaks along the way.

Our clinic is actually like one big sensory break, since we try hard to provide whatever equipment is recommended for a child by our Physical Therapist and Occupational Therapist colleagues. We turn to them constantly for support recommendations for our kids, as almost all of our kids are in one or both therapies. We would not be successful in what we do without them.

In Bevin's case, physical therapy (PT) had become a smaller part of his school life, but he was a growing boy, and his body and its needs were changing dramatically. I knew extra PT would have to be a part of the plan. Bevin benefited immeasurably, finding the proprioception he needed to deal with the over-alerting he experienced when seeking it himself. As Bevin announced one day, "**Bumps are bites**," and I appreciated the fact that I had been forewarned that the latter would follow quickly on the heels of the former if we both weren't careful.

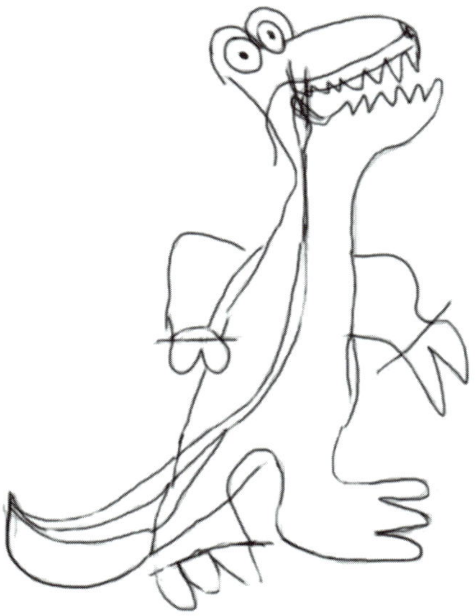

Self-regulation and sensory integration are two key concepts here. In Bevin's case, the need for intense proprioception has waxed and waned over the years, especially when the stresses of his school day have challenged his auditory sensitivity and limited ability to self-regulate. This is an important part of Bevin's story and one that we will, in fact, explore later on in Chapter 15.

The current chapter of his story is mostly about language, however, because at this time, elementary school still provided Bevin with a fairly manageable environment. In our clinic, as he worked on his language process, Bevin had access to any of the equipment and materials he wanted, which made the flow of activity work for him. He manned the TV remote from his lycra hammock and could fast forward to his heart's content. He could assemble the animals and Disney characters to illustrate his ideas and could direct me to draw whatever would complement his thoughts.

It took many months before I got to see that Bevin could draw much better than I could. It was only when I was clearly unable to draw something he wanted that Bevin grabbed the marker from my hand and made the humble illustration come to life. Bevin's mother noted that Bevin usually only drew in private, because he had become so used to other people dictating what he was to draw. As you can see on the previous page, Bevin was an artist!

Bevin's language growth over the next twelve months took many twists and turns. We had a few stalls, also, and there were times we explored an idea or a subject in depth and forgot about grammar for a while. We shared some important time together and forged a life-long friendship in the process.

But throughout that year, I kept my clinician's hat on all the time and kept track of the threads of development that Bevin's language was going through. That development divided into three time periods.

The first period of time was spent completing the mitigation process: leaving Stage 1 gestalts behind and emerging completely in Stage 2 of NLA. Once we were there, we hung out in the world of short phrases and experienced combinations and recombinations for several months. As with Dylan and all the other kids I have worked with, this period of time was powerful. Bevin reveled in being able to say things that were previously outside his grasp. It helped him understand that the language from each book, movie, or poem wasn't a completely separate "whole"—they didn't all have to be committed to memory in order to comment on their ideas. Fortunately, there were short-cuts!

At about six months into our process, Bevin was almost 11 years old. He was able to use a nice mix of short Stage 1 and 2 phrases for about 30 minutes at a stretch. The following sample followed 15 minutes of intense jumping and proprioceptive activity on a large trampoline. Bevin was very excited about planning a sleep-over and was well set up to advocate for himself. Only after this 30 minutes of using nice mix-and-match utterances did he lapse into quiet self-talk that was not intended to communicate. Half of the 79-utterance sample is included here. The entire sample is in Appendix F .

1	**B**	**Sleep over.**
	M	Sleep over for Halloween.
2	**B**	**Night—play on Halloween night.**
3	**B**	**Dump it out.**
	M	Yeah, (etc.).
4	**B**	**I'm so glad.**
5		**Stop it—**
6		**It's scary** (re: a spider book)
7		**x x sister's x x.**
	M:	Sister's books—
8		**These are stinks.**
9		**These are x x x.**

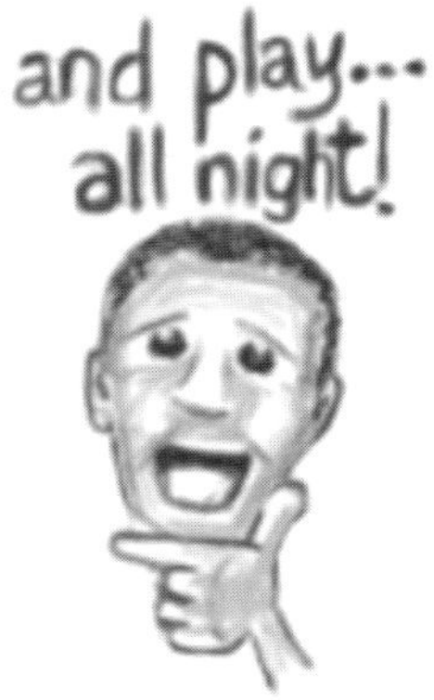

10		**Here, Hulk, here is for you, for you, for you, for you.**
11	**B**	**We are just gonna x x x.**
	M	We are just gonna have fun.
12	**B**	**I'm gonna just play over night x x x.**
13	**B**	**It is the only x x x.** (meaning 'the only way')
14		**And play all night.**
15		**And sleep.**
16		**And clean up all the toys.**
17		**And wait for Mom and Tori.**
	M	Let's play all night.
	M	Let's clean up in the morning.
18	**B**	**How about—**
	M	How about Papa?
19	**B**	**How about—**
	M	How about Tori.
20	**B**	**Princess stories**. (reading from a new Disney collection)
	M	Do you want some princess stories?
21	**B**	**No, thank you**.
22	**B**	**These are—** (handing them back)
23	**B**	**Iguanodon, where is it?**
	M	Iguanodon, you found it.
24	**B**	**Read it.**
	M	Read it.
25	**B**	**No.** (B had isolated 'no,' but it was not quite what he wanted to say)
	M	Not yet.
26	**B**	**Not yet.**
27	**B**	**Read—Velociraptor.** (looking at a new dinosaur book)
	M	Let's read about Velociraptor.
28	**B**	**No.**
29	**B**	**No—don't touch it.**
	M	OK.
30	**B**	**OK—I can x x x.**
31	**B**	**He's so big.**
32	**B**	**He's big.**
33	**B**	**He's big.**

	M	He's fun to read about.
34	**B**	**x x fun to read.**
	M	It's fun to read. It's fun to see.
35		**Oh, look.**
36–40		x x x x x x x x x x x x x x x x x x (to himself for the first time in the half hour; actually several utterances)

This sample represented amazing growth. I knew we were on our way, and, as Bevin approached 11 years old, he was also on his way to isolating the building blocks of original language. We were all thrilled.

The second period of time was spent further mitigating down to the single word (Stage 3 of NLA) and then spending several months practicing two-word combinations of all kinds. This was conscious practice and experimentation for Bevin, and my role during this period was to model some possibilities so that Bevin didn't limit his. For example, I would play with combining two concepts in our little pillow world in many ways. I would use Bevin's animal 'world' and some of his selected animals, such as 'bumble bee,' 'iguanodon,' and 'wolverine,' and produce two-word combinations such as 'iguanodon world,' 'world iguanodon,' 'iguanodon bumble bee,' etc. This is the two-word stage of every child's language development, where anything goes. It isn't about grammar. Rather, it's about combining concepts and seeing how relationships of all kinds can be contained in two-word combinations. Try it yourself, and see what I mean.

Stage 3 isn't about grammar. It's about combining concepts and seeing how all kinds of relationships can be contained in two-word phrases.

There's only one caveat here. Unless you're a toddler, two-word phrases are unusual to use for communication. People don't expect 'bumble bee iguanodon' or similar exclamations from 11-year-olds. So, during this time period, Bevin practiced short phrases but returned to using some short gestalts and mitigations to communicate. This way, he could continue to communicate while still spending time combining two words for his language work.

Included here is a language sample taken about six months later, or a year into our process. At this point, Bevin was almost eleven and a half years old and solidly at Stage 3. Even though there was the usual quiet self-talk some of the time, Bevin used two- and three-word phrases about 70% of the time, demonstrating that he was solidly at Stage 3. It was all so mundane-sounding compared with his usual, flowery gestalt language, but he played with two-word combinations very deliberately. Of course, nothing says it like the right gestalt, and he chose a few, very selectively, to communicate special things.

As you read this sample, please remember that Bevin was eleven and think about how hard it is to say two-word phrases when you are used to talking non-stop for hours with a flowery mix of soliloquies from every Disney character known to children. It helped, I think, that Bevin was not in middle school yet, where his age-mates were. He had another year of elementary school to go, and his language development benefited from the relatively lower pressure.

The first six utterances are Stage 3 combinations of single words:

1	**Now animals.**
2	**Pajama world.**
3	**Animal pajamas.**
4	**Treasure map.**
5	**Get map.**
6	**Get treasure.**

The next is a combination of two Stage 2 mitigations: "Where's" and "the pause" (button).

7	**Where's 'the pause'?**

The next four utterances are Stage 3 single words:

8	**No, no, no, no!**
9	**Suddenly—**
10	**Oh—**
11	**Hurry—**

The next is a Stage 1 gestalt:

12	**Will you knock it off—**

The next is a Stage 3 single word again:

13	**No.**

The next utterance is a Stage 2 mitigation:

27	**Stand back.**

The next seemed to be Stage 3 combinations where Bevin was mixing and matching from among the single word pieces, although each might have been a mitigation.

28	**Ran fast.**
29	**Get it.**
30	**Get going.**
31	**Run back.**
32	**Go back.**

The next utterance is clearly a Stage 1 gestalt, but one that's hard to match with grammar until one is a much more advanced stage of linguistic development:

49	**In a land far away, your dreams can come true.**

Yes, until you read the gestalt at the end, this language sample sounds surprisingly simple coming from a boy who was eleven and a half and could recite entire movies. So, please remember that what a child gives up in the floweriness of echolalia, he gains in communicative flexibility. It is simply a part of children's language growth. Granted, that's easy to understand when a child is 2 and 3 years old. We recognize this stage in toddlers, applaud it, and realize how flexibly kids can express a great variety of concepts with short phrases constructed of a growing vocabulary. Even when a child is 4 or 5 years old and his speech sounded like gibberish up until then, two-word phrases sound delayed but typical. In an older student, however, one whose language was usually long monologues, these two-word phrases sound truncated and quite surprising. They certainly did to Bevin himself, also, which is part of the reason I was so proud of him for allowing himself to play with conceptual combinations this way. He didn't talk this way all day long, of course, but certainly for a few hours a day: enough to learn the principle.

Developmental Sentence Types

Here's a wheel we don't need to invent at Stage 3: the varieties of two-word phrases we look for in all children. Published in *Developmental Sentence Analysis* (Lee, 1974), these sentence types have stood the test of time, as each provides the foundation for the kind of sentence that children develop next. With this list in mind, I encouraged Bevin to play with a wide variety of concept combinations and to create all of these phrase types for himself over a two-month period. The following is an extraction from Developmental Sentence Types, the pre-sentences Laura Lee outlined as preparation for the grammar she measured with Developmental Sentence Scoring, which we will examine in Chapter 5.

Developmental Types of Pre-Sentences	Examples
Nouns and Noun Elaborations	ball, a ball, balls, more balls, this ball, my ball, now ball, Daddy ball, big ball, baby ball, ball truck, not ball, another ball? what ball? and ball
Designators and Designative Elaborations	here, there, this, that, it, those, these, this? here? here ball, these balls, there now, there one, not there, that ball? who that? and here.
Verbs and Verbal Elaborations	imperatives (eat!), basic elaborations (eating, ate, can't, eat?), eat cookie, eat now, eat it, not eat, eat it? what eat?, and eat, wanna eat
Other vocabulary items and phrase fragments	OK, hey, Hi, bye-bye, oh-oh, what? in car, for me, plurals, adverbs (all gone, too big, up here), sentence modifications (to you, in it, not big, in here?), conjunctions (and, but)

Table 3: Developmental Sentence Types (Lee, 1974)

It's important that kids acquire grammar when their overall language level is ready for it. Grammar without content is pretty empty.

Before kids have the opportunity to create Stage 3 conceptual combinations, we risk oversimplifying their language with grammar, making it all form and no function.

The third period of time in Bevin's first year was spent with beginning grammar, and it represented a welcome change. Adding beginning grammar to his phrases made them sound so much more complete, both to Bevin and to others. Having spent months combining concepts at Stage 3, Bevin was ready for grammar, which at the beginning stages is less about word order than about efficiency. So, instead of combining specific words in every conceivable phrase combination (such as 'animal world' and 'animal pajamas'), Bevin could use grammar to take some shortcuts. A few examples would be: 'he has a world' and 'he has pajamas,' or 'got a world' and 'got some pajamas.'

Bevin was ready for grammar, and it is important that kids acquire grammar when their overall language level is ready for it. Grammar without content is pretty empty. It's tempting to teach 'He has a …' or 'I have a …' as sentence beginnings, for instance, too soon. Before kids have the opportunity to create Stage 3 conceptual combinations, we risk oversimplifying their language with grammar, making it all form and no function. Grammar provides some shortcuts, so it's important that kids learn the shortcuts only after they have something to shorten. It serves them well in their on-going development to have plenty of experience with the 'long version' (Stage 3) first.

Because this part of Bevin's story involves grammatical development, and we have not yet explained how grammar develops, we will postpone telling more of his story for a few chapters. But Bevin's story will continue in Chapter 13, as he leaves elementary school, and we will then follow him through middle school in Chapter 15.

For now, let's just say this: it was hard, but there was no stopping Bevin in his pursuit of his dreams. By sharing his story, we can share some of the lessons he learned along the way. Quite simply, extreme gifts come with extreme challenges. Bevin's extensive mental encyclopedia just kept adding entries. Parsing it all down—again and again and again, over and over—was a mammoth undertaking. Through elementary school, Bevin could manage, and his grammatical development continued as long as he remained self-regulated.

Once he was faced with the sensory demands of middle school, however, he shut down. His supersonic ears just couldn't keep the constant noise out, and his self-selected words, **"Me hurt everywhere,"** communicated his distress. Moving from elementary school seemed like innocence lost, until we were able to finally address Bevin's sensory defensiveness with a focused sensorimotor program that restored his faith in the world and his openness to what it had to offer.

That part of our story will have to wait for another chapter. But in the meantime, please keep in mind the goodness of childhood and how we want to continue to tap into that "inner child" of our echolalic students. It's in there, just like it is in the little boy illustrated below: deep in thought in his sandbox story world and ready to emerge into language.

Let's continue by summarizing what we have learned so far.

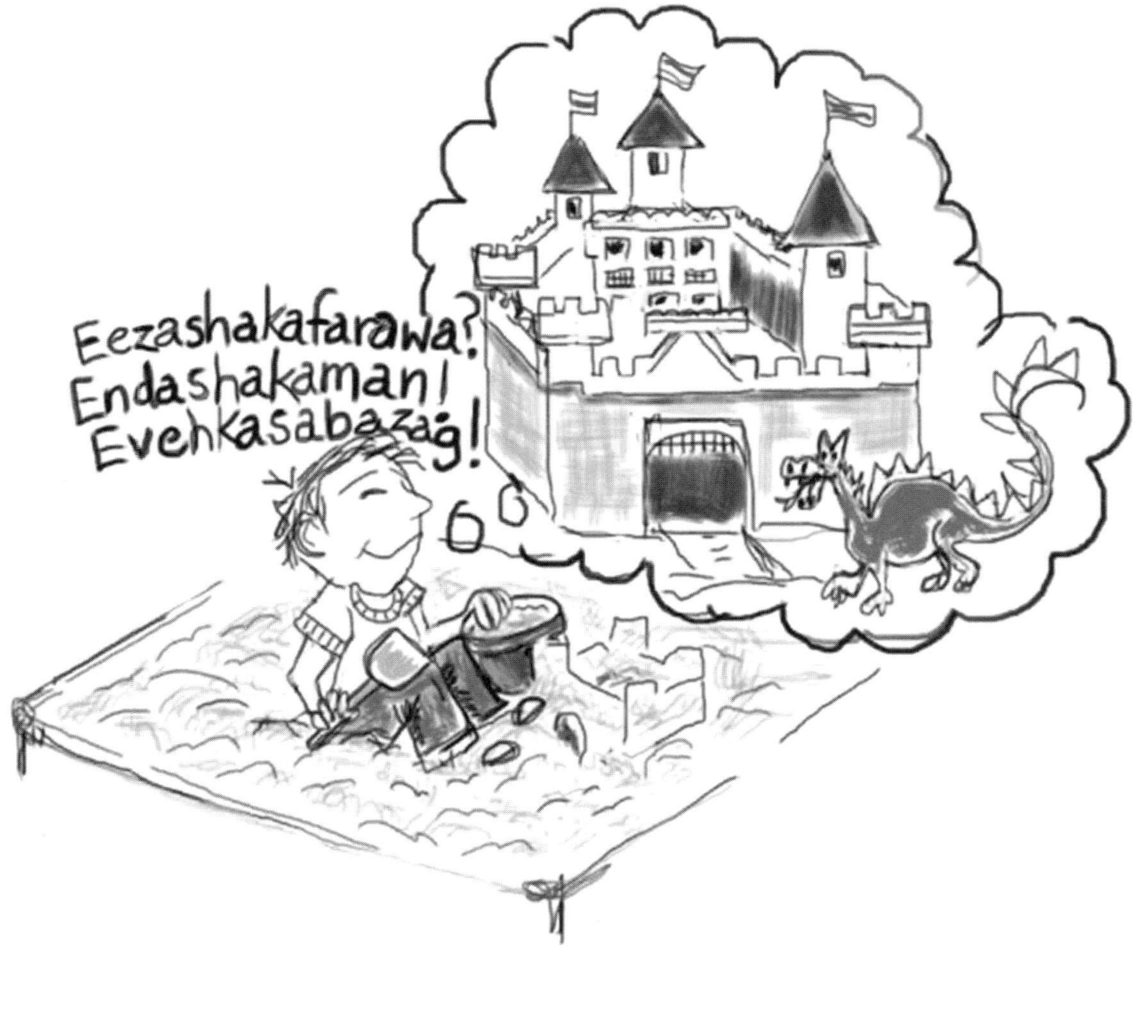

Chapter 3
Summary: What We've Learned So Far

Let's take a breather now, and review what you've learned so far. First, you know that echolalia is OK. Better than that, you know that it's good. You know that echolalia matters to our kids' language development and that it belongs there. You've learned, also, that the term 'delayed echolalia' should be re-framed as Stage 1 of Natural Language Acquisition, since it is the time when kids use language gestalts to communicate.

You know that Natural Language Acquisition is normal. It takes longer than the other way, the analytical way, but you know it's the natural way for most boys and most of our ASD kids. You know the process can be time-consuming, but it leads to flexible language use. So it's not only worth it, it's critical! You know the process can be relatively fast and seamless when kids are younger, and that even when kids are older they can move through it in a predictable fashion with our help. You know, too, that even our older kids can come out on the other side with productive, original sentences that communicate intentionally.

Obviously, we need to cover more territory, and even though you probably feel excited and hopeful about the potential for your own child's language development, you may feel somewhat unclear about what to do. And if your child is young, you might be feeling encouraged. But if your child is older and seems just about as complicated as Bevin, you may be wondering how it will be possible to help your child move through the stages Dylan did so easily, and Bevin did with sheer determination.

Section 2 of this book will help considerably. It will give you a respite from emotions involved in real kids' stories for awhile. It is designed to be a side journey into some of the theoretical underpinnings of language development and to give you confidence that people have thought about this process for a long time. You can relax now, for a little while, and drink in what researchers discovered about language development and how this matters to our particular population of kids.

You won't have to apply anything from this section. It is here to give you a sense of what's gone on before. It will be comforting, though, because it will help you understand where it all fits: where gestalts fit in linguistically and where grammar fits in as well. And it's an exciting side journey, so let's get started.

section 2

Theoretical Background: Echolalia and Grammar

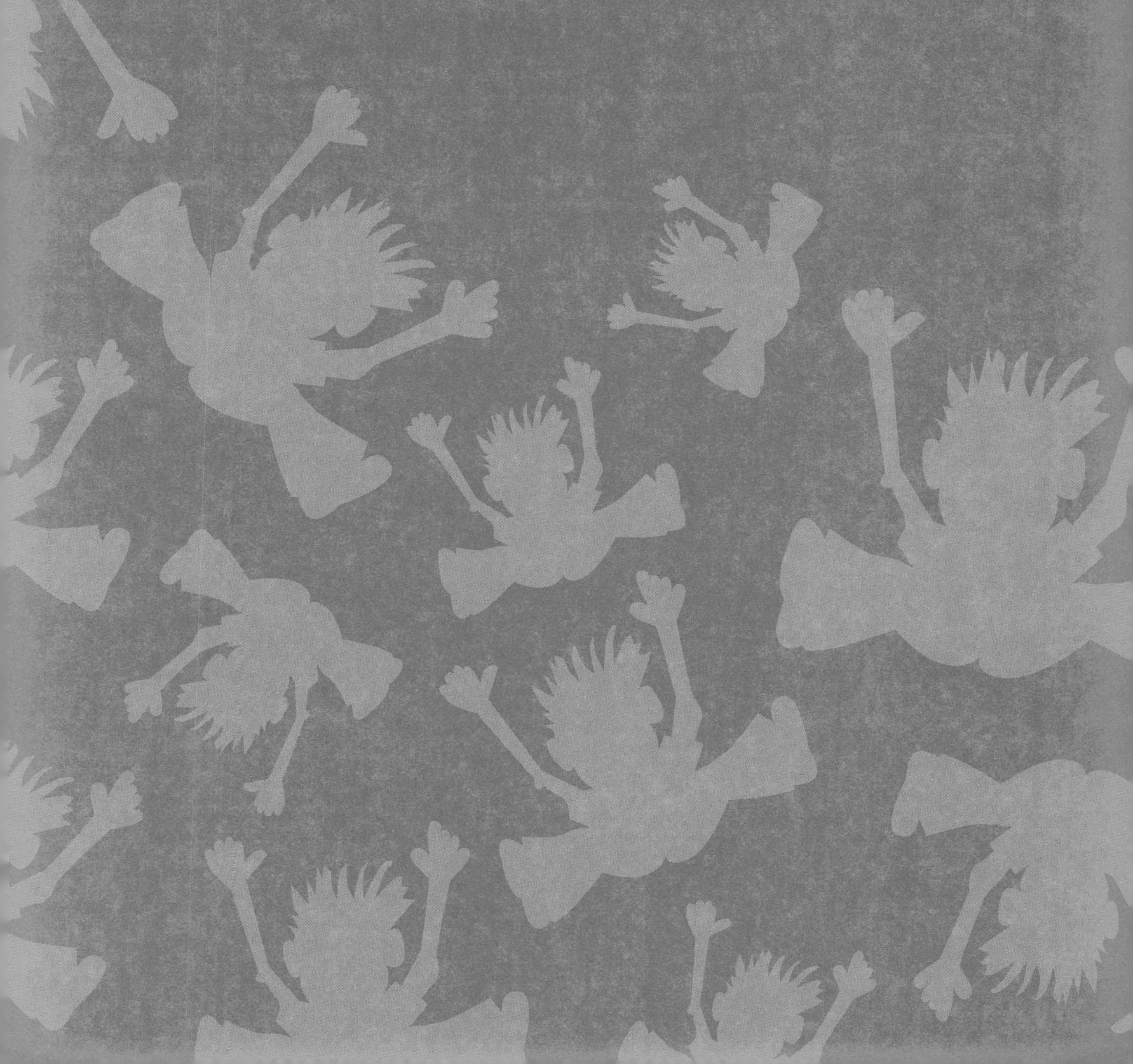

Introduction

You were promised a little respite in this section. You were told you could just sit back and read what language researchers have found out about our kids and their particular style of language development. If you thought our kids' learning style was unique, you will be pleasantly surprised to find out how typical and ordinary it is. That's why Chapter 4 will provide such respite.

In Chapter 5, you will learn more detail than you ever wanted to know about grammar. While this part of the book will seem pretty unsurprising to you, it will serve to validate how typical and ordinary your child's language development really is.

In Chapter 6, you will review what you have learned by then and be ready to either read about Preschoolers in Section 3 or go on to Elementary School Kids in Section 4.

So, without further ado, let's begin this journey from a place we already know but which deserves further elaboration: how our kids do communicate with echolalia. Once you fully understand how much the research validates this, the more you will begin to appreciate how much our kids share with other gestalt language processors off the spectrum. So, let's begin at that place we already know a little about: echolalia.

Chapter 4
Echolalia Isn't Just About Autism

How echolalia communicates on the spectrum

The 1960s and 70s were the era of grammar study in child language research. Researchers set up home recording studios in their children's nurseries to record the soliloquies of their offspring as they nodded off to sleep. Some of the most cherished examples in our language textbooks come from these impromptu "language labs," and the early research on echolalia is no exception.

Several early researchers in child language acknowledged the place echolalia played in normal development, describing echoed phrases that were situationally-important and that usually remained in kids' repertoires only a few weeks or so.

When examples of the delayed echolalia in autism were reported, however, they seemed more extreme and more enigmatic. The odd utterances reported were more like the classic one from Leo Kanner (1946), "Don't throw the dog off the balcony" (p. 262). Idiosyncratic delayed echolalia seemed like a dead end, communicatively. Because the original source of echoed language was often hidden in the past, delayed echolalia was hard to understand, to generalize, and to consider as a serious attempt at communication.

In 1981, however, Prizant and Rydell presented findings of some exciting research to the American Speech and Hearing Association (now the American Speech-Language-Hearing Association). Using videotaped sampling of kids with autism, these researchers discovered that their echoed utterances did communicate. Summarizing their findings in 1982, Prizant noted that they had "identified 14 functional categories in over 300 delayed, echoic utterances of autistic children and adolescents. Like immediate echolalia, delayed echolalia was used for seven communicative purposes (e.g., requests, protests, providing information) and two other interactive ones, as well as to serve cognitive functions (e.g., self-directive, rehearsal)."

Research found that echolalia serves communicative, interactive, and cognitive functions.

One example cited by Prizant in 1982, taken from his 1978 dissertation, was the child who often said, "Mom's washing the clothes," when he saw, through an audiocassette window, the audiotape turning around. This child was applying the words he first heard as he watched through a washing machine window clothes tumbling around.

In their 1984 article on this research, Prizant and Rydell included several examples, each seemingly spoken to the children on earlier occasions: "Hey, don't put that ring in your mouth," "Don't do that; that hurts," "Put the vitamins away," and "On top of your desk, chump." While none of us likes to hear our less-than-admirable remarks repeated by our kids, we can only hope this one was a fluke: "I'm gonna tie you up."

Prizant noted, "Although all subjects in the delayed echolalia study exhibited patterns of emerging spontaneous, analytic language (one- and two-word utterances), delayed echolalia was a functional tool for communicative and cognitive purposes. This notion of a two-language system (gestalt and analytic) co-existing in an individual child was proposed independently by Peters (1977) for a normal child and by myself (Prizant, 1978) for autistic children" (Prizant, 1982). As we will see again and again, this progression from one language system to another is important as we look at how our kids grow in their communication skills over time.

How echolalia communicates off the spectrum

Historically, linguistics and language development literature have contained numerous references to echolalia as a part of gestalt language development, one of the two normal ways of acquiring language. Normal speakers were observed as naturally dividing into two groups: analytic language processors and gestalt language processors.

Analytic language processors are much more familiar to us: they start with single words, naming things with lots of labels. These first words catch our attention because we understand them. We were, in fact, the ones who taught them to our children. We expect kids to point to things and label them—doggie, kitty, spoon—and we can easily keep track of this language growth, partly because kids are good at pronouncing these first words. Our literature calls these children 'word babies,' and it has norms for them and lists of the usual first 50 words.

Language development researchers also describe gestalt language processors, or 'formulaic' or 'intonational' learners, and Amy Wetherby summarized the characteristics of the two styles (1992). Her description of 'word babies' sounded like the little girls in our lives, the ones who named things we pointed to, and 'intonation babies' as the little boys in our lives, the ones who played in the sandbox and produced the sound effects of the Battle of Gettysburg with their action figures. On the next page is a summary, offered by Amy Wetherby, but credited to Ann Peters (1984) and Barry Prizant (1983).

As we ponder this chart, we can think about what processing gestalts implies at the earliest stages: that the earliest gestalts in the sandbox are more like 'sound gestalts' and not 'language gestalts' at all. We think about the meaning of these sound gestalts and recognize that the meaning isn't linguistic, but situational. Remembering renditions of the Battle of Gettysburg we have watched on TV, we think of the soundtrack. It had no words, but the meaning was there in the sights and sounds of the battlefield. For the boys who can visualize it, meaning is there, but not in words.

'Word Babies' (Analytic Processors)	'Intonation Babies' (Gestalt Processors)
Focus on referential use of utterances (i.e. labeling objects) and semantic relationships of language	Focus on intonation and social interaction structure of language
Basic units of language are single words	Basic units of language may be words, phrases, and/or complete sentences
Language use is generalized to relevant objects and events quickly	Language use remains specific to situational contexts for longer periods of time
Language is productive and generative early on in the language acquisition process	Language is relatively inflexible in the early stages
Early language acquisition moves from single words to two- and three-word utterances	Early language acquisition involves multiword phrases functioning as single words
Rule induction of language forms allows for increased grammatical complexity	Increased language complexity is achieved through recombinations of established gestalts
Most common in girls	Most common in boys and ASD children

Table 4: Individual Differences in Language Acquisition (A. Wetherby, 1992)

Those of you who have known some intonational learners will recognize how different they are from the little word learners. And you remember how misunderstood they can be when they try to talk about what they feel, think, and know. When these children start kindergarten, they are often identified as "speech delayed" and spend time with SLPs. This was the case in my family, too, as the story of my nephew, Andy, will illustrate later in this chapter.

Right now, as you think about the "typical" little boys in our lives, you might be considering how much like our echolalic ASD kids they actually are—the big difference being that our ASD kids are much older, much more echolalic, and much more misunderstood. If this is crossing your mind, you are where I was when I first saw this chart of Amy Wetherby's eighteen years ago.

I was, in fact, first introduced to the concepts I've just described in 1994, when I first began working at the University of Wisconsin teaching clinic. Amy Wetherby's handout was the gift of a colleague there, as I embarked on my first clinical opportunity to work with little kids with ASD diagnoses. I had worked with only a few kids with ASD in my 20 years of public school work, and this chart was a God-send to me. It presented a framework for seeing our kids among all the kids acquiring language, and this made intuitive sense to me.

A linguist's view of gestalt language processing

The field of Speech Language Pathology spent several decades looking at the normal development of grammar, or syntax, in kids. In the 70's and 80's, as we were exploring concepts such as 'deep structure,' proposed by Noam Chomsky, Ann Peters completed her doctoral dissertation in linguistics (1973) and revised and published it in 1983.

All kids' language development begins with a unit of language: a word or a whole string of sound.

Peters' *The Units of Language Acquisition* was made available electronically in 2002 and represents an enormous contribution to our thinking about language development, especially language development among gestalt language processors. In her work, Peters studied the literature, synthesized it, and explained it. She found that, regardless of the path kids took in language development, they began with a 'unit' of language. This 'unit' is a perceptual marker, varying in size but always the beginning point for auditory processing and language acquisition. A child who is an analytic processor perceives little units of language: that is, words. A child who is a gestalt processor perceives larger, intonationally-defined units of language: gestalts.

So, at the first stage of language acquisition, a 'unit' is whatever children are able to extract from the continuous stream of sound around them. It is a word for some children and a stream of sound to others. In typical language development, analytic processing and gestalt processing are simply descriptors of the type of the units kids extract from running speech around them. Depending on their own style, kids might hear one-word naming going on around them or they might hear intonational contours, punctuated by exclamation points.

When Peters wrote *The Units of Language Acquisition*, the language environment for gestalt processors was most typically the sounds of conversation around them. This was the case for Temple Grandin, who refers to her internal "grammar check" she runs by replaying her childhood mental movies of her parents talking. But not all of Temple Grandin's age-mates with ASD had enough exposure to language to extract its commonalities. Individuals whose echolalia consisted of a few enigmatic comments of the variety "Don't throw the dog off the balcony" and "On top of your desk, chump" obviously had precious little opportunity to mitigate.

What's "typical" about "typical language development?"

By the time young gestalt processors utter their "first word" they have done an immense amount of language work and know quite a bit about the world.

Reading Peters helps us work through old biases that analytic processors are the normal and typical ones. We have all called the language development of these analytic processors "typical," and we are generally guilty of comparing everyone else to them. This includes the seemingly delayed little boys whose language often sounds behind that of little girls as they enter kindergarten. As young analytic processors begin to use the basic constituents of language, words and word parts, to move through the stages of increasing linguistic complexity, we take comfort in how much like little adults they sound. Peters addressed this propensity among linguistic researchers as well and cautioned that by the time young gestalt processors utter their "first word," they have done an immense amount of language work and know quite a bit about the world.

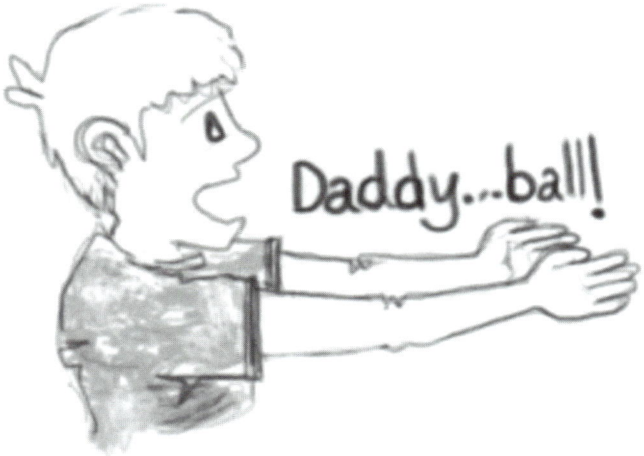

To add to our bias, the speech of little analytic processors is considerably easier for us to understand than that of their often-unintelligible gestalt counterparts. Single words are infinitely easier to say than long sentences and movie scripts, and as little analytic processors start to put words together, their motor skill seems to keep pace with their sentence length. We understand "first words" in our young analytic toddlers and recognize their initial attempts at two- and three-word phrases. Generally, they are the very phrases we have exposed them to and, thus, recognize.

Young gestalt processors present a very different story. We generally have difficulty understanding their long, poorly-articulated and echoed sentences. All too often, we dismiss them as babbling or "gibberish." But after they have been talking for quite a long time and manage to isolate a single word or two, we typically recognize it and think that they have just begun to talk. As we call their first isolated words their "first words," we underestimate how much talking it has taken to get to this stage and how much knowledge of language patterns got them there. In retrospect, often years later, we look back and recognize that our kids were actually talking all along. And as we think back, often for the first time, we recognize what they were saying years before.

With this context in mind, think now of the dilemma for our ASD kids who have never had any success with mitigation or the isolation of a single word. If they are still attempting to articulate long gestalts and did not achieve a measure of speech clarity until they were 4 or 5 years old, we may well have called them "non-verbal" up until then.

Can we call our kids "non-verbal" just because we don't understand them?

It's not only our dyspraxic children whom we erroneously judge as without language when their speech is halting or absent. We call many of our ASD kids "nonverbal"—because we don't understand them. More often than we'd like to admit, kids can have an amazing amount of language in their heads—and even on their lips—but because we don't understand it, we call it "babbling."

The roadblocks are thus set up to stop our kids' natural development. Without some listener validation, children can remain echolalic far longer than if we are able to help. We haven't ignored them deliberately, of course, because we didn't even realize they were talking. To add insult to injury, if we didn't know they were talking, we might have presumed they didn't understand and talked down to them, making them feel like babies.

What to do? First, let's look at the larger population of all kids so we can put our kids in perspective.

Gestalt language processors among us

We find children all around us who are gestalt language processors. Many of them are neurotypical little boys who tell long, complex stories, mostly with their hands and action figures, and whose lengthy "jargon" is completely unintelligible. By the time these children are four and five years old, they have successfully broken down their long story chunks (that were word strings, not jargon at all) into phrases and single words, have learned to say these shorter sound-sequences correctly, and have built up a sizable repertoire of original, generative sentences. They may appear delayed compared with their more analytic kindergarten peers (usually girls), but we have learned to expect that of boys.

My great-nephew, Andy, was one such story-teller. I remember when he was four years old and, except that he was unintelligible, was a perfectly typical little boy. He was such a good story-teller that his grandfather, my brother, insisted he knew just what Andy was saying. GrandPaul, as he was known, then received this challenge from his wife, Tara: "Well, GrandPaul. if you are so sure what Andy's saying, then tell me!" "OK," stuttered GrandPaul, "it's all about those guys, and how they went up there, and they got in a huge battle, and—" "Yeah, Paul," countered his wife, "but what did he actually *say*?" "Well," Paul replied," I don't know exactly, but—" You get the picture: Andy began speech therapy.

So, what was going on? Andy was talking a blue streak, but he was only four, and his tongue didn't quite move fast enough to tell you the entire complexity of "Green Power Ranger meets Ninja Turtles III" or whatever combination of stories his active mind was creating. Whole sentences from one met whole sentences of the other, and it would have taken an auctioneer to decipher the phonetics (Please look back at the drawing on page 43 for an illustration).

Gestalt processors have huge units of meaning in their heads that are impossible to say.

And that's the problem. Gestalt processors have huge 'units' of meaning in their heads that are impossible to say. It is amazing that strings of sound can roll off their tongues at all. And the more a child like Andy puts into his brain, the more impossible it gets for him to try to say what he wants to say.

Whew! That GrandPaul got it, even somewhat, is a tribute to him and probably a statement about the kind of units of meaning that are natural to GrandPaul too. That his wife didn't get it at all tells us something about her as well. Hmm. Could we be onto something? And how many women like Tara are the teachers of kids like Andy—and Paul? And who writes the books about them?

Boys' brains

In 1997, Michael Gurian wrote *The Wonder of Boys*, which was a good reminder that boys' brains are different from girls' brains. Gurian's description of boys is particularly useful to us as we think about our kids with ASD. To begin with, his description of child development includes several important points: that the cortex of girls develops more quickly than the cortex of boys, that in both sexes the left cortex develops somewhat later than the right, and that "in males … there is an even greater lag" (p. 50). This perspective provides a useful context for thinking about gestalt processors in general and our ASD kids in particular, the little ones who tend to process their first experiences as visual ones, largely devoid of language.

Gurian goes on to describe boys' language development, reading skills, and hearing. He points out that boys develop verbal skills up to a year later than girls and tend to have three times more reading difficulties than girls. "Boys from very early on are reported to ignore voices, even parents' voices, more than girls do. In some of these cases, they are simply not hearing …" Gurian notes that boys tend to hear less background noise and differentiate less, and he urges parents and educators who feel unheard by boys to replace some of their frustration with an understanding of how the boy's brain is working. Gurian suggests, "If he's not hearing, try another sense—especially the visual, which is the boy's best sense on average. Also try to get the message to him through stories, games, objects that move through space" (Gurian, 1997, pp. 16–17). As we think of our parenting and education of kids with ASD, these descriptions and strategies sound quite familiar. Taken together, these reminders about developmental differences that have only to do with gender help us put our own ASD kids into a larger context.

Boys' brains at school

Boys' learning style was taken into the classroom in Gurian and Henley's later book, *Boys and Girls Learn Differently!* (2001). Gurian and Henley's comments about boys seem to echo what we know about our ASD kids. They note that "Boys tend to hear less" and even find jargon and coded language more interesting than everyday language. These authors comment that boys "get bored more easily than girls" and need more input and more variety to remain attentive (pp. 45–46).

" … try to get the message to (a boy) through stories, games, and objects that move through space."

The Gurian and Henley book also describes boys' sensorimotor needs in a way that sounds similar to how we describe them for our ASD kids. "Brain-based gender research has taught us something fascinating about the need for movement in the male brain. It appears that the male brain does not as quickly move neurotransmission in the upper limbic areas; nor does it as naturally direct emotional material between the right and left hemispheres for analysis and verbalization. But engaging the whole body in the task of emotional processing seems to enhance neurotransmission to limbic (emotive) and left-brain (verbal) areas. When we think of boys punching a bag or doing karate or riding their bikes fast through the bike trails when they are angry, sad, or frustrated, we are seeing this theory in practice. The boy is naturally moving energy through his

"The boy is naturally moving energy through his own brain by making his arms, legs, and whole body move."

own brain by making his arms, legs, and whole body move" (Gurian and Henley, 2001, pp. 150–151).

As we ponder this paragraph and think about how our ASD kids are not naturally good at moving their bodies in space and integrating their brain hemispheres, consider how Gurian and Henley talked about the gender bias. "Statistically, the majority of ... disorders have been and will continue to be related to the male brain because it is not as good at self-development. Normal growth of the male brain typically requires additional external help" (Gurian and Henley, 2001, p. 187).

External help—that is what we know we must provide our ASD kids. Whether cognitively, linguistically, or physically, they have a propensity to "get stuck" often, until we supply the appropriate external help.

But what about the girls with ASD? How is their learning similar and different from the boys with ASD? In our clinic, as in most, our experience is relatively limited. This does seem to be partly because of the relatively fewer number of girls, of course, but there seems to be something else. Ratey and Johnson wrote in *Shadow Syndromes* (1997) about a phenomenon they dubbed Autistic Echoes, in which they speculated about girls: "... perhaps the celebrated female advantage in language and social intelligence protects some women born with the genetics for autism, nudging them up out of the diagnosable category of 'high-functioning autism' into the undiagnosed and unsung shadow syndrome of the disorder. Perhaps in women, mild autism, like mild attention deficit disorder ... is masked by other strengths" (p. 219).

Learning styles

This is where the concept of multiple learning styles fits in. They are a significant part of educational strategies and deserve to be considered more frequently among our ASD kids.

A classic system that teachers have used for looking at their students' learning preferences is Howard Gardner's "theory of multiple intelligences" (*Frames of Mind*, 1983). In this view, learners might approach material through any combination of these 'intelligences': linguistic, musical, logical-mathematical, spatial, bodily-kinesthetic, intrapersonal, interpersonal, and naturalistic.

Another way of looking at cognitive styles comes from Mel Levine, who described learning styles as eight "neurodevelopmental systems": attention control, memory, language, spatial ordering, sequential ordering, motor, higher thinking, and social. Through the mechanism of a neurodevelopmental profile, Levine described how particular patterns might be more successful within particular times and environments, but less so in others. So rather than thinking in terms of 'learning disabilities,' Levine would prefer to think about a match for a child's particular profile (Levine, 2002).

In 2005, Temple Grandin wrote a column in the *Autism Asperger's Digest* entitled "Different Types of Thinking in Autism." In this article, Grandin noted, "All minds on the autism spectrum are detail-oriented, but how they specialize varies. By questioning many people both on and off the spectrum, I have learned that there are three different types of specialized thinking: 1. visual thinking—thinking in pictures, like mine; 2. music and math thinking; 3. verbal logic thinking. Since autism is so variable, there may be mixtures of the different types."

"All minds on the autism spectrum are detail-oriented, but how they specialize varies."

Given the plethora of information out there, it makes good sense to apply all the information we have about learning styles, multiple intelligences, and differences in language processing styles (analytic vs gestalt). It also makes good sense to cross-reference these materials and examine how our kids' use of echolalia fits with other developmental and learning style probes we make. As Temple Grandin reminds us, each of our kids is unique and not to be treated in a 'one size fits all' manner.

Back to the basics of child development

A review of all the approaches to learning will help us in the autism community to get back to the basics of child development. This, in turn, will help us out of the dichotomy we seem to have created when we began to think of our ASD kids as different from other kids. Rather than begin our lectures on autism with the DSM listing of behavioral characteristics that define a syndrome, we might consider a very different introduction. It might start by describing the continuum of all learners and include the multiplicities of thinking styles, propensities, and language-acquisition characteristics. It might continue by looking at our ASD kids as simply kids on the larger continuum—with gifts, challenges, and a need for "additional external help."

Why haven't we approached ASD in this inclusive way? With the rapid rise in ASD diagnoses, most of us in the autism community have been too busy scrambling for ways to help our newly-diagnosed kids simply be safe, feel better, and then to function with some dignity. Figuring out what to do about echolalia and how it might fit into language development has seemed like a secondary concern.

My guess is that each of us has gotten a bit lost in the maelstrom, maybe because we work with many ASD kids on our jobs or because we have a child with ASD ourself. We all seem to get caught in the "rush to judgment" that autism tends to bring with it. Once a child is diagnosed, we are inundated with resources, programs, and fix-it solutions that seem, collectively, to trump any rational review of child development. In every area, we are quickly told what we must do. We must get a visual schedule; we must teach our children to request help; we must reinforce the behavior we want to see.

Once a child is diagnosed, we are quickly told what we must do.

Autism researchers Sally Rogers and Laurie Vismara commented on the "brand name programs" that tend to rise and fall over time: "The press for well-publicized branded treatments can become an economic nightmare for families and schools, and the high demand for a treatment may result in more and more providers providing poor delivery of the brand name program, compromising its possible benefits ... the packaging and publicizing of autism treatments may make it more difficult for parents and others to appreciate effective generic teaching practices. The desire for an effective treatment may become synonymous with a particular brand of treatment, and the brand name issue may obscure the strengths of a very well-designed generic intervention plan for an individual child built on empirically sound practices and solid data. It would be helpful to the field for treatment givers to point out commonalities between the brand name interventions and others, and to document empirically the specific generic efficacious practices underlying the effects in the brand name program" (Rogers and Vismara, 2007).

When speech and language programs are considered, parents are often told they "must" begin a particular program immediately in order to catch a child during his prime language learning years. Maybe it's PECS, or sign language, or manding, or learning to imitate sounds. Each comes with a plausible theory of its own, and some come with supporting data. Each is "evidence-based" in its own way. But, if we actually spend time looking into any one of these programs, we discover that one may actually be diametrically opposed to another. If one were chosen because of the individual characteristics of a child, that would be one thing; if one were chosen because it is the 'program d'jour,' that is another.

Regardless of the program, you can be sure it does not assess and work with gestalt language processing. So few people know what to do with echolalia, and, even more fundamentally, when a child is young, echolalia might not even be recognized.

Gestalt thinking

So far in this book, we have been looking at our ASD kids as part of a larger group of language processors. We now need to further broaden our conceptualization of our kids and see that their language processing style is a part of their thinking style. As gestalt thinkers, they join a whole group of thinkers generally referred to as "right-brained." Extending this picture further, then, our kids now have a place along an even larger continuum, that of all learners. Note below their place on the far right side, among children along the continuum—left-brained, right-brained, and everything in between.

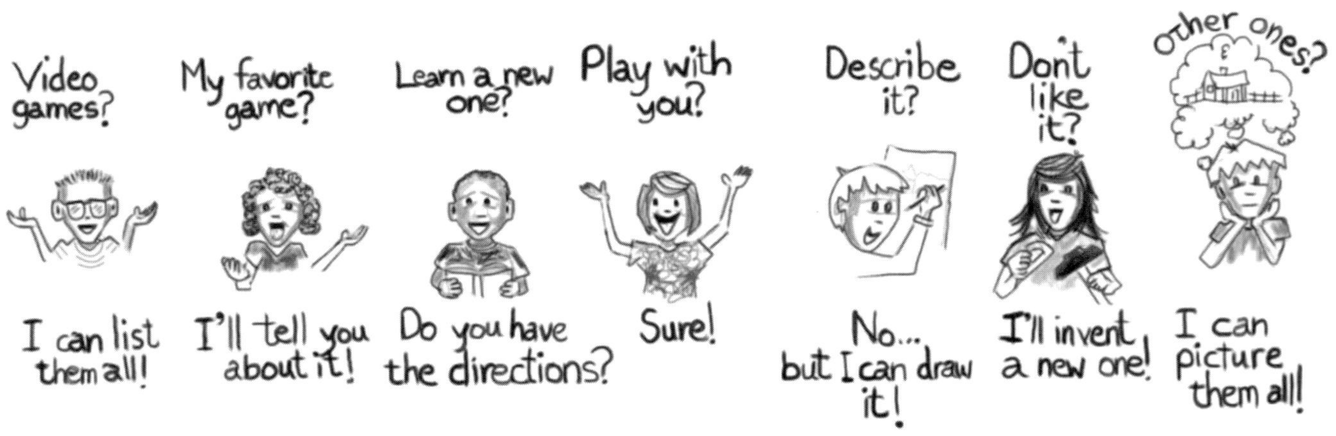

As right-brained thinkers, our kids are in good company, and to see them this way we need to step out of the comfortable surroundings of our ASD world and step into the larger, long-established world of learning styles in general. Let's take the classic definition of "learning disability" as a beginning point and note that learning disability specialists use a statistically significant discrepancy between auditory/verbal modalities and visual/spatial modalities to define a learning disability. Of course, testing our kids is difficult, because of the demands on motor responding. But just knowing how "learning disability" is conceived in educational literature is helpful when conceptualizing how our ASD learners compare.

Before looking at our ASD kids within the larger group, however, let's re-examine who we're talking about among our own kids. Classic autism and PDD are very different from Asperger's Syndrome, of course, even though these two groups of people share many behavioral features. By definition, one of the hallmarks of classic autism is a significant delay in the acquisition of language, while a defining characteristic of Asperger's is normal developmental language milestones. Truly, the two groups of kids could not be further apart on the entire spectrum of language learners, not just on the autism spectrum, but on the larger continuum of all learners.

A useful book in picturing a continuum of all learners is *The Right Brained Child in a Left Brained World* by Jeffrey Freed and Laurie Parsons (1997). The authors use a straight line to illustrate the relative place of all learners, including those with classic autism, on a left-brain–right-brain continuum. Their descriptors place classic autism at the extreme right end of right-brainedness. Although the book is primarily about ADD kids, whom the authors describe as right-brained, it is fascinating to re-read this chapter, mentally inserting the word 'autism' whenever 'ADD' is written.

"The farther right an individual falls on the continuum, the more intuitive and random in processing he will be and the more apt to store information primarily in pictures."

A sample from the book includes this comment: "The farther right an individual falls on the continuum, the more intuitive and random in processing he will be and the more apt to store information primarily in pictures … Being a visual-spatial thinker goes hand in hand with keen intuition because intuitiveness, or 'filling in the gaps,' is what the visual thinker does by nature" (Freed and Parsons, 1997, p. 66).

Also, Freed and Parsons (1997) write, "Right-brained people are holistic, whole-to-part learners. They pick up skills more easily by having them demonstrated than by having the steps explained. Instead of learning to ride a bicycle through trial and error (getting on and falling off), they'll study how others ride a bike, then jump on and do it when they feel confident they're ready" (p. 54).

The authors continue, "They are spatial and three-dimensional in their thinking; they prefer drawing and creating to writing and talking. They have a natural ability to hold images in their heads for prolonged periods of time … many architects and builders say they can 'see' in their mind an image of the finished product long before it's translated into blueprint" (Freed and Parsons, 1997, pp. 54–55).

And then, "They lack impulse control, have poor organizational skills, and are often clumsy … (being) late walkers (with) delayed gross and fine motor skills as toddlers and preschoolers … children with ADD tend to have problems with how they perceive their bodies in relation to space" (Freed and Parsons, 1997, pp. 55, 64).

And next, "Kids with ADD literally feel more than do other children … It could be said that ADD and very right-brained children have this 'super radar' … Next to hearing prowess, the most prevalent sensory characteristic of extremely right-brained ADD children is touch sensitivity … the more severe the ADD, the more intense the sensory bombardment will be. They solve the dilemma by shutting down" (Freed and Parsons, 1997, pp. 55–56).

"Autism is found at the extreme right end of my continuum; it's the most pronounced form of hyper-sensitivity and right-brainedness."

"Autism is found at the extreme right end of my continuum; it's the most pronounced form of hypersensitivity and right-brainedness … the senses of these individuals are so heightened and overwhelmed, they simply shut down to survive. The antennae of autistics pick up so much that they lack the ability to screen the often overwhelming stimuli from the environment" (Freed and Parsons, 1997, p. 71).

Temple Grandin endorsed the book, writing, "This book could help a lot of creative thinkers … make it through an educational system that is run by linear thinkers."

Although Freed and Parsons do not include Asperger's at the extreme left of their continuum, we can see how it would fit. Along with the "word salad" that is on the far left end, one can picture a child with Asperger's Syndrome reciting a train schedule or asking everyone in the room when their birthday is. Far from being language-delayed, the Asperger's kids are language-precocious, with right-brained deficits in the visual and/or spatial dimensions. Often considered the clumsy kids, our 'Aspies' quickly progressed through the stages of language development that we expect of all analytic children, and became the left-brained talkers we recognize them to be.

The continuum of all learners

But back to the subject of our book: our ASD kids who are language-challenged. It's the ASD kids with delayed language skills we are considering—and looking at how they fit along the continuum of all learners.

The children with classic autism and PDD are the visual/spatial kids, the kids who see the world in 'wholes,' whether they can talk about it or not. As we look at their place at the end of Freed and Parsons' continuum of learners, we see that they are the kids who are visual in the ways described by Temple Grandin, who naturally "think in pictures" and not in words. They are the kids who hear music when other people hear sentences; they are the "intonation babies" who hear the flow of sound, as opposed to the "word babies" who depend on the specific parts of it.

But they are not a separate class of thinkers. They are like the right-brained ADD kids in Freed's book, just more so. Besides being visual thinkers, many can visualize well; some see the world in their 'minds' eye' in exquisite detail; some are even visually gifted, like Grandin. If they were given Grandin's test of visual thinking, our classic ASD kids would excel. And they might not feel disabled at all; like Grandin, they might feel like quite competent thinkers. As Grandin wrote in *Thinking in Pictures* (1995), "I used to become very frustrated when a verbal thinker could not understand something I was trying to express because he or she couldn't see the picture that was crystal clear to me" (p. 11).

Grandin's view offers a nice complement to the Freed and Parsons picture: our kids are not a separate class of thinkers, but they are certainly at the extreme right end of the continuum. ASD kids are not different from other right-brained children in their style of language processing, either, but the results can be more pronounced. As the extremes among their peers, they might be quite gifted in their ability to visualize, to store visual media, and to recall them along with their sound track. Gestalt processing in this broader context is a useful concept, then, because not only do our kids need to learn to mitigate language, but they need to "mitigate" experiences as well, to pull out the individual trees from the forest.

Gestalt language development: the continuum of intent

The language development literature from the 1980s and 1990s noted ASD kids who were using echolalia communicatively—and naturally developing some generative language. In their 1984 article about their research, Barry Prizant and Patrick Rydell reported nine communicative functions of delayed echolalia in their three subjects with autism, seven of these intentional. These seven communicative functions were: interactive labeling, providing information, calling (calling attention of oneself or to establish/maintain interaction), affirmation, requesting, protesting, and directing others' actions. The two categories of non-intentional communicative functions were turn-taking in a verbal exchange and verbal completion of a verbal routine.

Perhaps our kids' communicative intent is delayed because others fail to understand their message.

One ingredient in kids' success appeared to be communication partners recognizing communicative value in echolalic comments, which helped kids develop communicative intent. Prizant and Rydell (1984) speculated on the development of communicative intent this way: "When a child begins to observe and realize that his or her utterances do have specific effects on the behavior of listeners and thus uses utterances more frequently and specifically for a particular effect, it can then be stated with some confidence that the child knows the relationships between his or her signal (e.g., request for food), the effects of the signal on the listener (e.g., listener provides food), and the desired goal (e.g., acquisition of food). It is at this point that the child's behavior can be said to show evidence of communicative intent. With autistic children, however, the production of nonconventional signals (utterances with "private meanings") may preclude a listener's ability to infer communicative intent; thus, reliable judgments on communicative intent may be difficult to make … When there is behavioral evidence that an utterance is used to achieve a particular result, it can be said with some confidence that the utterance is part of an intentional communicative act" (p. 190).

"With autistic children … the production of nonconventional signals … may preclude a listener's ability to infer communicative intent."

We all know about the rapid development of intent among analytic language processors compared with gestalt language processors. Universally, babies' first word is a variation of "Mama," which we reluctantly admit began as a simple biological juxtaposition of closed mouth, voicing, open mouth. But once we hear our baby say "mama," meaning is attributed and there is dancing in the street. Of course, the infant would like to recreate that joy and does, with increasing intent. This is the classic example of what Prizant and Rydell are describing and is perhaps a reason the gestalt language processor is delayed in achieving this glorious result—and in achieving communicative intent.

Prizant and Rydell analyzed the language of their subjects with autism and reported types of utterances and functions. For their three subjects, the percentage of echolalic utterances was 70% in the youngest subject (4 years 8 months), 38% in the next oldest subject (12 years 4 months), and 33% in the oldest (14 years 2 months). The corresponding percentage of generative ("creative") language was 7% in the youngest subject, 37% in the next oldest, and 40% in the oldest. Subjects' generative language was single words and short combinations such as "block away" and "a blocks" (subject 1), "wanna put away" and "book" (subject 2), and "mine" and "eat a cornflakes" (subject 3).

Assessment and intervention guidelines

In 1988, Prizant's assessment and intervention guidelines made up Chapter 35, "Communication Problems in the Autistic Client," in the *Handbook of Speech-Language Pathology and Audiology*. "Over time, changes in echolalic behavior relative to the emergence of rule-governed linguistic behavior can be used as an index of emerging linguistic competence … Baltaxe and Simmons and Prizant hypothesized that, for echolalic individuals, growth in expressive language abilities is predicated on the segmentation of echolalic "chunks" along with the acquisition of early semantic and syntactic structures, resulting in greater creativity and flexibility in language production" (p. 1031).

Prizant recommended strategies for responding to echolalic utterances to help break the linguistic code.

Continuing in the *Handbook of Speech-Language Pathology and Audiology*, Prizant referred to his 1983 article in which he discussed the importance of simplifying the language modeled and of specific strategies for responding to echolalic utterances in order to increase functional usage and conventionality of these forms. Among those strategies were: "helping echolalic individuals to break into the linguistic code and to begin to acquire more flexible and rule-governed linguistic abilities … Evidence of structural change, such as pronominal adjustments, telegraphic echoing, verb tense changes, and intonational changes, may be indicative of some degree of linguistic processing and may signal emerging linguistic competence."

Prizant and colleagues always recommended embedding intervention in a social-interactional approach, and Rydell and Prizant presented strategies as a chapter in Kathleen Quill's 1995 book, *Teaching Children with Autism*. "Increased flexibility in the application of word meaning and sentence structure (mitigated echolalia) may be initially demonstrated in gestalt learners in a variety of ways … Partial repetitions, reductions, replacements, and expansions have been documented as typical means by which these children combine and recombine semantic knowledge and linguistic chunks in new ways … mitigated echoic utterances of seven autistic children were characterized by similar modification strategies … children with autism may be using the similar modification strategies through mitigated echolalia as normal and language-disordered children use to modify their imitative responses" (p. 125).

Rydell and Prizant continued, "Intervention strategies should take into account the dynamic nature of autistic children's echoic productions in their attempt to move the child toward more conventional and flexible uses of language production. Interventionists should provide direct and systematic modifications of the child's echoic utterance through verbal modeling in order to foster increased creativity in language production. Depending on the goals of therapy (semantic or syntactic flexibility), the interactant can provide systematic modifications that serve to reduce, replace, or expand constituent parts of the child's echoic utterance that more accurately reflects the current referent or activity" (Quill, 1995, pp. 125–126).

The place of echolalia

Research found only 4.5% of echolalia to be "nonfocused."

Echolalia has another, quite different, historical linage, however. From the time of Leo Kanner, the communicative value of echolalia has never been an open and shut case. In 1979, Lovaas, Varni, Koegel, and Lorsch collected what they termed "self-stimulatory" delayed echolalia, believing this "psychotic speech" was under control of intrinsic rather than extrinsic reinforcement. But in the Prizant and Rydell study, almost 50% of subjects' echolalic utterances were found to be communicative, and another 25% judged interactive in some other way. Only a small portion (4.5%) were classified as "Nonfocused" ("may be self-stimulatory"). In spite of this finding, however, the term "verbal stim" seems to have become firmly rooted in the autism community. Even though the old Lovaas admonition, "Don't echo," may rarely be heard any more, the checkered past of echolalia and the mixed feelings about it remain.

So, even now, the developmental place of echolalia is sometimes lost among the fears of "self stim." As the number of children with autism has risen, programs of all kinds have emerged to try to meet the challenge. Applied Behavioral Analysis (ABA) programs have proliferated; within them, language is approached as a set of skills taught as "verbal behaviors." Echolalia often falls under the rubric of "stimming," which is often seen as interfering or at least non-functional.

Echolalia fares better in developmental models, however, and as newer autism programs have become more available, Stanley Greenspan's developmentally-grounded "floor-time" model has offered families a clear alternative to ABA models (Greenspan and Wiedner, 2006). Even so, developmental language intervention, as seen from the discipline of Speech-Language Pathology, is secondary in all psychology-based models.

Thus, while children with ASD are routinely treated by SLPs in schools, clinics, and Birth–Three programs, the percentage of a child's day or week devoted to moving his gestalt language to more generative language seems to pale in comparison to the rest of his time. The SCERTS program certainly helps this dynamic, but, in most settings, it is up to Speech-Language Pathologists and childrens' families to bring the rest of a child's team on board with the developmental language progression children are capable of achieving.

The challenge to Speech-Language Pathology

Speech-Language Pathologists thus find themselves working in myriad situations, from integral, to collaborative, to consultive, to "trying to get a word in edgewise." The most challenging are in programs lead by behavioral psychologists, where teaching "functional speech" as behavior ignores the research from Speech-Language Pathology about the communicative functions of echolalia and the natural progression from gestalt to generative language. Targeting "verbal behaviors" (Lovaas, 1981) implies that its proponents believe language does not develop naturally but that ABA can teach it. A well-publicized 1987 ABA study (McEachin et al., 1993) sounded convincing, with its impressisve, but controversial, results. For a while, Lovaas-style programs were widely seen as the only ones with "evidence" to support them. These programs proliferated.

Replication studies didn't support the 1987 results, however. In reviewing the relevant research in 2007, Rogers and Vismara noted some conflicting results in later studies. The 2000 study by Smith, Groen, and Wynn showed nice gains among its PDD subjects, but no gains (and language loss) among its subjects with autism diagnoses. Rogers and Vismara (2007) noted that an explanation for the differences seen between the 1987 study and the 2000 one was the differentiation of PDD, which did not exist at the time of the earlier study (pp. 13-16).

In the second replication study (Sallows and Graupner, 2005), bimodal results emerged. On the one hand, eleven of the children did very well (attaining IQs over 85 and succeeding in the classroom), while the other thirteen demonstrated "poor outcomes" (little developmental acceleration and little decrease in autism symptoms) after four years of 30–40 hours of intensive daily treatment. As in the other replication study, "pretreatment measures associated with poor outcomes included initial low IQ (below 44) and lack of language (no words at 36 months)" (pp. 16–18).

The lessons are apparent only to those who are aware of these results.

Back to the future

It's time to raise the bar on language programs and rediscover language development.

Speech-Language Pathologists do need to reinvent one wheel that has rolled away from us. From a developmental perspective, ABA programs are anathema to natural language acquisition. When the birthright of natural, flexible, self-generated, intention-based language development was never considered, and instead some version of the simplistic goal, "Johnny will produce 'I want ___'," is written, we might conclude that we've set our sights too low or maybe been blindsided completely.

Language researchers with expertise in ASD have proposed raising the bar. In a 2009 article in the *Journal of Speech, Language, and Hearing Research*, a team of language researchers recommended using a developmental framework to report studies about language intervention in kids with ASD. Challenging the autism community to "move away from the commonly used term *functional speech* as the outcome goal for intervention studies," these researchers proposed the following framework for reporting intervention outcomes with ASD kids: Preverbal Communication, First Words, Word Combinations, Sentences, and Complex Language. Significantly, these researchers also recommended analyzing spontaneous language samples as one of the sources of data (Tager-Flusberg et al., 2009).

What support looks like

Instead of taking language out of a developmental context, much less a social-communicative context, true help for our kids would look more like understanding the natural process and supporting the developmental nature of that process. Fairly simple support like listening and modeling is enough for some kids, while for others, only direct, appropriate language development intervention is enough to help kids get unstuck in their language systems.

Kids are often reluctant to leave certain gestalts behind because using them conjures up the experience of first hearing them.

In 1982, Prizant described aspects of the stuckedness some of our kids experience: "… it often seems to be an effort to conjure up the whole situation in which the utterances were first heard … such unanalyzed units are often produced as a partial fulfillment of a situational gestalt, possibly as an attempt to replicate the situation in which the utterance was originally heard." In our clinical experience, kids are often reluctant to leave certain gestalts behind because using them does conjure up the experience of first hearing them. Using the exact words of the movie character, for example, may bring to mind the child's feelings at the time he first heard them. Formulating a more mundane linguistic expression just isn't the same.

Recall the examples of Bevin's utterances in Chapter 2, when he was using such a nice assortment of Stage 3 single word combinations, and remember how refreshing the insertion of just the right Stage 1 gestalt sounded, even to us. Bevin had just produced a series of two-word combinations ("**Run fast**," "**Get it**," "**Get going**," "**Run back**," "**Go back**") and then burst into a beautiful gestalt: "**In a land far away, your dreams can come true.**"

When any of us wants to make our best points, we tend to quote from the literary masters. Our kids do the same thing, just more often!

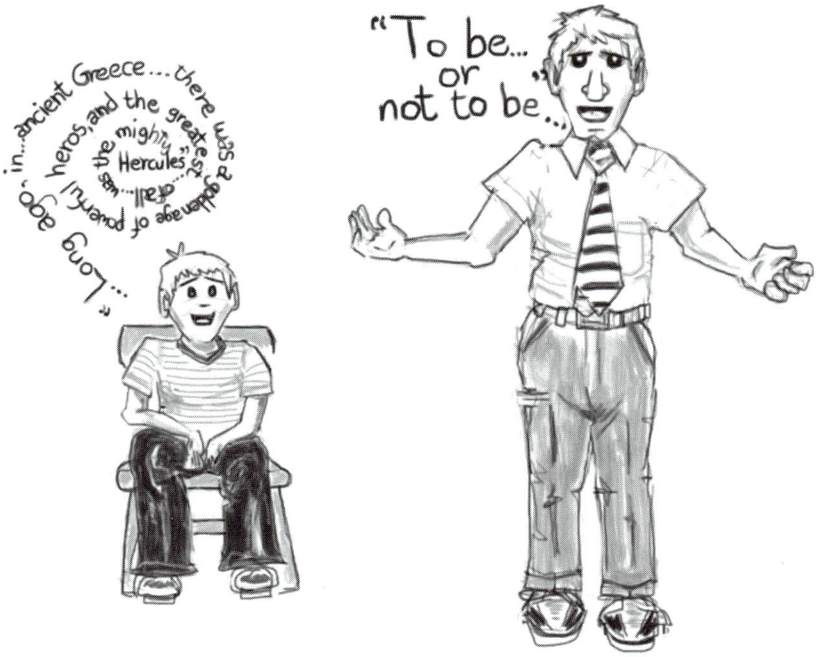

The "Aha!" moment is the quantum leap of the gestalt thinker.

When the whole seems bigger than the sum of its parts

The stories are as numerous as the kids themselves. Gestalt thinkers seem to just absorb wholes—not part by part, but whole gestalts. Temple Grandin often describes a pivotal personal example. She was trying to understand blueprints and their relationship to structures. She said she looked and looked and looked at a blueprint. And she walked and walked and walked around the structure—until, bingo: the quantum leap happened, and it all became crystal clear!

Parents often describe their child's "Aha!" moments, which might come unexpectedly after long hours of watching over and over and over again. Stories such as the following illustrate the logic of gestalt thinking.

The first story comes from the mom of a brilliant boy named Andrew, whose brilliance was hard to see when he was little. Andrew just sat, and even though he was watching, no one knew it. He would just observe and observe and observe until one day, a leap of faith occurred, and Andrew tried out the whole process he'd been examining. His "learning curve" seemed pretty flat until it was showtime, and Andrew demonstrated what he'd learned. In the words of his mother, "Andrew just sat at the bottom of the stairs but never attempted to walk. We didn't realize he was watching us all the while until one day, he got up and ran all the way across the room! Even before his 'first step,' Andrew was running!"

Another story comes from the mom of a little boy named Aden. Aden's mother understood Aden's propensity to keep sets of toys intact, because, she recalled, she had this same gestalt propensity when she was a child. But Aden was gifted in a way his mom was not. As she recalled the story, "Aden never did put together any baby puzzles. He just studied the 200-piece puzzle his father had put together, and, later, when all the pieces got put back into the box and dumped back out again, Aden just put it all together!"

But, eventually, kids need to find the parts

Eventually, kids need to discover the parts of their wholes. If the whole is running across the room, one part might be stopping mid-way across to get something. In this case, some extra sensory feedback helps a child know where he is in space in relationship to the room. Another 'part' might be slowing down the motion, grading it more precisely, and isolating portions of it enough to deliberately walk.

We can look at language gestalts in a similar way. If the child is only aware of a moving stream of sound, realizing the ways that sound is segmented in music, in verse, and in breath groups might provide the key. Maybe the formula for making each part salient is to give it form, shape, color, or other visual/spatial qualities. Something like the ABC song, for instance, makes so much more sense when looking at a visual display of the alphabet.

Segmenting any behavior is consistent with our larger objectives: helping kids become aware of movement, aware of timing, aware of the social environment, and aware of their speech so they can begin to coordinate all their actions: gesture with speech, body proximity with eye gaze, reaching with looking, language output with their partners.

If we want our kids to derive useful language that is their own, we need to model contextually-meaningful gestalts that have that language as constituent parts.

Our best help also comes with our selection of learning targets. If we want our kids to learn to reach with purpose, for instance, we want our action gestalts to be about reaching in functional ways so that useful "parts" can be "mitigated" from the whole. So, too, if we want our kids to be able to say useful words and phrases communicatively, we need to introduce contextually-meaningful gestalts that have those words and phrases as their constituent parts.

All this is to say that mitigation of wholes can and does happen. Our kids are quite capable of it, and even though their "learning curves" can appear quite flat for a long time, the immediate quantum leap can be quite startling and exciting. So, regardless of how long it takes and the types of support individual kids need, our echolalic kids are on a learning trajectory that leads to grammar, and, ultimately, to flexible, creative communication.

We have come to the end of our chapter. Supported by a conceptual framework that puts our kids on the same continuum as their peers and establishes a template for their individual maps, we are ready to continue our journey into another area.

Our next chapter will rejoin our friend Bevin at the point where we left him in Chapter 2 and take him on his next adventure. Having ventured through Stage 1 (communicative echolalia), through Stage 2 (mitigation), and into Stage 3 (isolating single words and recombining them), we are nearly ready to look at Stage 4 for Bevin: grammar. Up until now, the process has been deconstructing wholes and combining their constituent parts in creative ways. Now at Stage 4, we are ready to combine parts using the formula that is grammar. Yes, it has been a long road to get here, but we are here.

Chapter 5
Readiness for Grammar

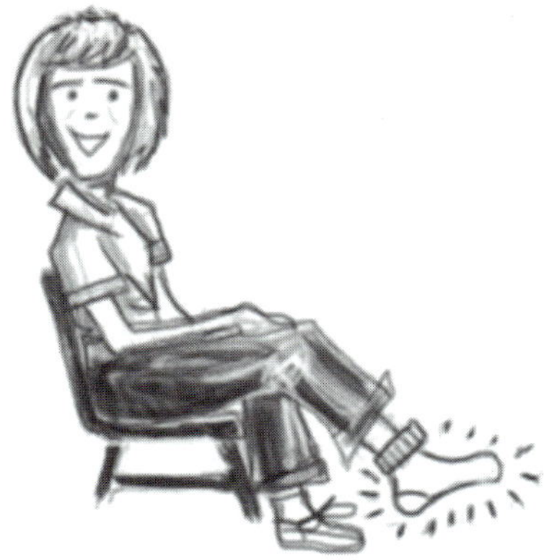

Taking stock

Before we delve into grammar in earnest, we need to first revisit the Stage 3 word combinations we talked about when Bevin learned to construct them back in Chapter 2. We recall how easily little "word babies" put words together and even how smoothly Dylan could play with two-word combinations when he was ready. Both these images contrast sharply, however, with the deliberate process Bevin used, since he had to whittle down an oversized encyclopedia of gestalts to find the kernels he could eventually put together.

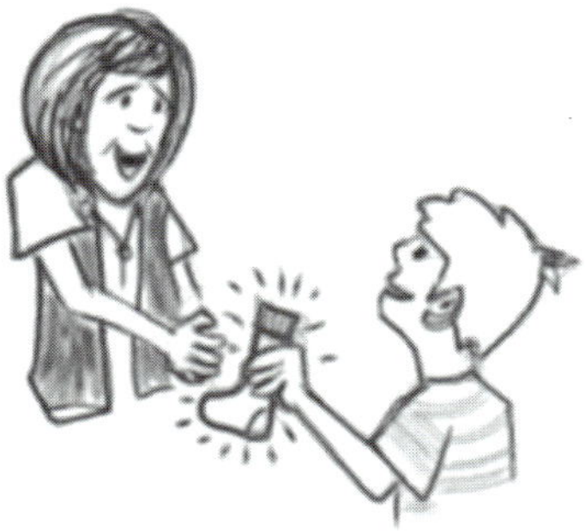

Our kids are clearly up to the challenge. Stage 3 is a cognitive task as much as a linguistic one, and once kids have successfully isolated single words from the contexts that gave them meaning, two-word phrases represent creative combinations of ideas, and it can be quite fun. It really is a learning experience for our kids and for us when we consider what can be combined in our minds.

A classic example in speech and language textbooks uses the phrase "Mommy sock" to illustrate the immense number of relationships between two words or two concepts. Consider how toddlers talk, and think about how we need to know what they're referring to in order to understand the meaning of their sparse phrases. This particular phrase could mean any of a dozen or more things, yet we usually know which one a child means because we're there with our child and we're both looking at that little pink sock together.

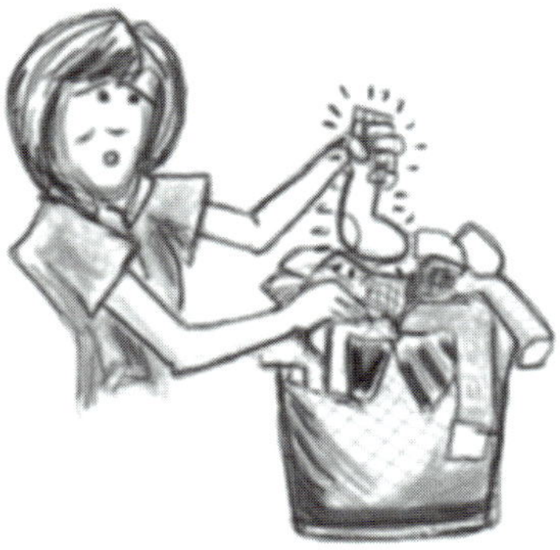

Think for a moment about how many ideas that phrase could express, and you'll get the idea. That single phrase can mean any of the following, and probably does, at different times: "Mommy, you have a sock," "Mommy doesn't have any socks," "That's Mommy's sock," "Mommy, can I have new socks?" "Mommy, where's my other sock?" "Mommy, where is your other sock?" etc. Consider, too, that the true meaning of the phrase might be any of these as well: "I'll give my dirty socks to Mommy," "Your socks are clean, Mommy," "These socks are my mommy's," etc. The word order of the original phrase could as easily have been "Sock Mommy" at this stage of development, and all the meanings listed above (and then some) could have been possibilities.

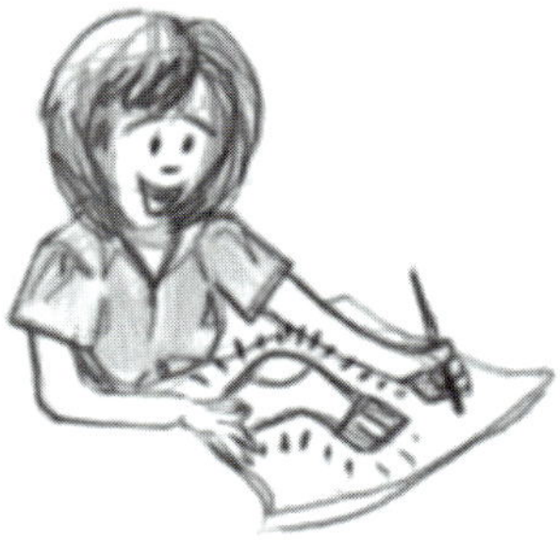

The point here is that at the two-word phrase level, word order simply doesn't matter. Word order would imply a correct sequence, and that implies "grammar" or "syntax." The two-word level is about combining concepts such as "Mommy" and "sock" in all the myriad ways these two concepts can be combined. The possibilities are so vast that we realize how fortunate we are to have that sock in front of us so we know what our darling child is referring to.

Referencing is important at this stage. Our literature is filled with information about "joint referencing" and how important it is for children to share references with their communication partners. When trying to understand something so elusive as "Mommy sock," that little sock you can both see at the same time is terribly important for the words to have communicative value. Considering the motor challenges our kids have with reaching and pointing, it is no wonder that referencing is one of the defining challenges of autism.

Two-word combinations at age five—or twelve

First of all, is combining words harder or easier if you're a five-year-old gestalt processor or a two-year-old analytic processor?

On one hand, when a child is five years old and combining words on his own for the first time, it's easier, because he already knows so many words. Dylan, for instance, had a huge variety of vocabulary words embedded in his gestalts and his mitigations. Once he was ready to isolate single words, he could do so quite readily, and he began to combine them with relative ease. His first conscious success was quite surprising to him, however. It was **"I—toy,"** clearly a combination of words rather than a familiar sentence, something we could tell from the lack of dramatic intonation Dylan usually used. It was original, and the surprised look on Dylan's face was priceless.

On the other hand, at five years of age kids realize that two-word phrases are not expected of kids that old. Their short phrases sound funny to them, and they know they sound funny to others. Five year olds need a little private practice time with you and the reassurance that this is just part of the process. Yes, two word phrases are valuable in the whole scheme of things, and we'll have some fun playing games with them. But we need to reassure our kids that they won't sound like this forever.

Combining words for the first time is harder for an older child than a younger one.

If five year olds need a little privacy for practicing, kids who are older than five need even more privacy and huge doses of encouragement. You will be able to give them this at home. It's helpful to set aside a time and place to practice and play with combinations of ideas and concepts and to explain to kids that this is a game that challenges and trains their brains. It is also extremely helpful to play the game with them and even to enlist other family members to play it too. It's interesting and fun for all of us as we imagine the possibilities of combining objects and concepts.

It's time for you to practice

Try it yourself right now. Looking at the array of objects in front of you, how many ways can you combine two of them? For example, I can see in front of me glasses, a highlighter, my calendar, post-its, a lamp, and my computer. I can say, "Highlighter calendar" or "Calendar highlighter." I can say, "Highlighter glasses" and "Glasses highlighter." You get the idea. It's easy at one level but hard at another. Without the support of grammar or context, it can be a challenge in word-finding, which will help us empathize with our older kids who are doing this for the first time.

Now, listening to yourself, you realize how odd an eleven-year-old feels making such phrase combinations. But Bevin did it with enthusiasm and pride. When we left Bevin's story, back in Chapter 2, he was firmly engaged in Stage 3 word combinations. I actually think that it was fun and relieving to him to speak deliberately and to engage his whole brain in the task. I speculated at the time that the concepts might have been triggered by his right brain but the words themselves were housed in his left brain, and that the whole-brain process was an engaging one. Bevin certainly didn't talk this way all day long, but, with his family's support, he spent hours at it daily for several months. Please look back at Chapter 2, if you'd like to review the kinds of phrases Bevin was making at Stage 3.

The trick to doing Stage 3 well when a child is older is to stay there long enough to use every type of word combination known to the English language.

The trick to doing Stage 3 well when a child is older is to stay there long enough to use every type of word combination known to the English language. Older kids have spent years saying long sentences—but without the benefit of left-brained grammar. As they emerge into grammar for the first time, it will work if they get adequate practice with all the varieties of ways words can fit together. But please remember, it's not easy for an eleven-year-old to feel "smart" doing this; he needs lots of social praise for doing so or he will try to leave it prematurely and end up back with his familiar gestalts.

Here's your practice material

Your job at Stage 3 will be much easier if you learn to rely on the Developmental Sentence Types (DST) chart introduced to you in Chapter 2. As you may recall, the chart follows every way of combining two words there is and shows how each track leads to particular grammar. A slightly-shortened version of the DST chart is included below. To take one sentence and the roads to getting there, consider "Mommy gave me the sock," where "Mommy" is the subject, the sock is the direct object, and "me" is the indirect object. "Noun elaborations" are all about the relationships between Mommy, me, and the sock, and "verb elaborations" deal with the relationships among all of us, and "giving," itself.

The DST also includes three-word combinations, each an elaboration on a two-word phrase in one of the five categories listed below. We've not included all those possibilities here, but suffice it to say that we want our kids at Stage 3 to do lots and lots of two-word and three-word combining that doesn't have anything to do with grammar. At the end of the complete chart of two-word phrases are a few examples of three-word combinations so you can get the idea.

Table 5: Nouns and Noun Elaborations

Single words, such as:
Mommy, Daddy, kitty, truck, cookie, book

Single-word elaborations and modifications, such as:
cars, me, nobody, book? car?

Two-word noun phrases including articles, possessives, quantifiers, adjectives, and attributes:
a truck, the car, Daddy car, Josh car, more ball, other doggie, two kitty, big slide, dirty bike, blue book, baby bear, police car

Two-word elaborations, including plurals, additives, adverbs, subject-objects, and subjective-locatives:
the trucks, more balls, Mommy Daddy, kitty doggie, now truck, truck too, truck again, doggie bone, Josh doggie, car garage, Mommy home

Two-word sentence modifications, including pronouns, negatives, questions, wh-questions, and the conjunction 'and':
this one, my truck, her cookie, not car, not truck, not this, a car? another car? which one? and car, and truck, and this

Table 6: Designators and Designative Elaborations

Single words, such as:
here, there, this, that, it

Single-word elaborations and modifications, such as:
those, these, this?, that?, here?, there?

Two-word elaborations and modifications including plurals, adverbs, pronouns, negatives, questions, wh-questions, and the conjunction 'and':
here car, there truck, this car, that truck, it car, it truck, these cars, there trucks, there now, here again, here something, there one, not this, not here, not there, that truck? this truck? what this? who that? and this, and here, and there.

Table 7: Descriptive Words and Predicative Elaborations

Single words, such as:
big, pretty, broken, fixed, one, two, more, on, off, up

Single-word modifications, such as:
my, his, red? big?

Two-word elaborations and modifications, such as noun + descriptive word, plurals, pronouns, questions, and wh-questions:
car broken, truck dirty, light off, tv on, car there, truck here, cars here, lights on, that pretty, it big, something here, another one, car broken? it gone? where car? what here? who there?

Table 8: Verbs and Verbal Elaborations

Single words including imperatives, such as:
sleep, eat, walk, fall, look! wait! stop!

Single-word elaborations and modifications, including verb elaborations, negatives, and questions:
going, fell, can't, won't, don't, see? eat?

Two-word elaborations, including verb + object, verb + locative, verb + particle, noun + verb, verb elaborations, plurals, and adverbs:
hit ball, sit chair, fall down, saw car, eat cookies, eat now, fall too

Two-word sentence modifications, including pronouns, negatives, questions, wh-questions, conjunctions, and infinitives:
see it, find one, not fall, can't go, see it? go home? where go? what take? what find? and sleeping, wanna go, gonna go.

Table 9: Other Vocabulary Items and Phrase Fragments

Single words such as:
yes, no, OK, hey, hi, bye-bye, night-night, oh-oh

Single-word elaborations and modifications, including adverbs, questions, wh-questions, and the conjunction 'because':
again, now, too, huh? right? OK? what? who? where? when? how? why? because

Two-word elaborations, including prepositional phrases, plurals, and adverbs:
for Daddy, in car, on chairs, in cars, too big, all gone, up now, here again, right here, over there

Two-word modifications, including pronouns, negatives, questions, and conjunctions:
to you, in it, not big, not here, in here? all gone? and big, but dirty, and here

Table 10: Three-Word Combinations

Noun example (pronoun sentence modification):
his other truck

Designator example (negative sentence modification):
that not car

Descriptor example (adverb sentence elaboration):
light off now

Verb example (wh-question):
what take out?

Vocabulary example (conjunction):
and for me

Beginning grammar as Stage 4 of NLA

We now know how concepts can be combined into two-word phrases in order to form huge numbers of conceptual creations. Once we have supported our kids through all of these possibilities, with lots and lots of different vocabulary and concepts in real life play, they will be ready for grammar. Thought of this way, grammar is nothing more than making concept combinations more specific and relationships among concepts more precise. So, taking our "Mommy sock" combination of two words, we can be more specific about the types of combining we are doing. As we begin Stage 4, we use just a few classes of words: simple verbs; simple pronouns such as "it," "this," "that," "I," "me," "my," "you," and "your"; the negative "not"; and beginning questions made through word reversal ("It is" becomes "Is it?). So when we apply our first-level grammatical operations to "Mommy sock," for instance, we can now model: "I got a sock," "You got a sock," "That sock's yours," "Mommy's sock is pink," and "Is that my sock?"

After you have spent some time playing with the possibilities at this level, you will begin to wonder why we need any more advanced grammar. There is so much that can be said at this level that, after a little practice, you will likely have little trouble modeling sentences and engaging in fun Stage 4 conversation with your child. Please give it a short try right now before we take a little side trip.

Language development vs. language learning

One side trip needs to be taken right now, because it will help you feel good about the overall journey you are taking. The goal of our side trip is to reaffirm that our kids are **developing** language in the same sense that they are developing motorically. In the field of Speech-Language Pathology, we talk about language development or language acquisition for all kids, with and without disabilities. Language is a natural part of our humanness, and language development is a birthright. We want to support all children to achieve language development to the maximum level of their capacity.

Language development is a birthright. We want to support all children to achieve language development to the maximum level of their capacity.

As we have already noted, the term "language learning" is sometimes used to mean the same thing as language development. When an SLP says it, it is just an improper choice of terminology that was intended to mean the same thing. But when used by behavioral psychology, it means something else: learning a set of verbal skills as "behaviors" that may or may not support natural language development.

To parents hearing about "language learning," then, there is a risk of thinking they are one and the same or that language learning necessarily promotes language development. Neither is true. In some cases, language learning does no harm; in others, it can impede the language development process. The following is one example that illustrates a child learning something he was not developmentally ready to learn: After months of practice, a young friend of mine could recite a blurry version of the Pledge of Allegiance along with his class. He was proud of himself. That was good. But, this impressive language learning did nothing to promote his grammatical development. Not only did his spontaneous language lack any examples of prepositional phrases ("to the flag," "to the Republic"), but his pronoun reversal meant he had not developed the spontaneous use of the pronoun "I" which begins the pledge. Learning the Pledge of Allegiance didn't change that or set him up any better. It did nothing for his language development.

Learning is powerful; we have an enormous capacity for life-long learning. But development is another matter. Our competencies in motor development and language development happen during our childhood years, to the level of our potential. The developmental order is related to maturity, and the natural course of maturing defines the developmental progression. We watch our youngsters sit, stand, toddle, and walk in a predictable order. Language development has a predictable order, too, and you are reading about it in this book.

But learning particular behaviors or skills is something different. Any one of those behaviors or skills is easier if we are developmentally ready for it. My little friend wasn't ready, but after working really hard on the Pledge of Allegiance, he conquered it. Learning is that way. Our kids are capable and often very tenacious. But the pledge didn't help my friend's language development because he simply wasn't developmentally ready for truly acquiring language that advanced.

Verbal behaviors come in many forms. Counting to 10 is one, singing the ABC song is another, naming the colors or the days of the week are yet others. But even when we add up all the behaviors we can think of, they do not equal language development. Some of them can't hurt. Some can even help, if they are developmentally appropriate. But none of these behaviors, taken singly or collectively, is the same as language development.

To develop to his language potential, a child needs sufficient communicative opportunities and developmentally-appropriate language models.

Developing language is part of our potential, part of our humanity, and it happens naturally in the proper environment. We might never learn the capitals of the states or we might quickly forget the Gettysburg Address, but our language development is something different. As we grew up, it was our preverbal referencing, our use of single words, our juxtaposing of words in first phrases, and our beginning sentences that supported our continued development of grammar and vocabulary as we acquired more and more complex language. When we match our own potential in the areas of form (vocabulary and grammar) with pragmatic functions that communicate our ideas and intentions to others, we achieve our own best language development.

Here is the caveat, however: even though language development is natural, it doesn't happen in a vacuum. A child who develops to his language potential lives in an environment that provides communicative opportunities and developmentally-appropriate language models he can incorporate to express his communicative intentions. Understanding the premises and stages of Natural Language Acquisition is part of that support, and, once it becomes integrated into our lives, it provides each of our children a foundation for continued development and for life-long learning.

Splinter skills

Language learned out of context puts the cart before the horse, however. When development precedes developmentally-appropriate skill learning, skills are acquired quickly and easily. They become part of the "bag of tricks" a child can pull out to perform for fun, or to pass the test. But learning outside of development can take more time and effort, and the results are excruciatingly difficult to generalize and, paradoxically, to undo. Such "splinter skills" risk becoming "default" behaviors that kids say whether they mean to or not, because they have been over-learned. How many of our kids say, "Ready, set, go" or "Can I have a turn?" at all kinds of times they would rather say something else?

Splinter skills risk becoming default behaviors that kids say whether they mean to or not.

An even more serious risk involved in teaching words or sentences out of developmental order is that this set of verbal behaviors gets in the way of true language development. "Ready, set, go" doesn't really get in the way. It's no worse than annoying. But when a child is developmentally at NLA Stage 1, all language input is processed through the gestalt filter and heard as a gestalt. As we recall from Ann Peters, a gestalt processor at Stage 1 processes all auditory input as equally-indivisible chunks. This can be the ABC song, the Three Bears story, the word "No," the TV commercial, or a child's own name. Whether the gestalt is one word or twenty, it is all processed the same way by a Stage 1 processor. He cannot hear the individual words of the TV commercial. And while he can hear individual words like "No" or his name when they are spoken in isolation, they are not the "building blocks" of generative language we'd hoped. As gestalts, words like "chips" and "more" aren't any more useful to language development than is the trailer for *101 Dalmations*. When our child is operating at Stage 1, he is simply hearing language as gestalts: whole strings of sound he will eventually have to break down.

When a child is at Stage 1, he hears all language as a series of gestalts.

You can see the dilemma for the Stage 1 child. When we introduced single words, we thought we were teaching him a core vocabulary in hopes of giving him the building blocks for sentences. Instead, we were actually making it impossible for the gestalt processor to know what to do next, other than to learn more and more gestalts (words, phrases, trailers, movies, whatever). Then, if we ask him to go from "Chips" to "I want chips," as behavioral programs often do, he can do it, but it makes no sense to him. It makes no sense because the single word gestalt was already a complete request.

When we ask a child to go from saying, 'Chips' to 'I want chips,' it makes no sense because the gestalt was already a complete request.

The developmental alternative

Far more efficient, successful, reliable, and flexible, then, is to allow the horse to preceed the cart. If we help our child develop a language system, the one he has the innate potential to develop, he can then choose which carts he wants to pull. We have done our part by provide the nurturing environment; he can develop a flexible language system and then choose whatever facts, skills, and behaviors matter to him.

As we end this little side trip, a dictionary definition of "develop" is in order: "to go through a process of natural growth, differentiation, or evolution, by successive changes, as a blossom develops from a bud." (*Merriam-Webster's Collegiate Dictionary*, 2004). A nice reminder, and a nice metaphor for our children's blossoming language.

How grammar develops

Eventually our kids are ready for a grammar system.

NLA is about grammar, about the natural way a grammar system develops in our gestalt language processors. We have finally gotten to the part of our story where we are ready to look at beginning grammatical structure and see how it develops naturally in children—all children, including our children. It takes our gestalt kids a while to get to this stage, of course, but eventually they are ready to develop a grammar system just like everyone else's.

From now on, we will refer to this grammar system as "self-generated" or "generative," which will distinguish it from the grammar that shows up in our kids' language gestalts. When our kids use gestalts, even ones that include grammar, they were not generating that grammar, of course. That's just the way the gestalt came. But at NLA Stage 4, they are.

Grammar development has long been the subject of language research; the developmental chart presented here was compiled more than 35 years ago. Based on how children actually develop the components of a mature grammar, it has stood the test of time and has been widely used by language clinicians to assess and guide the grammatical development of spontaneously-produced language. It is called Developmental Sentence Analysis, or Developmental Sentence Scoring (DSS), and is divided by developmental levels 1–8. DSS Level 1 is the most basic, and Level 8 is the most advanced. There are eight categories, each representing an area of grammar that builds on itself as development progresses. The categories of grammar represented in each column are: indefinite pronouns, personal pronouns, main verbs, secondary verbs, negatives, conjunctions, interrogative reversals (where the subject and the verb are reversed, like 'Is it … ?'), and 'Wh' questions. When DSS is being used as a clinical tool to score a child's spontaneous grammar, a sentence point is also awarded if the entire sentence is correct, both syntactically (grammar) and semantically (vocabulary use). A DSS scoring guide is included as Appendix D at the end of this book, and a blank form is included as Appendix C.

DSS Levels 1–3 are presented here, because they form the foundation of basic grammar for young children. As such, they make up NLA Stage 4. DSS Levels 4–8 will be presented later in this chapter, and they constitute NLA Stages 5 and 6.

Unless you are an SLP, the scoring is more than you need to understand. What a parent or family member would want to gain from this chart is the order of development of various parts of speech and a feel for which structures develop in what order. Then, you can practice making up your own sentences at each level and, in that way, support your child's development by creating the right language environment.

	Indefinite Pronouns or Noun Modifiers	Personal Pronouns	Main Verbs	Secondary Verbs
1	it, this, that	1st and 2nd person: *I, me, my, mine, you, your(s)*	A. Uninflected verb: *I see you.* B. Copula, is or 's: *It's red.* C. is + verb + ing: *He is coming.*	
2		3rd person: *he, him, his, she, her, hers*	A. -s and -ed: *plays, played* B. Irregular past: *are, saw* C. Copula: *am, are, was, were* D. Auxiliary: *am are, was, were*	Five early developing infinitives: I wanna see (want to see) I'm gonna see (going to see) I gotta see (got to see) Lemme [to] see (let me [to] see) Let's [to] play (let [us to] play)
3	A: no, some, more, all, lot(s), one(s) two (etc), other(s), another. B: something, somebody, someone	A. Plurals: *we, us, our(s), they, them, their* B. these, those		Non-complementing infinitives: *I stopped to play.* *I'm afraid to look.* *It's hard to do that.*

Table 11: Developmental Sentence Scoring, Levels 1–3, Part 1

	Negatives	Conjunctions	Interrogative Reversals	Wh-Questions
1	it, this, that + copula or auxiliary is, 's + not: *It's not mine; This is not a dog; That is not moving.*		Reversal of copula: *Isn't it red? Were they there?*	
2				A. who, what, what + noun: *Who am I? What is he eating? What book are you reading?* B. where, how many, how much, what ... do, what ... for: *Where did to go? How much do you want? What is he doing? What is a hammer for?*
3		and		

Table 12: Developmental Sentence Scoring, Levels 1–3, Part 2

Basic grammar allows some flexible self-expression.

What you will notice as you look at the first three levels of DSS (equivalent to NLA Stage 4) is how much grammar is actually there. By DSS Level 3, a child can say almost any simple sentence he would want to express. That is comforting news, especially because we know of many students whose potential stops there, either because intellectual capacity is reached or because their age precludes development of more grammar. Even so, Level 3 includes enough functional grammar for basic communication, and with this level of grammatical competence, kids can be flexible communicators.

Colin was one such individual. At age 18, he had a few remnant Stage 2 mitigations he could only use in their original format, but otherwise, his language was moderately flexible and self-generated. Almost all of it depended on grammatical structures from DSS levels 1–3, with a smattering of higher-level structures. Here is a composite sample of Colin's spontaneous language, demonstrating how much can be expressed with just a DSS Level 3 competence and a few other structures (seen in the last five examples):

I'm so serious about my water.
I miss that Colleen.
Colleen was driving a blue dump truck.
Let's go to Shopko and Copps.
Are you a Blarge?
She's cute.
You closed your mouth on the driveway.
You picked me up from school.
I talked to you on the phone.
We saw Evan and Megan.
When will I see you?
Where else can we go? ("can go" is level 4)
What can I get? ("can get" is level 4)
Stop singing, Blarge. ("singing" as a gerund is level 8)
You're all done helping your mom. ("helping" is level 8)
What happened when I threw the fries? ("when" is level 8 when used to join clauses)

Colin still faced challenges with self-expression, to be sure. As a sensitive young man, Colin struggled with balancing self-advocacy with pleasing others. But at least he had the basic tools of grammar to meet most of his communication needs.

Allow grammar to build

One of the biggest lessons in grammatical development is that each level naturally supports the next as children continue to progress. If we keep our DSS chart handy, we can remain cognizant of the order of development within a category and also of which structures develop at about the same time. When we have a sense of our child's level, we can focus on that level as we talk with our child.

I carry a chart on my clip board, and we have several posted in our clinic. I always suggest that families put one on the fridge so everyone in a child's environment is aware of the language level we want to support and encourage at any particular time. The appropriate structures at any one time can be highlighted, and the whole family can make sure the child is hearing—and using—all the structures at a particular developmental level with a variety of vocabulary words. When a child has achieved competence at one level, everyone can begin modeling a small assortment of structures from the next level. A slightly-abridged DSS chart, on two facing pages, is included in this book as Appendix D.

How to assess grammatical level

Now that you know the structures at DSS Levels 1–3 and have read some sentences using them, you are ready to learn the steps in assessing your own child's grammar and ways of supporting his grammatical growth. We then will move on to the higher levels of grammar and explore the greater variety of sentences that can be constructed when children gain competence with them.

And, by the way, please don't worry if all this is "Greek" to you; you can turn the job over to your child's Speech-Language Pathologist. But if you are excited about the prospects of doing it yourself, here are the steps in assessing the grammatical competence of your child:

1. Find a time to just listen to your child and to write down a sample of his original phrases and sentences. Don't worry if the phrases are correct or not; we just want to see what he is attempting that is not a gestalt or a mitigation.

2. Look at your list and highlight the grammatical structures he uses or tries to use. Look at Level 1 on the DSS chart and move across as you look first for pronouns, then simple verbs, the negative "not," and the question form (interrogative reversal). That's all there is to Level 1.

3. Now do the same thing for Level 2, noting the more advanced pronouns "he" and "she," the more advanced verb forms (past tense and "to be" verbs: "am," "are," "was," and "were"). Continue with the secondary verbs: "Let's," the simple future tense: "wanna," "gonna," and "gotta," and then the "wh" question forms: "what," "where," and "how."

4. Continue with Level 3, noting the great variety of pronoun forms, the secondary verb "to …," and the first conjunction "and."

5. Your next step will require more time to listen to your child. This time, you will be listening for the variety of ways he uses each structure, and this will help you decide which forms he has had adequate experience with and which ones he has not.

6. Next, note which structures are just emerging and which ones show real competence. When a child is using a structure incorrectly or only occasionally, with just a few vocabulary words or in only a few contexts, the structure is not yet part of his competence. If he uses a structure routinely, within many contexts and with a nice variety of vocabulary words, it is part of his competence.

7. Mark your results on a clean DSS chart: yellow are the structures that are emerging and orange are those with which your child is competent. The yellow ones will be your first targets.

Now it's time to check in with your SLP to make sure your plan seems sound and that you are on the same page. If so, it's time to plan your program to support your child's development of grammar.

How to plan your support

For purposes of simplicity, we are going to look at only Level 1 now. But if your child is solidly at Level 1, this process will continue for every level where he shows at least one example of one structure used generatively. OK, here's the process:

Focus on an entire developmental level and watch it all emerge.

1. Scan your chart and notice your child's oranges: his competencies. Now notice the yellows at Level 1 (his emerging grammar) and then the structures he doesn't use at all. Make sure you listen for all of these structures during the weeks ahead because focusing on a single level will often help all the structures at that level emerge and solidify.

2. Look again at the gaps at Level 1 and pick one you might naturally target during your interactions with your child. For example, if your child says "I" and "it" in a variety of sentences, you have highlighted them with orange and know they are among his competencies. You notice, however, that he only says "mine" very occasionally (it is marked yellow) and never says "this," "that," "me," or "my."

Surround your child with a developmental level by becoming fluent in it yourself.

3. Think about the structures you have selected and think about some ways you could use them in a variety of sentences. Make sure it will be easy for you, and that modeling them will promote the structure's flexible use right from the start. This is the time to promise yourself that no one will "drill" your child on it or use a target within only one context or with just a single vocabulary word. All too often, one day's "script" becomes the over-learned "default" a week later.

4. Practice some of your language models until you know you can use them conversationally and playfully. Here's an example: You have decided to target "this," so you play a little game with a friend: you say, "Hey, Shawna, do you want that one?" and your friend answers, "No, silly, **this** one!" In this example, please note that your targets don't have to be sentences. They can be more like the mix-and-match of concepts and words we talked about at NLA Stage 3.

5. Once you are fluently able to converse with one language model, it would be good to add a second one from a different category. It's important to start to expand your repertoire of options so you can keep your language authentic and fun. A verb form is a natural, and you will quickly learn how important verbs are for early modeling, partly because they are so foundational to language development and partly because they provide instant conversation and variety. Let's take an example. Say your child uses "is" only with "it" and says, "It's red," "It's blue," etc. with several colors. You have marked the contracted form of "it's" as among his competencies. But you realize he never says, "It **is** red!" etc., so you decide to try to set up a game of naming colors where you say to a family member or friend, "Hey, it's blue," and he counters with, "It is not! It's red!" Just expanding on this idea, you might be able to lead quickly to a whole range of options and play games with your whole family: "Is it blue? Is it red? Is it yellow?" and one person pipes up, "No! "It's purple!"

6. You may begin to notice your child copying you, or "echoing." This is a good thing; it's his learning style and how he picked up language in the first place. You will want to keep mental tabs on what he echoes, though, and stay mentally ahead of him, giving him plenty of variety to listen to right from the start. Be careful not to let your language interaction become an inadvertent "drill." But, also, don't worry if your child doesn't start to echo you or use your models yet. He is a gestalt learner at heart and may need to amass enough examples before he's ready to take a leap. Plus, he has yet to learn to trust your judgment about what language might be beneficial for him. But once that happens, we have found that a child's progress is much faster. Once you and your child are a language team, your interaction can become a reliable place for language development.

7. As this process starts to become natural for you and you begin to expand your targets, keep in mind one to avoid early on. Until a time very much later, it would be wise to avoid "you" and "your." They are tricky to model and take another person to help you. Without that third person to label as "you," we find ourselves inadvertently stepping into the "pronoun reversal" trap. This, of course, has been considered a hallmark of autism, and various theories have been suggested over the years as to why. As a student of NLA, however, you know that it is simply comes with the linguistic territory. Gestalt processors process gestalts, regardless of the first person/second person form. We say to our kids all day long: "You got it"; "You did it"; "What do you want?"; "Use your words"; and "Where are your shoes?" What do we think they are prone to say, then, but: "You got it," "You did it," and "Where are your shoes?" when they refer to themselves and their shoes. An alternative is to speak for yourself, saying, "I got it," "I did it," etc. as you do something. Whenever you have another person to help you, each of you can use "I" statements; this illustrates the point that "I" is not synonymous with "Mom" or "Dad" but refers to the person making the statement.

Gestalt processors process gestalts, regardless of the first person/second person form.

8. You should also avoid, at least for now, question forms. Again, gestalt processors process gestalts, and every "question" we think we are posing might seem like a question to us, but to our child it is an inadvertent language model. Thus, it is not so surprising that some of the most intractable gestalts are some of the earliest learned and the most personal. One of my long-time friends, Russel, whom you will meet later in the book, still used an old gestalt even when his generative language was almost completely developed. "Where are your blankets?" he would ask (that is, comment) when he left the house as a way of saying, "I hope I have my blankets."

Every 'question' we think we are posing might seem like a question to us, but to our child, it is an inadvertent language model.

9. There is a wonderful strategy you can use, however, that circumvents the pitfalls of both "you" and questions: the use of "Let's." While it jumps up a bit into Level 2, this structure is so easy for all of us to use that kids usually pick it up readily. The only thing to be careful of, however, is to only use it for things your child truly wants, like "Let's get Barney!" or "Let's go to McDonald's!" The trick is to model it *only* when you know your child would like to be saying it himself. We have to be careful, as we can ruin the entire structure by using it with something the child would never pick, like cleaning up or going potty or putting on his coat. We might think we're

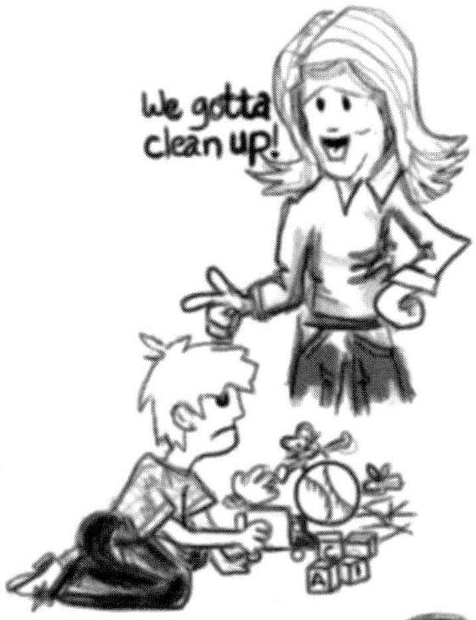

being polite and inclusive when we say, "Let's clean that up," but from the child's perspective, it's neither, and we have ruined the entire grammatical structure for the power it can have.

10. Not everything you say to your child represents an actual language target, of course. But any language you use with your child is really an unintended "model," so plan to use it in a good way. In the example we just gave, then, instead of ruining the inclusive, positive power of "Let's" by saying, "Let's clean that up," you can say, "We gotta clean that up," and then help so that it really is "we." Save "Let's" for something fun!

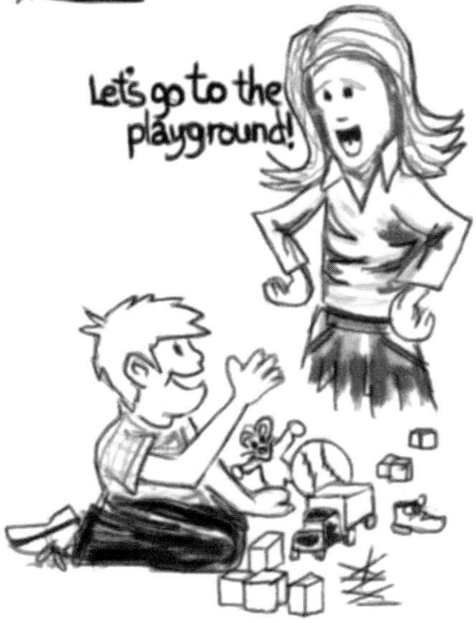

If you are reading this chapter to get an idea of the progression you will be able to follow one day, good. If you are reading it and applying it at the same time, that's good, too. But might we suggest that before you go much further, you consult your child's SLP and make sure you both are on the same page. Our kids hear language from lots of sources, and you want to make sure that everyone working with your child is in agreement about the process you have chosen to undertake. Besides the particular caveats mentioned already, if a child hears the same sentence modeled the same way more than a few times, it may well end up becoming an unintended "drill" and processed as just another gestalt, rather than an example of a grammatical structure as you had intended. You will want to make sure your team, starting with your SLP and then extending to the others, is working with you, and not in some other direction.

Advanced grammar at Stages 5 and 6 of NLA

As you continue your study of grammatical development, you will be impressed with how fine-tuned our syntactic system is and the specificity of time and condition that can be expressed with structures at DSS levels 4–8 (NLA Stages 5 and 6).

While I would love to walk you through the second half of the DSS chart, I'm afraid too many of you would simply fall asleep. A brief scan will give you the overview of what's possible. Truth be told, you have the basics now, and as your child is ready for more advanced grammar, you may decide to turn a good bit of the work over to your child's SLP. You will want to continue to model appropriate language at home, but it can become tedious to keep track of it all, and SLPs are well-trained to do this.

On the next page is the second half of the DSS chart, Levels 4–8. Levels 4–6 make up NLA Stage 5, and DSS Levels 7 and 8 make up NLA Stage 6.

	Indefinite Pronouns or Noun Modifiers	Personal Pronouns	Main Verbs	Secondary Verbs
4	nothing, nobody, none, no one		A. can, will, may + verb: *may go* B. Obligatory do + verb: *don't go* C. Emphatic do + verb: *I do see*	Participle, present or past: *I see a boy running. I found the toy broken.*
5		Reflexives: *myself, yourself, himself, herself, itself, themselves*		A. Early infinitival complements with differing subjects in kernels: *I want you to come, Let him [to] see.* B. Later infinitival complements: *I had to go, I told him to go, I tried to go, He ought to go.* C. Obligatory deletions: *Make it [to] go.* D. Infinitive with wh-word: *I know what to get, I know how to do it.*
6		A. Wh-pronouns: *who, which, whose, whom, what, that, how many, how much* B. Wh-word + infinitives: *I know what to do, I know who(m) to take.*	A. could, would, should, might + verb: *might come, could be* B. Obligatory does, did + verb C. Emphatic does, did + verb	
7	A. any, anything, anybody, anyone B. every, everything, everybody, everyone C. both, few, many, each, several, most, least, much, next, first, last, second (etc.)	(his) own, one, oneself, whichever, whoever, whatever: *Take whatever you like.*	A. Passive with get, any tense; Passive with be, any tense B. must, shall + verb: *must come* C. have + verb + en: *I've eaten.* D. have got: *I've got it.*	Passive infinitival complement: With get: *I have to get dressed. I don't want to get hurt.* With be: *I want to be pulled, It's going to be locked.*
8			A. have been + verb + ing; had been + verb + ing B. modal + have + verb + en: *may have eaten* C. modal + be + verb + ing: *could be playing* D. Other auxiliary combinations: *should have been sleeping.*	Gerund: *Swinging is fun. I like fishing. He staring laughing.*

Table 13: Developmental Sentence Scoring, Levels 4–8, Part 1

	Negatives	Conjunctions	Interrogative Reversals	Wh-Questions
4	can't, don't		Reversal of auxiliary be: *Is he coming? Isn't he coming? Was he going?*	
5	isn't, won't	A. but B. so, and so, so that C. or, if		When, how, how + adjective: *When shall I come? How do you do it? How big is it?*
6		because	A. Obligatory do, does, did: *Do they run? Does it bite? Didn't it hurt?* B. Reversal of modal: *Can you play? Won't it hurt? Shall I sit down?* C. Tag question: *It's fun isn't it? It isn't fun, is it?*	
7	All other negatives: A. Uncontracted negatives: *I can not go.* *He has not gone.* B. Pronoun-auxiliary or pronoun-copula contraction: *I'm not coming.* *He's not here.* C. Auxiliary-negative or copula-negative contraction: *He wasn't going, He hasn't been seen, It couldn't be mine, They aren't big.*			Why, what if, how come, how about + gerund: *Why are you crying?* *What if I won't do it?* *How come he is crying?* *How about coming with me?*
8		A. where, when, how, while, whether (or not), till, until, unless, since, before, after, for, as, as + adjective + as, as if, like, that, than: *I know where you are, Don't come till I call.* B. Obligatory deletions: *I run faster than you [run], I'm as big as a man [is big], It looks like a dog [looks].* C. Elliptical deletions (score 0): *That's why [I took it], I know how [I can do it].* D. Wh-words + infinitive: *I know how to do it.* *I know where to go.*	A. Reversal of auxiliary have: *Has he seen you?* B. Reversal with two or three auxiliaries: *Has he been eating?* *Couldn't he have waited?* *Could he have been crying?* *Wouldn't he have been going?*	Whose, which, which + noun: *Whose car is that?* *Which book do you want?*

Table 14: Developmental Sentence Scoring, Levels 4–8, Part 2

How much progress is possible?

> ***Kids can still work on grammar into their teens.***

The textbooks have warned us that it's not possible to learn rule-based grammar after the age of 6 or 7: that our left hemisphere is incapable of adding grammar after that age. Well, this might be true for kids who already have their entire grammar system in their minds by then, but our experience tells us that does not hold true for kids with language delays. If it were, our ASD kids wouldn't continue to integrate more and more grammar throughout their childhoods, and they do. The longitudinal data from language samples in our clinic shows kids' grammar developing to Stage 5 or 6 of NLA if they start the process by age 6 or 7. If they get started at age 8, 9 or 10, they can still achieve Stage 4 or Stage 5 grammar. In other words, kids can still work on higher-level grammar at age 12 and, depending on the child, into their teens.

This "grace period" in older students with Down Syndrome was documented by Thordardottir et al. (2002), who found that teenagers with Down Syndrome continued to develop grammar. Quoted in *Science Daily* (2002), co-researcher Robin Chapman noted, "… if an adolescent acquires the ability to understand complex grammar more slowly, he will also acquire the ability to speak that grammar more slowly … the study's findings suggest that there should continue to be language work in both comprehension and expression throughout teen-age and young adult years" (Chapman, 2002).

In personal conversation, Dr. Chapman offered some thoughts about the discrepancy between the literature and what she found. She hypothesized that children who have a complete grammar by age 6, when it would be expected, could not learn more grammar rules in the usual way. When they try to learn the rules of a second language, they have to learn through immersion and use their whole brains. Chapman theorized that kids without a complete grammar system in their left hemisphere, however, could continue to build one for many more years.

A 2009 article published in the *Journal of Speech, Language, and Hearing Research* acknowledged something similar among kids with autism: "… children with ASD continue to make important advances in language well into the school years …" (Tager-Flusberg et al., 2009). The researchers challenged the autism community to "move away from the commonly used term 'functional speech' as the outcome goal for intervention studies" and noted that this singular term is inadequate to reflect the development of language achieved by children with ASD.

This research team recommended describing language acquisition more completely and using the following framework for describing spoken language acquisition in ASD: preverbal communication, first words, word combinations, sentences, and complex language. While not including guidelines for echolalia, these researchers acknowledged its use at the early stages of language acquisition for ASD kids, but, lacking "clear criteria for defining delayed echolalia," they recommended echolalic and imitative language be omitted from analysis within the research framework they proposed.

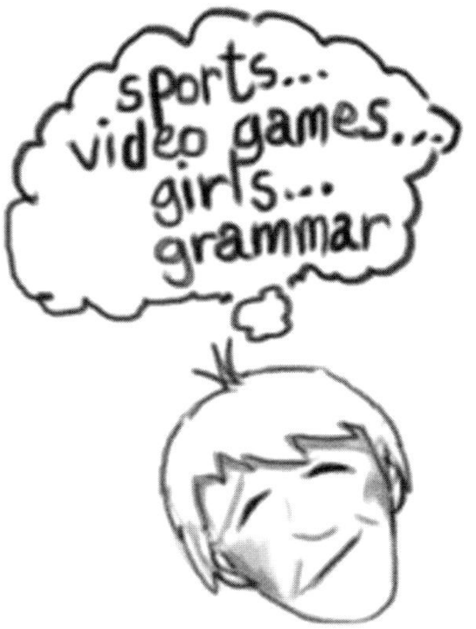

Challenges to language development for teenagers

The teenage years are notoriously challenging, not only on the spectrum but off the spectrum as well. In the experience of our clinic, these years are difficult ones for continued grammar development. For kids who started late, grammar continues to develop, but the process slows down considerably. The interference between old language gestalts and new grammar is strong, with the new grammar sounding so close to old gestalts that it is tempting to resort to the old language. The larger factor, however, is that the demands on teenagers' energies increase exponentially. Middle School is socially challenging, and physical, sensory, and emotional interferences often dominate. Kids who could live with their sensory systems in elementary school suddenly find the chaos of packed hallways and gymnasiums overwhelming. In addition, kids' bodies grow quickly, and the core muscles that once housed a place of self-regulation become difficult to find in a tall, gangly body. Unfortunately, it is also difficult to re-engage OT and PT services after they were withdrawn when kids were younger and doing well. Our teenagers are often expected to survive without OT/PT support. And grammar? Well, it seems to runs a distant last place in the priorities of this time period. The bottom line is that until a teen's grammar is complete, developmental potential may still be there, but life conspires to make it more difficult to address.

So, besides grammar, what else is there to work on?

Yes, we continue to work with our teens towards higher level grammar as long as we can see it still developing. But, at the same time, there is much more to communication that we can successfully address. After all, grammar is just a tool; it is how grammar is used for self-expression that matters.

Chapters 16 and 17 will explore the use of language for story-telling, self-advocacy, and developing friendships. All through the journey described in this book, we support children to use their developing language, including grammar, within interactions and for a wide variety of communicative purposes. As you continue the journey of this book, you will learn how to support your child in all these ways.

So, here's your first exercise. It's about you. Please stand back from your child for a moment and think about the life-long learners we all are, the life-long learner you are. Please pause for a moment and truly think about this. We are acquiring new words all the time and learning to talk about new concepts. We are using words in new, creative ways—all the time. Think about your last explanation to your boss, your last plea to your family, your last mental blog post, or the letter-to-the-editor you composed in your mind but never sent. As Barney would say, "The fun and learning never ends." That's life-long learning.

We all grow in our sense of conversation too: how to converse with our family members as they grow up or age; how to converse with new work-mates, new customers, and new bosses; how to converse in different groups and maybe even larger groups. And in our relationships, we are perfecting our turn-taking so that our turns don't trip over the other person's and sound like "Yeah, but ..." We learn to become better communication partners referentially as well, as we learn to use exact points of reference when we give directions and explain how to do things. We learn to use the other person's knowledge as a point of reference and realize how much easier it is to communicate when we begin where the other person already is.

Throughout our lives, we have the capacity to get better and better at perspective-taking, too; in our growing circle of acquaintances, we learn to address the points of view of others. Finally, there's the internal "contingency" of conversations: the way one person's comment is contingent on the one(s) before it. This sophisticated sense eventually allows us to build group ideas and even consensus as each thought builds a new collective. "The fun and learning never ends."

Now step back into the dyad with your child and understand why our older kids can feel so lost as their social worlds expand. Conversational skills are endlessly-challenging. But, thankfully, our kids are life-long learners too, and we don't expect our teenagers to conquer everything. Like you and I, our kids have their whole lives to continue learning.

Chapter 6
Summary of Theory

It's now time to reflect, to take stock of what we have have addressed so far, and to summarize the key concepts:

We can provide the right environment for our kids to develop as communicators.

We know that echolalia is normal and natural. We know that it is part of gestalt language processing. We know that it's part of a natural language development progression: that kids learn to break down their gestalts, isolate the single word, build their own unique word combinations, and progress to phrases and sentences.

We also know that our kids are part of a larger group of learners, not unlike ADD kids but often more right-brained, more visual, more holistic, and more sensorimotor-involved. As such, our kids need our understanding plus some help and support to move through this natural language acquisition process.

We know that we will be extremely helpful to them, and we know that we will understand how. We will provide the right language environment for our kids, the right social environment, and the right sensorimotor environment for them to access the language in it.

We know that the natural developmental progression of grammar and the methods outlined in this book will help ASD kids to become more flexible, creative language-users.

We know that developmentally appropriate communication activities will help our kids use their grammar communicatively and creatively and that each level of competence will support the next to emerge.

We know that a child's age matters and that the younger a child begins the NLA process, the easier his task and ours will be. When kids start the process as youngsters, they have fewer gestalts in their encyclopedias, and we can plan for them to hear ones they will be able to mitigate most easily.

We know that children can start the process later, however, and if they begin the NLA process by the age of 6 or 7, they may be able to continue into the higher levels of grammar. Even if they get started by age ten, they still have the capacity to make good, useful gains in grammar.

We know that grammar is just a tool and that what we learn to do with what we have is what really matters to our communication.

We know that we are all life-long learners and will continue to grow and expand in our use of language for creative, intellectual, and social purposes all our lives.

With this summary in mind, let's now turn to the preschool population and examine the principles of assessment and intervention appropriate to their age group. This section will be useful to those of you whose child is older than preschool age, too, as the principles will be the same even if you are not able to complete all the preliminary work outlined here. The next chapters will be a useful reference for all readers.

section 3

Preschoolers: Assessing their Language and Planning its Development

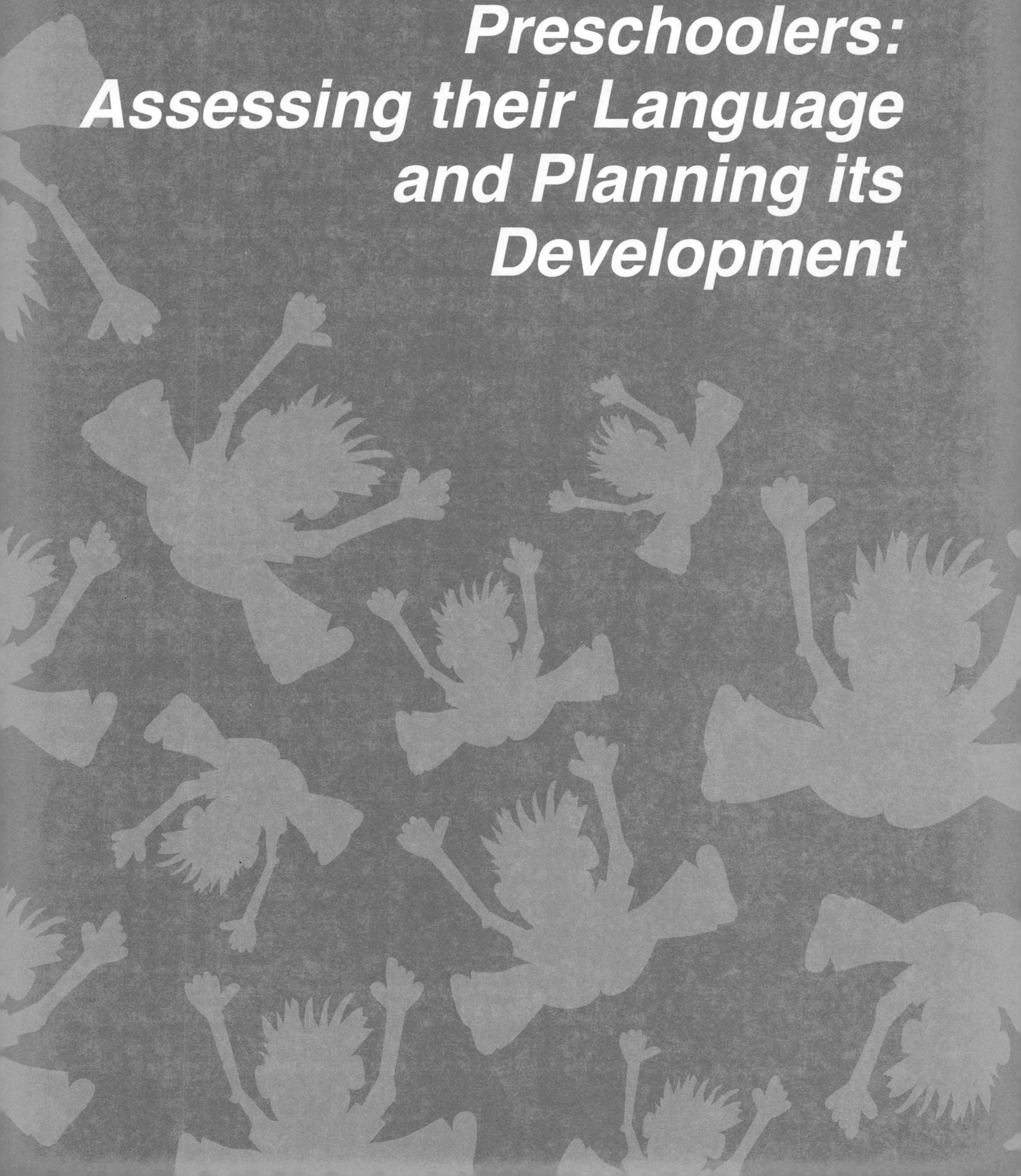

Introduction

We all know that early intervention is one of the keys to the best outcomes for our ASD kids. There are many reasons for this. Young children show the greatest brain plasticity, and, therefore, the greatest ease of learning new patterns. And that's good for those of us who want to help young children develop language.

Young children have less "on their plates" too. For the most part, they're not in school yet and are at home with their families, who can treat them like the individuals they are. Preschoolers have less on their minds, too—and less in their minds. Their language exposure has been limited, and their gestalts are less complicated and fewer in number. Recall Dylan at age four and how easy it was to plan nice, easy-to-mitigate gestalts to model for him. Plus, a four-year-old can only know so many movies by heart and thus has only a limited number of longer gestalts in his mind. Mitigation is usually easy for young children off the spectrum, who tend to accomplish it fairly seamlessly. But even with sensorimotor impairments, the process for young ASD kids is much easier than for older spectrum kids. We know that Dylan's library of gestalts was pretty manageable compared with the encyclopedia that was in Bevin's ten-year-old brain.

Early intervention is important, but it has to be the right one for your child.

Early intervention is an important key, but, not surprisingly, it has to be the right intervention. It has to be about language development as opposed to "language teaching," and it has to include acknowledgement of the communicative and linguistic value of echolalia. One doesn't have to completely understand the NLA process to acknowledge the communicative value of echolalia and honor a young child's intent when he uses it. Even if a good SLP in your community has never considered echolalia before, this book will give him or her ample information and guidelines. That piece of your search should not be difficult.

On the other hand, now that in-home intensive programs are available in more and more communities, your first decision may be much larger than simply enrolling your child in appropriate language therapy with a certified Speech-Language Pathologist. Within intensive autism programs, language programs are delivered by people other than SLPs, most notably in the form of language teaching under the rubric of ABA. Originally designed as Lovaas programs, such ABA programs are now often hybrids, but they still consider language something that is learned rather than something that develops. The foundation of ABA is behavioral, that is, it views what a child does as a set of behaviors learned through motivation and reinforcement that can be "modified" by others.

As a contrast, Greenspan-based "floor-time" programs are developmental in nature and see language as something that kids naturally develop. Echolalia will probably be outside the scope of a Greenspan team's understanding, however, so don't be surprised if the language curriculum for your child starts with single words. Parents would be wise to investigate their own community's version of floor-time and make sure that a Speech-Language Pathologist can be a part of the team or at least welcome to work with it.

Chapter 7 will delve into the issues of intensive autism programs, at least enough to help you look at them critically, and then will steer you back to the language development program you'll want to set up for your preschool child.

But first ...

Before you start, however, please pause—right now—and take stock of your child, your precious child, the individual person you care so much about. Think about this little person and formulate a picture of him or her—his loves, her passions, his fears, her concerns, his laugh, her cry, his scowl, her smile—and jot down some notes for yourself. Take at least fifteen minutes right now and draw up a little profile of your child, one you can refer back to as you begin to delve into the complexities of the outside world. As you step into the autism community, you will want to keep your child with you, in your mind and heart, at all times. You will want to ground yourself with that image again and again. You will hear all kinds of terms thrown about; you will be asked all manner of questions; you will feel that you need to choose a program, or an approach, immediately. If you take the time to formulate a picture of your child now, you will have much less tendency to leap into action, to act without a direction, to worry about something you don't need to worry about, and conversely, you will be able to pay attention to what you actually do need to pay attention to.

As you step into the autism community, keep your child with you, in your mind and heart, at all times. You will want to ground yourself with that image again and again.

As you meet people, you may be asked things like, "How many words does your child say?" And before you answer that question with something like, "I don't even think my child is talking at all," please consider what you know about your child's sound-making. Does she laugh? How does it sound? Does he make happy sounds or sad sounds? What do they sound like? Can you tell if she's pleased? Or distraught? Or hungry? How do you know? Remember that the "sound track" of gestalt language is a melody line. Is your child saying one? Or almost saying one?

Having thought about what your child sounds like, you can answer that same question a different way. Here's an example: "Well, in a way, I think my child is talking. She uses a high-pitched, rising sound pattern when she's delighted. I can hear a vowel sound in there that sounds like 'eee.' But when she's sad, her voice sounds sad, and she says something like, 'Awwww.' It makes your heart break. I don't know if there's a word in there or not, but maybe there's a sentence."

For some kids, however, the sound contours described here are impossible to produce, and some young children may be nearly silent. Many of our kids are unable to produce easy, fluent sound until they are somewhat older. It might be low muscle tone, limited breath support, and/or motor coordination challenges that make voicing or even sustained exhalation really hard. If this describes your child, you may want to skip to Chapter 9 right now. It will guide you through some thinking about sound-making that might be just what your child needs first.

Chapter 7
Intervention for Preschool Children: Applying the Principles, Looking at Individual Differences

Intensive autism treatment programs

Depending on the community, families of newly-diagnosed children might be considered for an intensive program, a choice of programs, or none at all. And depending on local information sources, families may not know what is available without doing some homework. It is important to research any intensive program in your community before choosing it for your child. Even a cursory examination of the possibilities out there reveals how different, and even diametrically opposed, they can be. Some intensive programs begin with "compliance," others begin by following the child's lead. ABA programs might prefer that a child sit at a table and respond to directions, while floor-time programs might prefer following a child's propensities in play. Some might approach communication by giving kids picture cards to use to make choices; others might ask a child to imitate sounds or words; others might begin with gestures.

As helpful as parts of all these programs might be, and as much "evidence base" as any one might claim, a particular program must work for a particular child in order to be appropriate. As difficult as this might be to figure out ahead of time, the veracity of this statement should be enough to alert any of us to do our homework and keep track of our child's progress ourself. Your personal assessment of your own child and the kind of progress he makes is imperative. As Rogers and Vismara pointed out in 2007, even the programs that can show significant results in a statistical sense worked for only half the kids in them.

As we mentioned in Chapter 4, these authors reviewed program outcome literature, including attempts at replicating the "recovery" purported by the original Lovaas study of 1987. Of the 28 children in the replication study (Smith, Groen, and Wynn, 2000), half were diagnosed with PDD-NOS and half with Autism. "When one examines the pre- and post-test scores in the published tables by child diagnosis, questions are raised about the effect of the treatment on children with the full syndrome of autism. The treated children with the full autism syndrome showed little developmental acceleration over the course of treatment. Their post-treatment scores were essentially the same as their pre-treatment scores, and they showed a 10-point loss on a standard language measure. Moreover, their post-treatment scores in IQ, language, and adaptive behavior were highly similar to the comparison group of children with the full syndrome of autism. In contrast, the experimentally treated children diagnosed with PDD-NOS demonstrated large increases in IQ and language scores from pre to post-treatment (including a 26 point IQ gain), though the differences were not statistically significant …" (p. 15).

A second partial replication study (Sallows and Graupner, 2005) was also reported, in which the ABA format was supplemented with a more naturalistic situation, use of picture cards for communication, more play time with peers, and part-time enrollment in preschool. After 3 to 4 years of treatment, almost half the children (11 of 23) had measured IQs over 85 and were reported to be succeeding in regular education classrooms. The other 13 children "showed no significant increase in IQ from pre- to post-test. Their pre- and post-treatment standard scores ranged from the 30s to the 50s … and their autism symptoms continued to be greatly elevated. Thus, half of the children in this study demonstrated poor outcomes, with marked delays in all areas, little developmental acceleration, and little decrease in autism symptoms, even after four years of 30 to 40 hours a week of intensive daily treatment. Pretreatment measures associated with poor outcomes included initial low IQ (below 44) and lack of language (no words at 36 months)" (Sallows and Graupner, 2005, p. 18).

So what do I do?

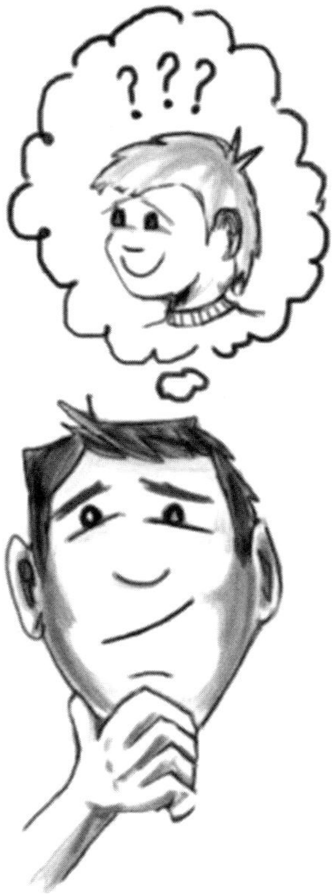

There are a good number of take-away lessons here, the first of which is to ask a crucial question before buying into any program even if it is "evidenced based," like the ones above. The crucial question to ask yourself is: Do I believe my child fits the half who made gains in this study as opposed to the half who did not, and who maybe lost language function along the way?

The second question is this: If I decide after a week, or a month, or six months, that this program is not a match for my child, will my insurance company and my program provider allow me to switch to something else I believe will be?

The third set of questions is about language development: If the program I'm considering teaches language as a behavior, and I feel my child is capable of natural language development, will the provider omit their typical language program and support the developmental one I choose? Or if the program I'm considering uses a protocol not intended for gestalt language processors, will the program provider be willing to substitute my language development program for theirs?

If the answers to these three questions is "yes," you may have a good package. If not, however, you may need to look for alternatives in your community or put your own together. As Rogers and Vismara pointed out, we can look for the best parts of various "name brand" programs plus add the "best practices" from the developmental therapies in our communities (Occupational Therapy, Physical Therapy, Speech and Language Therapy) and address our child's unique pattern of strengths and challenges.

Depending on your community, there may be other programs, available at centers, schools, and clinics, which address early intervention for kids on the autism spectrum. While a review of these programs is outside the scope of this book, one has only to glance at several of the newer, developmental models to see how much thought and longitudinal research have coalesced into these programs. The Early Start Denver Model defines itself this way: "Supported by the principles of developmental psychology and applied behavior analysis, ESDM's intensive teaching interventions are delivered within play-based, relationship-focused routines" (Rogers and Dawson, 2009).

The SCERTS model, too, was developed after years of research. The acronym stands for social-communication, emotional regulation, and transactional support, and SCERTS defines itself as: "a comprehensive, multidisciplinary, educational approach for individuals with ASD and related disabilities ... a comprehensive program for supporting children and their families that focuses on meaningful, authentic progress within everyday routines at school, home, and in the community." Its stated goal is to provide "a scope and sequence of developmentally grounded goals and objectives ..." Finally, it acknowledges the "continuum of echolalic to creative language," as some of its authors were the early researchers in gestalt language processing (Prizant et al., 2006).

Whether you embrace an intensive autism program for your child or not, your own language program for your child will be central to the progress your child will make. We are ready to turn to it now.

Your language intervention program

Now is the time to set up your child's language intervention program with the help of an experienced SLP and an experienced OT and/or PT who can partner with you. Let's examine some principles that are at the heart of why you are doing this:

- Our kids are language-delayed, first, because gestalt language processing is not well understood and our kids need support in order for their language to develop.
- Our kids are language-delayed, second, because their sensorimotor systems do not allow them the same opportunities to sift through the language available to their peers off the spectrum. Consider the sandbox monologues of unintelligible, but typically-developing, children. When kids feel no aversion to sand and can move their arms and hands to manipulate toys, they have the opportunity to use sound and language in a context and medium they like. The ASD child with tactile aversion and limited coordination of the upper body more often finds himself running away from sandboxes—and sitting in front of a TV or a book instead. Because our kids are not actively engaged with language and materials, they are more passive observers than active doers, and all development takes more time.

Our kids have unique interests. One size fits no one.

- Our kids, like all kids, have unique interests that are best understood by their families who can then help others understand what makes them tick and what they would likely want to talk about. One size fits no one.
- Our kids, like all kids, have unique learning profiles that need to be taken into account when programs are being set up.

Dealing with sensorimotor issues and learning styles

There are vast differences among our ASD kids, of course. While it might be tempting to apply a "one size fits all" program to our kids, it would be misguided. Not all our kids identify with, or even like, pictures. Not all our kids can, or should, sit still. Not all our kids can benefit from, or even tolerate, particular auditory input. Not all our kids can, or should be asked to, imitate sounds. Not all our kids are interested in, or benefit from, repeated drills.

The complicating factors are numerous, and you will find it helpful to ask an experienced SLP and an experienced OT and/or PT to help you sort it out. Some of our little ones may be operating with only one input channel, or one at a time. For one highly visual child, the auditory "sound track" of life may be too complicated for language to be extracted. For some who are very holistic in their thinking, the minutia of speech sounds may just not register yet.

Sensory challenges affect our kids in complex ways and must be considered when setting up a language program. We want to make real-life language experiences happen for our kids, and this is possible with appropriate PT/OT services and supports. Yes, it requires on-going assessment and ever-changing sensory diets, but this 24/7 sensorimotor support is key. And it bears mentioning here that even when one kind of challenge is attributed to many children, the manifestations are individual. Each of our kids is "a kid first" and a unique individual.

One child with an auditory aversion can tolerate conversational loudness at certain times; another can never tolerate it. The amount and timing of proprioceptive input is individual, too. While one child is able to be calmed under a weighted blanket, others are best served with "heavy work" activities. Registration of tactile input is equally highly variable, as are the effects of vestibular input. We know that some children can spin for literally hours without gaining the benefit they had hoped for, and others are not ready to tolerate even a little bit of turning in space.

For many of our kids, health and wellness come and go. Self-regulation fluctuates, and for some kids, "teachable moments" are so fleeting that registering language input during them is a chance thing. Motoric differences, too, run the gamut. Many of our kids are hypotonic, and getting them up off the couch is a chore. Some need to be up and moving for their muscles of respiration and phonation to coordinate. For some, it will take years before their torsos are strong enough to support their shoulders, neck, and jaw. Language may be developing, but its expression through speech may be delayed because of motor factors. For others, speech may precede writing and even keyboarding, because of challenges with fine motor strength and coordination.

No, it's not impossible to figure out, but it will be important to work with an experienced OT and/or PT who can help you set up your home to maximize the teachable moments and an SLP who can help you make them count.

What does your child want to talk about?

> *It takes a listener who attributes meaning to sound before a child uses it to communicate; it takes our understanding the communiqué before a child says it intentionally.*

There is one common denominator for all of us, including our kids: we all talk about what we care about. We sometimes hear it said that our kids lack motivation, but once we get through a child's sensory and/or motor challenges, we learn the truth: our kids are motivated to talk. Not only that, but our kids want to communicate, and what they want to communicate about is what matters to them. Our kids are often trying to communicate already, and it's their idiosyncratic means, unintelligible speech, and unpredictable timing that make it appear as if they don't. Recall the progression of intentionality that Barry Prizant brought to our attention: it takes a listener who attributes meaning to sound before a child uses it to communicate. And it takes our understanding the communiqué before a child says it intentionally!

All this is to say, first, that one size does not fit all. But it is also to say that there can be an appropriate, tailor-made program for each child once we figure out the child's unique profile of strengths, challenges, communicative desires, and motivations.

And here's the post script: once we get past the sensory and/or motor barriers and our kids are more easily able to talk fluently and intelligibly, we often realize that they already were talking. When kids slur long strings of sounds together, or whisper them so quietly no one hears, or say something several minutes later, it's hard for us to understand that they might actually be talking. But from the safety and wisdom of hindsight, we can finally see what we might have been blind to months or years earlier. Yes, it might be hard to admit we couldn't see into our child's heart and mind at the time, but once we finally do, we can try to keep our eyes and ears open from then on.

Know when to stand back

Language development is natural for our kids. And, knowing this, it is up to us to give our kids the support—and the freedom—to access that development. This may be quite surprising, but the greatest impediment we may run into is that so few people in the autism community or the larger educational community know what our kids have inside them and can develop further, if they only knew. Ironically, we may need to drum up the support our kids need to pursue this natural process.

You can start the ball rolling in your community, and this book will give you the tools you need to set up a language development program in your home. As you begin to bring your family on board with you, you will start to see change, and you will feel empowered to expand to your babysitter and others. You will even be able to hand-pick the people who provide language input to your child. They can watch you provide appropriate, mitigable gestalts and learn how to avoid language that inadvertently undermines the natural process of NLA.

Remember that when children are at Stage 1, everything they hear is processed as a gestalt. Even the canned phrases our kids are sometimes taught to say (think: "Ready, set, go") are all processed this way. Teaching language of the

"Can I have a turn?; I want more; I need help, please; Ready, set, go" variety is a roadblock to natural, flexible, self-generated language. You will make the development process easier for your child by not teaching him language that he processes—and overlearns—as gestalts. Know when to stand back.

Keep your language chart on your fridge

In our clinic, intervention has two main components: keeping up with kids' changing sensorimotor needs and keeping up with their language development so they can interact to the best of their ability. We know that as physical needs change, sensory diets need to change along with them (Biel, 2010), so our play time is spent providing our kids with the sensorimotor supports that will keep them feeling safe, comfortable, regulated, empowered, and wanting to interact.

During those teachable moments when kids are pain-free, self-regulated, and happy, we get to see all the things that make our kids tick. We get to see kids' interests, loves, and passions, and we'd not want to miss that for the world.

During those teachable moments when kids are happy, we get to see all the things that make them tick.

We have found that intervention that acknowledges the naturally-occurring progression of language makes all the difference. Then we can truly "be there" to interact, put words to experiences, and promote language development in our capable children.

Notice what your child notices

We need to pay particularly close attention during these magic moments, because kids' early interests provide the best starting place for language intervention. As parents, you should feel absolutely confident that you are the best detectives for discovering them. You are the ones who are privileged to catch glimpses into the heart of your child, and when you do, that sharing creates the very best place to start your language program. You are teaching yourself to look at the world through your child's eyes: first, because you want to, and secondly, because the sounds and language you eventually pair with your child's attractions need to be from his perspective.

You will catch glimpses into the heart of your child, and when you do, that's the very best place to start your language program.

To get started, you will want to make careful observations of your child's fascinations, joys, and favorites. Please start your observations today; jot down at least five things today and five more tomorrow. These favorites will become what you share, what you play with, what your child might want to refer to, what you will pair sound with, and, finally, what you will pair language with when the time is right.

Next, you will pay attention to the sounds your child associates with those favorites. How does the special song go? The special movie clip? The recurring refrain of the jingle? The sequence of words on that favorite page? The approach of Daddy's car? The rush of the bathwater? The squeak of the rubber ducky? The ring of the cell phone? The swish of the fabric? The tumble of the puzzle pieces? The flip of the page? Your child may not yet have the sensorimotor ability to explore space or even to visually scan the environment, so the modalities that come to him have real significance in these early years.

Honor gestalt thinking

Keep your child's cognitive style in mind as you plan his play and your intervention. Notice when he uses gestalt thinking with some motor accomplishment, some play routine, or some interest in collections or sets of things. Early interest in the entire alphabet, a set of story characters, or the completed circle of a train track are common among our kids and need to be honored so your child knows that you "get it." Make sure you write the entire alphabet on the chalkboard and assemble all the letters into a giant sidewalk around the room. Make sure you have all the characters before you take them to your child to play. Make sure you have all the pieces of the track before you assemble them with your child. The heartache of a "broken" whole undermines the beautiful language experience you had in mind, the one that never came to be.

To 'share' his set of pirates would be like asking another child, "Please share your doll with me. I'll just pull one arm out to play with."

I first learned this important lesson from an astute mom I know. Kieko understood gestalt thinking, because she recognized it in herself and could sympathize with her son's dilemma when he was asked to share his toys in preschool. Nicky had always lined up his toys from the time he was motorically coordinated enough to do so. His mother recognized how important it was to Nicky to see "sets" as whole entities. If another child tried to break up one of those sets, Nicky's world was literally shattered. Kieko explained her child's perspective to his teachers this way: "For Nicky to "share" his set of pirates would be like asking another child, 'Please share your doll with me. I'll just pull one arm out to play with.'" That poignant image will always stay with me.

In the next chapter, we return to Dylan to examine his story in depth and extract some principles for preschoolers. But before we continue, please look over the list of your child's favorites and make sure you have your own child clearly in mind. You will learn much from Dylan's extended story, but please make sure you have your own child solidly in mind so you can apply the lessons to him or her.

Look at your list, apply fun, and mix

Ready? You have a list of your child's favorites; you know the sounds he associates with at least some of them; you have determined that there's a good chance he is drawn to certain gestalts. You have the basics to play with, and you are ready to take off.

Let's return to Dylan's story.

Chapter 8
The Textbook Approach to Preschoolers: Dylan's Story in Depth

ASD kids echo what they hear

ASD youngsters often echo from movies. This is hardly new news, but when a child is young, it's often hard to see. Preschool children on the spectrum are often difficult to understand, and it may take a detective parent to recognize that kids are talking at all, much less what they're saying. That was the case with Dylan. Fortunately, he had a detective mom.

When Kathy first came to us, she told us that Dylan's language was all echoed from his favorite videos, especially *Aladdin*, *All Dogs Go to Heaven*, and *The Lion King*. Kathy was well aware of its origins, but until she met us, she doubted that Dylan intended to communicate anything with it. He did, however, occasionally take turns with her when they recited favorite movie dialogues together.

We played with Dylan at home and in our clinic and recorded everything he said during that second meeting. Most of what Dylan said was unintelligible to us, although his mother could catch much of it and even knew exactly which movie it came from. Even when it was intelligible, though, most of Dylan's colorful language was hard to interpret. Long strings of sound representing a slurred compilation of multiple sentences, such as **"Shh—look, there's Aladdin—quick!"** and **"Let's go find him, come on Spot, now let me think where are you,"** made up the bulk of Dylan's verbal output, but other, shorter comments like **"Where's the snowball?"** were simply confusing on this early fall day.

Dylan's mother knew a lot of the lines, and she even knew the preceding and following lines. This was the way she could create verbal interactions with her son. We applauded her, and Kathy knew it was important, but until she met us, she didn't really know **how** important it was. What she was doing was manyfold: she was confirming her child's interests and intentions by joining him; she was acknowledging his language as interactive; she was creating emotional and social reciprocity; and she was allowing her child plenty of practice with language at the first step of the gestalt language acquisition process.

Discovering evidence of communication

During our first clinic session, it was encouraging to realize that fifty of Dylan's utterances—almost half of what he said in an hour—were used in ways that had some obvious relevance to what was going on. The following dialogue took place at the end of our session, when Dylan attempted to keep us engaged by introducing a play sequence he had witnessed in a video (a snowball fight):

> "Helen, Tom!"

D	**Snowballs!** (Dylan reaches down to "pack" some "snow")
C	I'm gonna get you—ready?
D	**Helen, Tom!** (movie characters)
C	I'm gonna get you!
D	**Take that; take that!**

Dylan was having fun, and didn't want the play to stop. Granted, Dylan's peers would not have understood this with his opaque language. But we already knew not to take what Dylan said literally. That was our first rule of conversation. And, over the years, it has remained our first rule with almost every ASD child we have met. This is comforting and freeing, but not always easy to remember. We adults struggle when we don't understand; we panic, and, to make matters worse, our feelings get hurt. When our child says, "Go 'way!" or yells, "No! You're hurting me!" it's not easy to see past the literal and remember that we are witnessing an early gestalt. But if we all do our parts, that rough-around-the-edges language will later be replaced by phrase recombinations like "Not yet, thanks," and even more nuanced language like "Wait a minute, OK? I need time to chill."

Returning to the dialogue with Dylan, you will notice that he used obvious gestalts like **"Take that!"** and had also learned to mitigate, or break down, some movie gestalts, such as when he said, **"Helen, Tom!"** As we began our therapeutic relationship together, we first planned a series of Stage 1 experiences with a variety of useful, non-Disney gestalt models. Even though Dylan had demonstrated he was doing some Stage 2 mitigation and even Stage 3 single-word isolation, we wanted to give him a greater variety of useful language gestalts to work with. The language experiences Dylan had had so far were too limited to assure he'd mitigate enough "building blocks" for generative language construction. Single words like "Helen" and "Tom" wouldn't work with anyone but the most savvy play partner.

We needed more gestalts before we could expect fewer

> *All the language that surrounds a child provides language models, whether we intend it that way or not.*

What we did was build more useful, flexible gestalt phrases and sentences into Dylan's life at home. We explained to his family that all the language that surrounds a child provides language models, whether we intend it that way or not. We wanted to make sure that Dylan heard not only Walt Disney's language but plenty of other language that would become useful in everyday communication. "Let's get out of here!" works only some of the time, but "Come on!" is more universally communicative.

Next, we created home-made movies Dylan's family could watch together. We made sure our language was fun and lively—like Walt Disney's—but more predictable and useful to ready mitigation. Repetitive games and stories were also created so Dylan could hear, "Let's play with the …" and "It's a …" a bazillion times a day. When Dylan was ready for Stage 2, he knew that "Let's play with the ..." could be extracted from the many examples he'd heard daily and that "It's a ..." could be mitigated from other examples he heard as well.

Before we continue, let's take just a moment to review the first four stages of NLA to prepare ourselves for this next part of Dylan's story.

Stage	Examples
1–Communicative use of whole language gestalts	"Let's get out of here." "Want some more?"
2–Mitigation into chunks (a) and recombining (b)	(a) "Let's get" + "out of here" "Want" + "some more?" (b) "Let's get + some more?" "Want + out of here."
3–Isolation of single words, and creating two-word combinations	"Get—more." "Want—out?"
4–Generation of first sentences with beginning grammar	"I got more." "I wanna go out."

Table 15: The First Four Stages of Natural Language Acquisition

As mentioned in the Introduction, our work with Dylan lent itself to this tidy "textbook" because in addition to Dylan's family, there were three of us in our University clinic thinking about him each week. We wanted to present our own gestalts to Dylan, of course, so he would have access to "kid language" from which to mitigate and amass the building blocks, the words, to use in his own phrase combinations and sentence generation.

Competing with Walt Disney

Walt Disney's animation and language make movies a hard act to follow, so our real life language had to be fun and lively just to compete. We had to make sure that our play style was active and exciting and that our language was delivered with enthusiasm and all the theatrics we could muster. Predictable, developmentally-appropriate language can be deadly dull, unless we make it otherwise. So instead, we created great movement-based games and accompanying language: "Let's play with the ..." and "It's a ...," etc. Voila! A few months later, Dylan routinely extracted these types of phrases from our language and produced his own recombinations.

Predictable, developmentally-appropriate language can be deadly dull, unless we make it otherwise.

Dylan knew that listening to us was entertaining, but he also learned to trust that we would give him language that would be developmentally easy to pick up, socially rewarding, and useful to him. Dylan still used many of his movie gestalts and mitigated them, too, but they were increasingly transparent and easy to interpret. Here are some of the utterances from our sixth session:

Let's get outta here!

Whoa! That was close!
Here I come!
I'm the king!

Evidence of mitigation

By our ninth session, Dylan was mitigating routinely, using, **"I got it,"** a gestalt we had modeled, but also changing it to, **"We got it!"** Dylan produced the following sentences during a paper-cutting activity, and they clearly illustrate Stage 2 recombinations, using "cut out" as their foundation:

Cut out Buzz Lightyear.
Cut out dinosaur.
Cut out the Slinky.
You cut out Slinky.

After three months, Dylan showed further progress with mitigation and, in the process, created some "errors" that verified that his utterances were not gestalts, but mitigations. When Dylan used the phrase from our tag game, "You're it," in various mutations, he created not only the recombination **"I'm it!"** but a combination of combinations, referring to the game itself as **"It's 'I it.'"**

During his sixth month of therapy, Dylan was producing far less colorful language, in general, but it was almost all "transparent" and easy for familiar partners to read. Following is a short excerpt from a session about that time. The two clinicians are labeled C1 and C2:

"You bubble!"

C1	Let's blow bubbles.
D	**Bubbles?** (getting the bag of balloons)
C2	I want to play with the bubbles.
D	**Of balloons.**
C1	There's a lot of balloons.
C2	I'm blowing a big balloon. (blowing one up)
D	**You bubble.**
C2	What? What to do?
D	**You try.**

Single words emerge

During his seventh month, Dylan fully embraced Stage 3 single word isolation and beginning combinations. On the surface, it sounded like a step backwards when he went from "Let's play with the monsters" to **"I—toy!"** We witnessed the startled look on his face as he clearly isolated two important words and put them together in a completely different way from anything he'd ever heard. It was surprising to Dylan and thrilling to us, because we knew it signaled that Dylan could now generate his own unique phrases. Interestingly, we rarely witnessed single words being spoken in Stage 3; rather, their isolation in Dylan's language competence led immediately to two word combinations.

At that point, having isolated the building blocks from real-life language, Dylan began building his own unique phrases from scratch. His utterances had the ring of an analytic two year old, and sounded a lot less colorful than his earlier gestalts did. On the other hand, his short phrases were quite transparent to his partners, as they literally meant what they said. And we'd known Dylan "before," so we also knew that his thinking went way beyond how he sounded.

In our next sessions with Dylan, we tried to help him make the most of Stage 3 by setting up situations where all kinds of conceptual categories naturally bumped into each other. When Dylan was at Stage 3, a typical conversation sounded like the following, in which D is Dylan and C is a clinician:

D	**Basketball.** (making a ball out of play dough)
C	Basketball.
D	**All right, basketball.** (finding a "basket" to throw into)
C	Throw it in the basket.
D	**To basketball.**
C	Oh, basketball.
D	**We to basketball.**
C	Pass it! Pass it!
D	**One, two.**
C	One, two. Want more? Oh, ugly. (referring to some gray play dough)
D	**I—yuck.**

"We to basketball!"

At Stage 3, Dylan didn't use grammar. He combined words, and, more importantly, he combined concepts. And we really wanted him to explore, explore, explore—and to hear and use words in all kinds of combinations before he tried out grammar.

When he was ready, Dylan moved on, as have the scores of children in our clinic over the last fourteen years. And we still spend plenty of time at Stage 3, knowing that kids will naturally move on to Stage 4 when they are ready.

The wisdom of putting words together

In hindsight, it's easy to believe in this process, because we have seen it unfold so many times. But even seventeen years ago, we could see how Stage 4 happens when it is time. Once kids have had plenty of experience combining words in every conceivable order, grammar is just the next logical step.

Generative grammar doesn't happen in a formalaic way. It doesn't have scripts, because it doesn't need any.

Generative grammar doesn't happen in a formulaic way. It doesn't have scripts because it doesn't need any. We don't teach kids to use particular sentences, because we don't need to. In fact, if we did, our gestalt processors would quickly over-learn them as just a set of Stage 1 gestalts. Rather, we model particular grammatical structures with lots and lots of different examples so that the

Beginning grammer is more about trying things out than learning rules, and that's how creativity and flexibility are kept alive.

flexibility of Stage 3 is carried over to Stage 4.

Please glance back at the Developmental Sentence Types chart one more time, just to remember the utter breadth of variety—mostly about a ball and eating cookies. Study these word combinations and conceptual combinations carefully and see how we can refer to practically everything in our environment with two-word phrases. Then, think how much we miss if we make the mistake of jumping from single words to grammar prematurely. We would be wise to step back and apply the lessons from typical language development and let our kids experiment with two- and, later, three-word combinations the same way. Beginning grammar is more about trying things out than learning rules, and that's how creativity and flexibility are kept alive.

We also need to remember the distinction between language development and language teaching again. If we introduce a common sentence starter like "I want" or "I see" before a child is ready for Stage 4 grammar, the child has just another Stage 1 gestalt or Stage 2 mitigation to try to break down.

But there's another reason for spending ample time at Stage 3.

Conceptual ordering may be universal

There may actually be a "grammar" that is common to humanity, a cross-cultural ordering of concepts we use regardless of the grammar of our own language. Research in this fascinating area looked at the spontaneous ordering of hand gestures in adult speakers of four different languages when asked to non-verbally describe simple events presented on videos. In a 2008 article in *Science Daily*," lead author Susan Goldin-Meadow noted, "Not surprisingly, speakers of different languages describe events using the word orders prescribed by their language. The surprise is that when the same speakers are asked to 'speak' with their hands, they ignore these orders. They all use the same order when they gesture." Three of the four languages studied use this grammatical order: subject, verb, object. But with gestures, all the speakers of all four languages used this order: subject, object, verb.

"There appears to be a natural order that humans use when asked to represent events nonverbally ... The ordering seen in our nonverbal tasks may shape language in its emerging stages."

The researchers noted, "... there appears to be a natural order that humans use when asked to represent events nonverbally ... The ordering seen in our nonverbal tasks may shape language in its emerging stages." The article also referred to spontaneously-created sign languages among deaf children not previously exposed to sign language, and these also followed this same subject-object-verb ordering.

How this matters to us in relationship to our language-delayed children is many-fold. First, if a natural ordering juxtaposes the subject and the object and then the verb, then Stage 3 mix-and-match employs perfect conceptual logic. That "Mommy sock" has been an icon for SLPs carries more universal wisdom than we realized. Also embedded in this logic is that watching the natural development of language in our youngsters carries "evidence" that our formal studies have a hard time keeping up with.

Practicing process over particulars

In our desire to help our kids and teach them things to say, we have inadvertently short-changed our ASD kids time and time again. With nothing but the best of intentions, we have presumed they needed to be taught particular sentences to survive. We have wanted them to have some functional sentences, but built into this good intention was the untested assumption that they are not capable of developing normal language. We felt we had to give them something they could use: "functional speech." The unintended upshot is that kids are inadvertently taught one of the toughest gestalts and mitigations to ever get past. Our kids still say, "I want ..." year after year, in a robotic fashion that hints of the non-generative quality these rote patterns have.

We have wanted to teach our kids some functional sentences, but built into this good intention was the assumption that they are not capable of developing normal language.

In our clinic, we refer to these over-learned patterns as "default utterances," and we try to plan ahead so that we don't inadvertently reinforce a particular utterance or set up a situation where a child says something more than once and gets stuck there. What we have found is that this constitutes a drill of sorts, one that we had never planned on.

We find that once a child has said the exact same utterance twice in a row, there is the distinct possibility it will become a pattern. If he says it three times in a row, it may be so well-practiced as to become a default. This is how scripts come to be, we find, and while some children may need repetition, we want to make sure that a particular child is one of those before we lock into a pattern he then needs to work hard to get out of.

Once a child has said the exact same utterance twice in a row, there is the distinct possibilty it will become a pattern.

In the section below, you will learn the alternative supports we use and how they lead to natural use ("generalizing"), without locking in particular utterances. You will learn the intervention principles we used with Dylan, ones that you can modify to fit your preschooler and his life. After that, we will temporarily leave Dylan's story, to return to it in Chapter 12 where we will talk about his grammatical development at Stages 4–6. But first, we will talk about the intervention principles we can use with preschoolers.

Intervention principles with preschoolers

Dylan's story became a textbook example partly because Dylan loved to play and loved all the language we introduced to him. We suspect, too, that his story makes sense to you and sounds logical and valuable. But we also suspect that you may be wondering how you will ever set up a situation that promotes language as well as Dylan's did. You might be thinking that your child just wants to sit in front of the TV and hates to try new things, so how will you get him up and moving enough to want to throw a basketball or discover yucky play dough?

Use your knowledge of your child's loves and his sensory motor system to structure an environment that promotes playful interaction and language development.

A solution might be relatively easy to imagine, but putting it into practice is usually complicated. The first step involves combining your intimate knowledge of your child's loves with your understanding of his sensorimotor system. This is necessary in order to think about how an interesting environment might promote playful interaction and language development. You will need an OT and/or PT to assess your child, look at your home environment, and help you reconfigure it for fun—the kind of fun your child wants and needs. Next, you will need your family or friends or an intervention team to help you think, plan, write things down, and take some movies of your play so you can keep track of what's working and what's not working. Finally, you will need an SLP to help you learn to listen closely to your child, notice his intonation, notice his gestalts, and think about what your language models might be.

Here are some of the principles involved:

Redefine relevant play.

1. Redefine relevant play: it is whatever is fun and engaging to your child, not anybody else's. It won't look like anybody else's picture of play because it's designed for your child. Let me give you a few examples: If one child loves bubbles, baths, and music, his language time can revolve around bubbles, baths, and music. If another child loves squishes, jumping, and mud, her language time can revolve around squishes, jumping, and mud. Fun is in the eyes of the beholder, nobody else.

Redefine relevant language.

2. Redefine relevant language: the language of bubbles, baths, and music might include whatever catches the attention of your child. It might include: "It's a huuuuuge bubble!" and "It's gonna pppppop!!" and "I got it; I got it!" and "I can't geeeeet it!!" and "Whoooooops!" and "Wheeeee!" The "language" of your language activity might not even be language yet; it might be sound contours, songs, or squealing laughter.

Redefine "language teaching."

3. Redefine "language teaching." What you are doing to support your child's language development isn't actually "teaching" at all, but "language modeling." Language modeling exactly matches your child's learning style. Your child was built to echo; you're just giving him appropriate sounds and language to echo.

Your child was built to echo. So, give him appropriate sounds and language to echo.

4. Redefine success: It's what your child says or doesn't say the *next* time you play with bubbles or mud that gives you your feedback. Don't expect instant results. Remember that we are talking about "delayed echolalia," and you may not hear your pearls again till the next bubble play, or play in the mud, or after your child gets to watch the movie version a few—or a bazillion—times. And if your child only uses one or two of the sentences you said, great. Now you have a clue about what to use for the next selections. Dylan used our language models during the same play session, but that wasn't until he learned that what we said would be relevant. It takes time.

Once you have sensorimotor supports in place, autism takes on another, hopeful face.

5. Redefine support: It is whatever your child needs to be able to engage in playful language time. As I have said before, our clinic is set up with this in mind, so we can individualize the environment with each particular child in mind. We might have a trampoline, a bank of mirrors, dozens of crash pillows for one child, a hidden Barney character for a second child, and a climbing maze with Ninja characters at every level for another. Support is only support if it supports—end of story.

6. Redefine autism: Remember, as a diagnostic category, it's a set of behaviors, which until we can provide appropriate sensorimotor support, can look discouraging. But we can tell you from the delightful place of hindsight that once we have supports in place, autism takes on another face. Then it's fun, playful, full of hope, and full of happy sound-making and, we dare say, language.

Summary

So, before we leave Dylan's story for a while, let's summarize what we have learned. Two decades ago and in a single year's time, Dylan had taught us most of what we needed to know about the process Prizant, Wetherby, Rydell, and others had described. He had gone through Stages 1, 2, and 3 like a little trooper. It was fun and almost effortless for us and, we think, him.

We have given you some of the intervention strategies we used with Dylan because they provide a nice template for children in this age group. Preschoolers love to play; they love to be physical. If your playroom is the most interesting and motorically exciting one in town, your preschooler is sure to want to engage with you and develop language at the same time.

If, however, you can see that the intervention strategies in this chapter are simply not enough for your child, then please do not give up. We will return to intervention many times again in this book, and we will recommend some supportive and supplementary strategies that will help you with the foundational pieces you need.

Before we leave this chapter, it would be good to think about where we are with our preschoolers in relation to where we will be heading. The description of NLA on the following page includes definitions of each stage and a progressive example to illustrate the process from stage to stage. You will notice that the example presented earlier in this book is now followed from its original gestalt origins through mitigation, single-word isolation, and then into the successive levels of grammatical development. Please glance at it before you move on and consider that it might be a nice handout for your child's team.

We are now ready to move on from Dylan's very general example and to explore some other strategies that are appropriate to subgroups of preschoolers. Chapter 9 introduces Jake, a little guy who was nearly silent—until he discovered where his breathing came from.

Stage	Examples
1 - Echolalia: Use of complete gestalts (sound tracks, intonational contours, sentences, scenes, episodes, or other wholes processed as a unit) taken directly from the child's environment and used moments, hours, or days later.	**"Let's get out of here."** **"Want some more?"**
2 - Mitigated Echolalia: Use of partial gestalts that have been mitigated from the whole; Mix-and-match of partial gestalts or constituent parts in semi-unique phrases and sentences.	"Let's get" + "some more" = **"Let's get some more!"** "Want" + "out of here" = **"Want out of here."**
3 - Isolation of the single word: Use of single words that have been isolated from mitigated phrases; Mix-and-match of single words to create original two word combinations	(1) "Let's get" + "wanna get" = **"get"** "Some more" + "No more" = **"more"** (2) **"Get more!"** and **"More get!"**
4 - Beginning generative grammar: Use of original sentences using beginning grammar, both correctly and incorrectly (Developmental Sentence Scoring levels 1–3)	**"I get." "Get more no." "No get some."** **"I wanna get some more toys."** **"He got toys and books."**
5 - Advanced generative grammar: Use of original sentences using more advanced grammar (DSS levels 4–6)	**"I used to want more toys, but now I don't. I know you never got any more of those because they always break. Can you just get me something new?"**
6 - All sentence patterns: Use of complex sentences that incorporate DSS levels 7 and 8.	**"Why don't we try to buy some more wooden toys with the money we saved when we gave up plastic ones?"**

Table 16: The Six Stages of Natural Language Acquisition

Chapter 9
When Motor Development Lags Behind, It All Sounds Like Jargon

How do I work on language when I can't tell if it's there?

If your child is minimally verbal, minimally vocal, or even mostly silent, you may want to read this chapter before some of the others. Even if your child is becoming verbal but has been called dyspraxic or apraxic, you may want to read this chapter now in order to put speech, particularly "praxis," or motor planning for speech, in context.

For too long, we have thought of our minimally-verbal children as "low functioning." We never actually defined the term, but we used it anyway. And the tragedy is in how we have tended to treat these kids as cognitively challenged. Admittedly, some of our kids may be cognitively challenged, just like some of the kids who are not on the spectrum are cognitively challenged. However, demonstration of cognitive ability is clearly not the same as cognitive ability. Motor coordination and motor planning challenges can mask many things, and kids thus affected can look uninvolved, disinterested, and, yes, cognitively challenged. But looks can be deceiving. We now realize that the 40% of ASD kids who have been considered "non-verbal" are the kids who are severely challenged with motor planning (Richard, 1997). Speech is coordinated motor movement, so all speech is "motor speech" and requires motor planning as it develops.

With dyspraxia, groups of muscles fail to work well together, especially when kids try. Kids affected by dyspraxia often also lack purposeful use of their arms and hands and the ability to get their bodies to perform coordinated motor patterns like riding a bike. They may be unable to perform activities of daily living like gathering their toys and getting their own food. When they are young, they might lack varied facial expression and may not laugh, or even cry. As they get older and gross motor function improves, motor planning for fine motor and speech may lag behind; children can display dyspraxia of phonation (voicing), and some can have dyspraxia of speech articulation. These kids can even get physically "stuck" and may find themselves unable to sit down at the top of a slide, or to stop running in a particular direction, or to come when called.

With dyspraxia, groups of muscles fail to work well together, especailly when kids try.

If this is your child, you will definitely want to meet Jake, a little boy who was a year and a half old when we first met him. That first day at his house, Jake was silent until he nearly spat out a mono-toned "Aaaa." I remember asking his mom what else Jake might say. She replied, "Not much." Mostly, Jake was absolutely silent, and it was just this occasional raw sound that suggested to me that his speech was "stuck" somewhere, clearly somewhere beneath the level of his mouth.

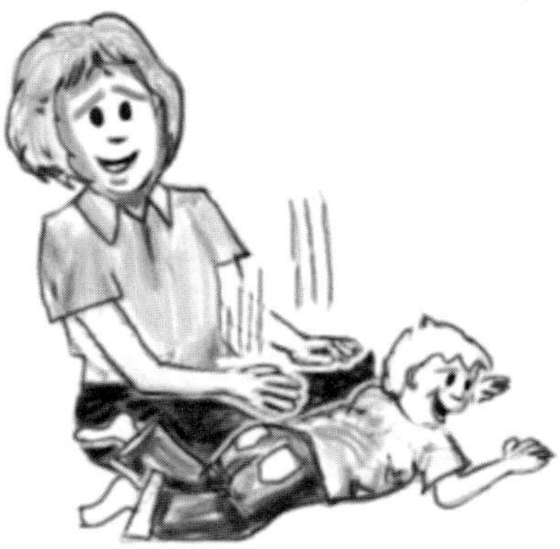

Jake didn't look interested in communicating. He fit the stereotypical profile of an 'uninvolved' child with ASD: arms at his side, minimal eye contact, walking around seemingly aimlessly, avoiding touch, occasionally screaming, and throwing himself on the floor in a tantrum.

That Jake screamed was a good sign, though, because at least he could use his voice at this reflexive level. Mostly, however, Jake was silent, and he looked content to push his truck back and forth as he lay on his side, not communicating distress—or anything else—at all.

Sometimes when he was moving, however, Jake could produce a little sound. As he bumped along behind his push cart, he could say "Uh uh" once in a while, and this obviously made him happy. Jake had successfully found a way he could force air out through his vocal cords, and when he did, his voicing was automatic. The key to Jake's speech was deep down in his belly. And once he discovered more ways to produce exhalation, Jake found his voice.

Over the course of the next year, Jake became a true speaker, one whom everyone acknowledged was talking and communicating. Our therapy program started at the "bottom"—the base of support for breathing and prolonged exhalation—and, finally, coordinated that air with his voice. Through lots of gross motor activity, Jake learned to coordinate his body better and to be able to find situations that promoted his speech.

At first, to promote deep breathing, I played with Jake in a high-energy way he enjoyed: running around his basement together and landing in the ball pit. The resulting laughter was happy voicing, a more flexible alternative to the voice of screaming.

Then we started running down the hill in front of his house, bumping behind the push cart. We huffed and puffed and, again, laughed at the involuntary sounds we made. Later, I played invisible "drums" on his back, and Jake produced involuntary sound that became more extended as he learned it was funny. Over time, Jake's laughter turned into a continuous "Uh uh uh uh uh uh," a string of sound that he could keep going until he stopped to take in another breath. Jake learned much in the process: laughing wins you more friends than screaming and sets you up for turn-taking with other people. Also, laughter seemed to give Jake a positive sense of himself and provided him a way to get used to the sound of his own happy voice. Along with laughter and shared hilarity came eye contact. This just added to the fun, as, invariably, I did something funny whenever Jake looked at me.

Jake's parents continued to play in the same ways we had modeled, so he was getting lots of voicing time. And his voice gradually began to show variation in tone. He could maintain it for longer periods, not just saying, "Uh uh uh" in fits and bursts, but "Uuuuh" for an entire second. And with one second of sustained vocalization, one can say "Uuuuh" with rising tone, or falling tone. This sounded just like an intonational question and then an answer. While we couldn't claim this was language yet, it was certainly the support for expressing language, and Jake used intonation more and more often.

We then started to play with intonational contours as we ran around the basement or I drummed his back. Because Jake wanted to play the game again and again, he gained some ability to start and stop the sound, which gave him a real sense of power. Our work with Jake was through the local Birth-Three program, so at the same time we were working with Jake, he was receiving OT and PT supports as well. His body was moving better, and his access to deep breathing was a part of that.

Jake's moments of sustained vocalizing were now predictable enough and long enough for his mouth to open, close, and begin to change shape as he exhaled. With those different mouth shapes came different vowel-like sounds and Jake began to sound like he was talking. For example, when Jake started laughing, his jaw dropped open and he produced "Ah" without even trying. As Jake gradually got used to more and more textures, his chewing and tongue control allowed his mouth to develop more and more shapes, and with them, more vowel sounds. Jake was no longer limited to grunts and screams; he actually sounded like he was carrying on mini-conversations, at least the way they sound to us when we're in the next room.

Jake even sounded like he was using "jargon" now, but we didn't conclude that this was all it was. We had certainly had plenty of experience with "jargon," and because Jake was such an engaging, bright little boy, we suspected it was probably language—unintelligible, but real echolalic language. It took a while to find out for sure, though, because Jake needed some more time with supported voicing to get all his vowel sounds in place. By then, however, it started to become clear that Jake was saying phrases.

By the time he was two years old, Jake's parents and I had long been talking to him as if he understood "everything" and engaged with him as if he was communicating. Finally, after six months of doing this, we found out we were right. Jake rewarded us with some of his first intelligible sentences. They sounded almost like "I did it!" and "I got it!" but without the consonant sounds or the diphthongs (the vowel slide that makes up words like, "I").

And as Jake began talking more and more, we started hearing lines from his *Thomas the Tank Engine* movies. As he played with his own train set, we could hear Sir Topham Hat talking to the engines in the unintelligible voice of Jake. Jake began demonstrating that he had plenty of language gestalts in his young repertoire and a nice assortment of mitigations he could use to mix and match.

By age two and a half, Jake was indisputably a talker, had obviously learned to mitigate further, and could isolate the single word. He could yell, **"No no no!"** and **"Mommy—Mommy!"** as plaintively as any other child. He only had a smattering of consonant sounds, though, and could not say, "Daddy" or "Christian," the names of the others in his family, and he could not say his own name. But Jake was a talker.

And once Jake's voice was no longer stuck in silent mode, he found it more and more often and became very vocal. Jake loved to talk, in fact, and kept his

Kids seem to understand what adults forget: dyspraxia is a disorder of trying, and automatic vocalizing is the way to jump start talking.

voice going for as long as he could at a stretch. Like other children with praxis challenges, Jake didn't like "losing" his voice and having to start it all over again. But, like many other smart, dyspraxic children, Jake also learned reliable ways to start it up again spontaneously. Jake knew that force never worked and just made him feel bad about himself, but any way he could find to fall into a giggle fit worked. He liked tickling, and he could always get people to do something funny that would make him laugh. Kids seem to understand what adults forget: that dyspraxia is a disorder of trying, of volition, and that automatic vocalizing is the way to jump start communicative talking.

There is more to Jake's story, which was originally published in the *Autism Asperger's Digest* and is available at the author's website ("Finding the Words … When It's Hard to Find Your Voice!" Jan–Feb 2006 and Mar–Apr 2006). You can also download the original article series, When Speech Gets Stuck (Sept–Oct 2004 and Nov–Dec 2004), which describes the hierarchy of supports for dyspraxia we have introduced here. The articles also include specific suggestions for children who are like Jake.

Here is the eight-step hierarchy for supporting speech with dyspraxia. Each level is supported by all the ones below it and involves coordination with those levels. The level of vowel sounds, then, is what we described in Jake: using prolonged voicing with intonation along with the different mouth shapes that make up the vowel sounds. Next come the consonant sounds, involving further refinement of mouth shapes. Once enough consonants emerge, it is possible to coordinate sounds into sequences that make speech more intelligible. All this remains somewhat automatic, though, until kids are practiced enough to speak more purposefully, or to motor plan.

Level 1 – Deep Breathing / Exhalation
Level 2 – Voice / Vocal Production
Level 3 – Intonation
Level 4 – Starting, Maintaining, and Stopping Voice
Level 5 – Using Vowel Sounds
Level 6 – Consonant Sound Development
Level 7 – Sequencing Sounds
Level 8 – Purposeful Speaking

Table 17: Hierarchy of Practical Supports for Dyspraxia in Children with ASD

Summary

To summarize, Jake offers us a look at a child who had praxis challenges that were identified early in his life. He had support from his family and his Birth-Three team, and he loved experiencing the progress he was making. Having been able to follow Jake for many years, I can tell you that his encyclopedia of movies, games, conversations, and stories grew to be huge. His progress with language development followed the predicted stages at a relatively young age, considering his early speech challenges. As time went on, Jake's speech fluency increased until it finally caught up with his language. After that, there was no stopping him in story generation—or in life.

Now, as we continue with our story of preschool intervention, we will look at other young children and how individual differences create differences from the textbook approach we first devised for Dylan. You will see that there is a strong similarity in the general order of events but many differences in execution, as each child is an individual first and a gestalt processor second. Our hope here is that you will find some qualities about individual stories that you can identify with and, in that way, think about how your own child's program can be individually tailored—for your child!

Let us continue.

Chapter 10
Variations of the Preschool Story

Our ASD kids are as varied as are all kids. And each has his own desires, propensities, strengths, and challenges. Dylan's textbook progression through the stages of NLA provided a template for approaching language development on the spectrum, but individual styles tell the individual stories.

In this chapter, we will look at four different preschool children with four different styles. From their very different profiles, you will be able to get a sense of the variety of paths children take and then to develop some ideas about how to approach your own child's language future.

The first child is Josh, who we dubbed "the linguist" because of his ability to use language on the spot and to mitigate it. Josh was such a master of "immediate echolalia" that it was not always apparent that he had any difficulty generating language.

The second child is Izzy. She was a story-teller and so adept at echolalia that she could learn an entire script almost as easily as a single sentence. Her rate of learning was so fast, in fact, that story lines had become overlearned by the time she'd said them twice, and sometimes, it seemed, once. While this was clearly a gift, it painted her into many a corner, stuck.

The third child is Andrew, who was certainly a gestalt processor of life. It was hard to see his gestalt processing of language, however, because he had so little understandable speech as a preschooler. His parents knew how gestalt he was, however, from the time he decided to walk. As we described earlier in this book, Andrew had watched and watched people walking, but never attempted to take a step. Then, one day, from the bottom step he was sitting on, Andrew got up and ran.

The fourth child, Russel, defied early description. His capacity for gestalt language processing wasn't even on the radar when he was little, because he was too busy processing all the other gestalts in his environment, particularly the alphabet. It took us a while to bridge a chasm most people don't think of: letters are beautiful in their own right and form an artistic composite, and that they should have symbolic value seems superfluous. Alphabet did not equal language to Russel, and it took us a while to even get to language at all.

Josh, the linguist

When we first met Josh, he was three and a half years old and able to maintain a nice, reciprocal conversation. And to the casual observer, Josh appeared to be generating his own sentences and using grammar expected for his age. Two assessments, at 35 and 36 months of age, found that his expressive language was at or above age level. But his astute parents could see something else: Josh could only talk about the topic at hand, and although his sentences seemed like they were coming from him, they seemed to be heavily reliant on the words his partner had just said. Here are a few examples from our first session with Josh. Notice his "mix and match" strategy, using his partner's grammatical models, and the limited vocabulary of the play. (C = clinician; J = Josh)

C	She's yellow.
J	**He's black and white, too. He's black and white, too. And he's black and white, too.**
C	Yeah, you're right. They're all black and white.
J	**Wow!**
C	Cool!
J	**He's black. Lots of cars.**
C	Yeah, we got our cars.
J	**We got our cars.**

The next sample took place as Josh, the clinician, and the *Cars* characters slid down a slide. The question form "What's your name?" used here was also used throughout the session whenever Josh wanted to greet someone.

C	Here I come from the top. Wow.
J	**I am the top.**
C	OK, come down super fast.
J	**Wow.**
C	That was fun. Let's try it again.
C	This time it's my turn.
J	**What's your name?**
C	Hello, Blue Lightning McQueen. I saw you go down. It was awesome.
J	**Hello, Blue Light McQueen.**
C	Hey there.

The third sample illustrates Josh's reliance on his partner's language but then his ability to mitigate when he really needed to!

C	Oh no, a washer.
J	**A washer.**
C	It broke.
J	**It broke.**
C	Our washer broke.
J	**Our washer broke.**
C	But we can fix it.
J	**But we can fix—no, you can fix it!**

As this compilation shows, Josh was a master at staying in the conversation and taking the language around him and blending it. It was difficult for his partner to tell exactly what was going on during these conversational exchanges, however, as she was busy keeping the conversation going herself, trying to understand Josh's intentions and help him express them.

Josh's language assessment

But this session and the others during Josh's diagnostic therapy period were all recorded and Josh's language transcribed. In our clinic, we allow anywhere from one month to three months for this process to be completed. During this time, patterns emerge, and enough progress takes place that we are able to plan effectively for a child's future growth. In Josh's case, his patterns became clear after a few more sessions. Following are some of the findings from our assessment of his language level.

Josh used very few gestalts, the exception being sentences such as "What's your name?" and "That's a good idea," the latter used often to Josh's social advantage. Josh used Stage 2 mitigations extensively, but these were primarily "immediate" as opposed to "delayed." The mitigations Josh held in his mind were limited but did include a variety of pronoun + verb phrases. Josh could say sentences with "He's," "They're," and "You're," but he had not isolated the pronouns individually to be able to construct completely unique sentences. Instead, his Stage 2 combinations sounded like this:

He's fell.
He's has a get all the jellies out of his engine.
Yes, he's got under the tunnel.
He's go to car.
You're eat a—you're eat a spoon.
They're don't say 'cheese'

"I Henry. I Josh. I just Edward."

Josh did have some Stage 3 isolated words and word combinations, however, most notably, "I." His constructions sounded like this:

I Henry.
I Josh.
I just Edward.

Josh also combined some Stage 2 phrases and Stage 3 single words, for example:

I think that way. [2 + 2]
Maybe that way. [3 + 2]
I think I can't—how 'bout maybe Lightning McQueen? [2 + 2 + 2 + 3 + 3]
What a mess with this. [2 +2]
Hey, maybe Topham Hat. [3 + 3+3]
Maybe how 'bout James—that's a good idea. [3 + 2 + 2+1]
Then maybe slow—lots of slow. [3 + 3 + 3 + 2 + 3]

Josh produced a few Stage 4 grammatical constructions such as "She sinked them," when he occasionally took the time to work on them. But it was clear from the small number of such constructions how laborious this process was for Josh and how little language he had to work with. It was simply not yet time for him to be trying to construct sentences. It would be much better to meet him where he was and give him some tools he could use to get there when he was ready.

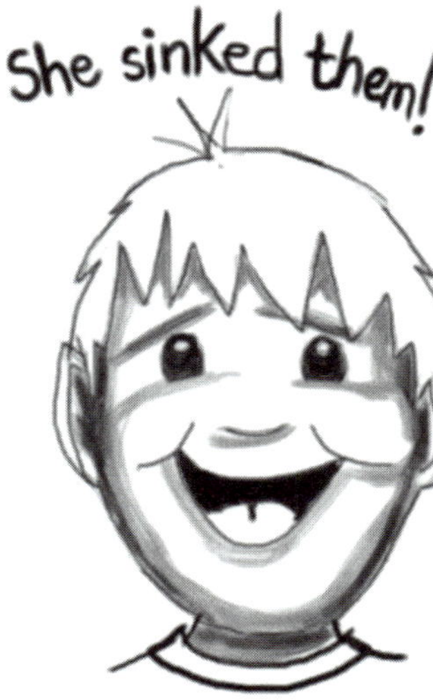

Recommendations for Josh's family were predicated on this mutual understanding: Josh was not self-generating sentences, nor was he ready to. Our work was to help him develop a foundation for this task, and that involved giving him plenty of opportunities to hear and use Stage 2 mitigations so he could develop a repertoire he could use independently. Specific recommendations were made to his family, including structures to model and others to avoid. Josh's family was also asked to help others refrain from introducing even more grammar to Josh yet, since this was only delaying the task he was developmentally ready for: solidifying a set of mitigations he could use communicatively.

Josh's language progress

Josh's progress was a joy to watch. In two months' time, Josh was developing some confidence with his Stage 2 combinations, producing a great variety during each session. Here is one day's compilation of similar utterances that illustrates Josh's discovery process:

> **I found the cars.** [2+2]
> **I found 'em.** [2+3]
> **I found them.** [2+3]
> **I found a truck and a car.** [2+2+3+2]
> **I found one truck.** [2+2]

While single words were rare two months after treatment began, in four months' time, Josh had moved from Stage 2 phrase combinations to Stage 3 word combinations, as seen in the following dialogue. Notice that the clinician had modified her utterance length and type to match the target constructions we were after.

C	It's stuck.
J	**Wow.**
C	Lots of toys.
J	**There's dinosaurs.**
C	And lots of trains.
J	**Trains.**
J	**And Teletubbies.**
J	**We'll play this.**
C	There's some animals in here.
J	**Yeah. Which animals?**
C	Who's going to drive those?

J	**The tractor is going to come in.**
J	**Cockadoodledoo.**
C	Wake up.
J	**Green pig.**
C	Farmer has to move the cow.
J	**Yeah and that too.**
C	Move the pig too!
J	**Chickens!**
J	**Watch out!**

By the time he was four years old, Josh had progressed further, into Stage 4, and was able to use basic grammar to express himself. He had enough of the tools by then to begin to explore an area that had eluded him up until then: pretending and make-believe. The following sentences were produced as Josh began to play catch with some balls but turned the game into something else. In this sample, his partner's comments are not included, but the notations will indicate whether or not Josh was imitating her.

I put two—
I'm gonna throw a ball at you.
Yes.
This ball got me out. (Josh used the ball to get out of a hole in the pillows)
And it got me out. (Josh seemed to want to add something, but could not)
It must be magic. (Imitated the clinician)
I pretend it's magic. (Refined the previous comment.)
Disappeared. (The word was hard for Josh to use in a sentence.)
Now it's gone! (The clinician supplied an alternative, which Josh imitated)
The magic earth.
Can't get the sun, because there's no earth.
Where is the earth? (The ball was lost in the pillows behind the trampoline.)
Maybe my purple rope can get the sun! (A rope was used to pull Joshua out of the pillows.)
Now I need the magical ball.
Now I'm going to try the magical ball.
When I say, "one," I'll make some music and I'll get the the the the—
Ah, it's bright!

The clinician's progress note that day was telling. She said, "I was struck by this dramatic play for a number of reasons. First of all, we did not play out a story from a movie, which we used to do last spring. We did not even start from an identified story and then branch out, which is what we did over the summer. Over the fall, we've spent a great deal of time playing out stories that were original but were strongly grounded in physical props. But today, we played out a seemingly original story with a ball and a rope. I think Josh was free to explore this kind of play because his language is starting to catch up with his ideas. The last several sessions, Josh has explored all kinds of creative language (concepts, descriptors, cause-effect), and I think this development ushered in a new kind of play."

Grammar was clearly providing Josh a personal linguistic tool. When it is self-generated and flexible, grammar becomes a way for kids to do what they want with language: express what they want to express, invent the verbal parts of what is forming in their minds, and share it with their family and friends.

When it is self-generated and flexible, grammar becomes a way for kids to do what they want with language.

Josh at age five

Josh's linguistic adventure continued steadily. A year later, when Josh was five, he was able to share the complex inventions in his head. His grammar was not complete yet, as the progress notes for this day showed, but Josh was able to socially engage in a way that was fun for everyone: "Josh initiated a new version of Pokémon today. Usually we play with no reward for the winner, and we keep score by winning rounds. This time, Josh suggested that we use the necklace as a prize and that we have an overall winner of the game by counting the cards at the end." Josh worked on explaining his idea:

J	**Whoever wins the game gets the necklace.**
C	Oh, this is a new way to play.
J	**But if there is a tie, one gets to wear it and one gets to wear another one.**
J	**But there can't be three winners, right?**
C	There could be, but I don't think that will happen.
J	**Or we can play until xxx.**
J	**Count it at the end of all other battles games.**
C	So, we keep playing games, and count it at the end?
J	**Count it at the end.**

The notes continue, "Josh was able to explain the new variations to the games by taking several conversational turns. We were impressed by his versatility and creativity within the game. Mixing up the rules added excitement to today's game."

During the game itself, Josh tried to complete the explanation of his idea and use the complex grammar this would take. While he never quite got both elements of the syntax together, he got them one at a time at various junctures during the play. If he used "not," he omitted "until," and vice versa:

> **We're** (not) **counting our cards 'til the game is over and whoever has the most cards wins.**
> **But remember, we're not counting them at the end.**
> **But remember, we're** (not) **counting them 'til the game is over.**

A few months later, Josh was working on story-telling, as up until that time, Josh's most typical story line involved the characters introducing themselves and having an epic battle. The progress notes from that day said that the characters included a porcupine, a baby elephant, a herd of elephants and a T-Rex. In order to keep the characters straight, Josh used three distinct voices: a baby voice for the baby elephant, a deep voice for the dinosaurs, and a kind of Sean Connery impression for the army of elephants. Josh also "paused" the game to make comments of his own, using his own voice.

The story began with introductions:

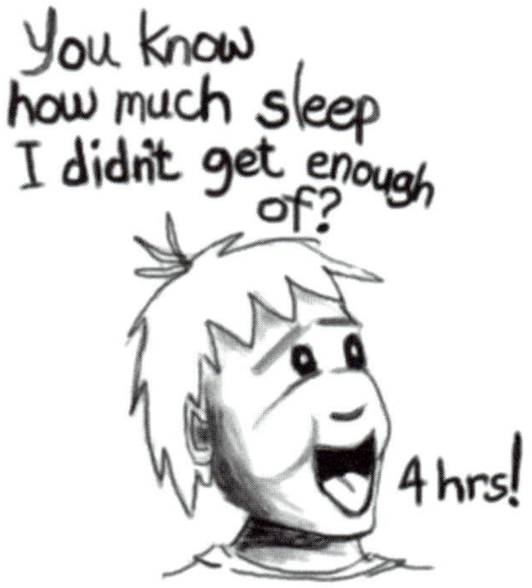

C	Who's there?
J	**It's just me.**
C	What's your name?
J	**Porcupine.**
C	How can you help us, Mr. Porcupine?
J	**I would certainly like to help protect the other dinosaurs from the other emenies, enemies.**
C	Oh, like a cannonball?
J	**Cannonball. But I'm pokey. Well, I can jump, and squish them.**
C	You're on the team.

Later:

J	**I'm just a baby. Can I come in?**
C	What are you going to do?
J	**Just relax and sleep. I'm just a little tired because I didn't get enough sleep.**
C	We'll let you sleep for three hours.
J	**You know how much sleep I didn't get enough of? Four hours.**

Back to Porcupine:

J	**Wait guys, wait. Somebody wants to meet you; somebody wants to meet you.**
J	**I'm just Porcupine.**
C	What do you do?
J	**So they could throw me out the cannonball and poke all the enemies.**

Enter T-Rex, followed by the narrator:

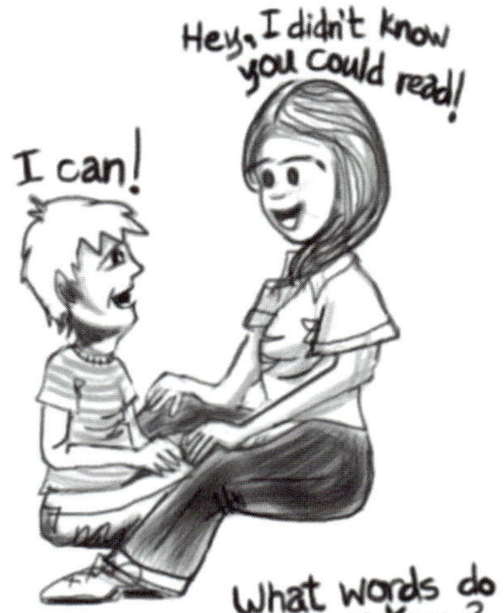

C	How's your breakfast?
J	**I can eat 500 pounds of breakfast in one bite.**
J	**That's where I learned about T-Rex—the iPad.** (switching out of the story)
C	You have an iPad?
J	**There's a little thingy like a marker. You put a black thing on each word then it tells you the word.**
J	**Some of the words I already know.**
C	Hey, I didn't know you could read.
J	**I can.**
C	What words do you know?
J	**Like "the." That's pretty much it.**

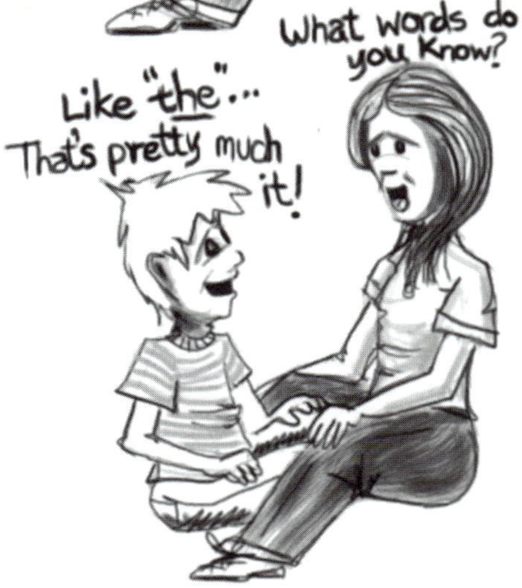

Finally, Baby Elephant came on the scene, and Josh and the clinician entered uncharted territory as the story evolved as a joint venture:

J	**I'm a little baby elephant.** (using a baby voice)
J	**I'm just a baby elephant; I'm not attacking the castle.**
C	I think you're trying to be sneaky.
J	**We don't want you to attack any more.**
J	**We don't want to attack any more.**
J	**Yes, it's true.**
C	You have a whole army down there.
J	**I think I want to live in a new family.**

As the story moved along:

J	**We know that Porky is actually in our family.**
J	**Well, we, well, tell us something.**
J	**When I was, I was, when I was born, I was actually in an elephant egg.** (as Porcupine)
C	Really?
C	Really?
J	**Yup.**
J	**Well, he was in our family.** (as baby elephant)

Now everyone was on-stage:

J	**I'm a henormaus t-rex.**
J	**I am sharp tooth.**
J	**Do you know who Sharp Tooth is, actually?** (in his own voice)
J	**He's in the movie with Littletooth's mother battles him but gets hurt by the T-Rex.**
J	**I am T-Rex. Want to battle me?**

Josh's therapy continued on from there, even though his formal language scores put him well within his age group. We knew that Josh's language was far from matching his potential, and that he had a long way to go in the myriad ways he wanted to put that language to use. Therapy during the next year of his life was able to provide Josh the opportunities to use his language to do what he wanted: to create, to socially interact in personal and complex ways, and to plan all the games and activities he had up his sleeve.

Izzy, the story-teller

We now turn to Izzy, who also came to us as a three-year old presenting a profile of challenges with speech intelligibility, language access, functional use of language, sustained interaction, and sensory modulation. Her first language samples included small dialogues like these below. Clearly, Izzy was demonstrating that she could combine words and even self-generate a little, but it was difficult.

I	**What is that?**
C	What is that?
I	**Walnut.** (pronounced "wahwumnut")
C	I love walnuts! Wanna try?
I	**Wanna try?** (pronounced "wahwaw twy")
I	**I take a baby pumpkin.**
C	What does the baby pumpkin do?
I	**It play.**
C	Is that one icky?
I	**No it's n—**
C	It's—
I	**—not icky.**

Izzy was much more fluent when she could imitate or use the language around her for support. Much of her language turned out to be parts of scripts she had been exposed to in her intensive autism program, and, unbeknownst to us, she learned them faster than she learned almost anything else. For that reason, it took a while to elicit enough spontaneous language to piece together a complete profile that reflected her true language level. Once we knew Izzy better, we could easily see the difference between her over-learned scripts and her struggling generative language. The following snippets of conversation illustrate Izzy's various forms of language production over the next several months.

The first example makes Izzy's language sound more sophisticated than it was. Izzy was using a nice sentence but repetitively and inflexibly, suggesting that the grammatical complexity was not her own but a combination of Stage 2 mitigations:

I	**I need some more pillows; I need some more pillows; I need some more pillows.**
I	**I need some more pillows.**
C	More pillows—hmm. (giving Izzy a chance to take another turn)
C	These pillows are around the trampoline—in case we're gonna jump. (trying to see what pillows Izzy wants)
I	**I need some more pillows—in there.**
C	How about the light blue one.
I	**x x the light blue one.**
C	(commenting on pillows)
I	**The light blue pillow.**

"I need some more pillows; I need some more pillows; I need some more pillows."

The next dialogue sounds less sophisticated with its absence of grammar, but since Izzy was only "borrowing" grammar through Stage 2 mitigation, the following is actually more original. It represents Stage 3 single word isolation:

I	**A balloon.**
C	What can we pretend it is?
I	**A spider.**

In the following dialogue, Izzy did a nice job forming a question through mitigation:

I	**What that ballon?**
C	That's a good question, what does that balloon look like?
I	**A dog.**

Izzy moved into a guessing game, which we quickly discovered was a learned script. Her utterances were deceptively complex:

C	You hid the fish somewhere?
I	**Yeah—do you want a clue?**
C	Sure; I'd like a clue.
I	**It's in something made of wood.**
C	He's in something made of wood—that is wood—

As the game continued, Izzy needed to generate her own language momentarily. Then, running out of scripted comments, she kept the play going with the clever use of "Whoosh," which quickly became "over-learned," however:

C	Need help up?
I	**Lift.**
C	(became a mermaid and swam in the waves)
I	**Whoosh!**
I	**Whoosh!**
C	Izzy, help me!
I	**Whoosh!**
C	I think I'm gonna turn into a mermaid—
I	**Whoosh!**
I	**Whoosh!**

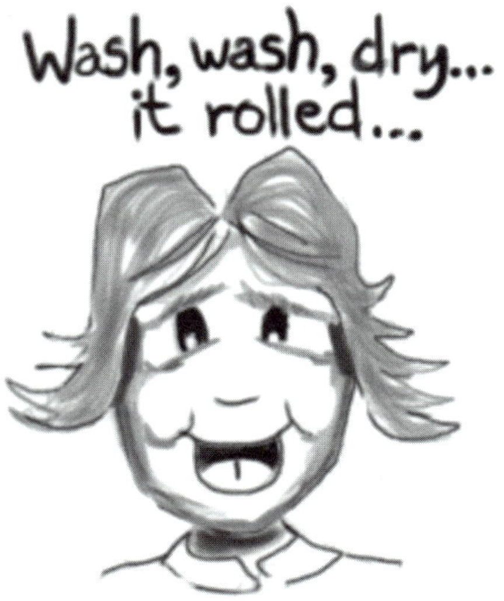

Izzy's therapy plan

Goals for Izzy were built around giving her an enormous variety of language models so she could extract certain commonalities that would help her move towards flexible language use. This plan included giving her maximal opportunities to use these target mitigations, which meant "preempting" her use of other automatic, script-line comments. The latter was hard, because once Izzy had said something a few times, it became ingrained. Then, it came out automatically, before she could give herself time to think and produce something more useful.

The following language sample took place after Izzy had been in language therapy for a month; it illustrates the way she was able to work on extracting "It's" and "It" from the language she and her partner were using. The following utterances were not consecutive, but were used in the span of a few minutes within dialogue:

It's all washed.
It's dried.
It's dirty.
It's to be a dirty.
Wash, wash, wash.
It dirty, it dirty, it dirty.
Wash, wash, dry—it rolled—

As the clinician continued to model a great variety of sentences with "It's" and "It" in conversation, Izzy continued to use the pronoun flexibly. Following is just one sample dialogue from the session:

I	**It turned into a starfish.**
I	**It's a towel.**
C	But it turned into a starfish.
I	**It turned into a beach towel.**

In this way, Izzy got to hear "it's" and "it" in a myriad of contexts and, because talking was a big part of her learning style, got to "mix and match" this pronoun with a great variety of mitigated phrases.

A month later, Izzy had isolated many pronouns and was on her way to mixing and matching a variety of semi-original utterances. Notice the difference between her "perfect" but inflexible utterances (labeled "1") and her imperfect, more flexible ones (labeled "2"):

I	**Is that the smallest pumpkin?** [1]
C	This is a pumpkin patch. (modeling something simpler)
I	**This is a pumpkin—I gonna put these—I gonna put these on them—too** **Pumpkin—these—put on—need some help?** **Miss—** **x x** [2; Izzy used her mitigations nicely, but abandoned a more complicated utterance]
I	**Do you want to go on the hay ride?** [1; Izzy then turned to a script]
C	It sounds like fun.
I	**Which pumpkin do you wanna pick?** [1] **Which pumpkin—wanna pick?** [2]
C	I want to pick—this one!
C	I picked a pumpkin!
I	**That squash—is a not pumpkin. It's a gourd!** [2; nice originality!]

Another month passed, and Izzy showed a combination of developmental stages: she was still in the mitigation process with some words and structures but combining some isolated words in flexible ways. Following are a few short dialogues, less-sophisticated on the surface but far more useful. The first is a combination of mitigations:

C	Where is the sleigh?
I	**It's pretend. It's not real. We need to get real ones.**

The second shows some combining of single words, then "growing" her utterance to become more grammatically correct.

C	Are you ready?
I	**Find me. Cover me. Cover me up. Cover me with pillow, Kristen.**
C	Okay, I need more pillows.

Progress notes from the session are quoted here: "Clinicians loved today's session … (because) it encapsulated so many of this semester's highlights. Izzy demonstrated the progress she has made in breaking down her former gestalts and the resulting flexibility and variety in expressing herself. Some of her utterances were quite original and thus contained grammatical errors, which is expected. The clinicians were thus able to support Izzy in all her endeavors: to express herself through novel utterances and then hear clinicians provide the correct grammar afterwards."

Izzy's own style

In her own unique way, Izzy continued with this mitigating—combining—growing process to move smoothly among Stages 2, 3, and 4 in the course of each session. Izzy was very attentive to all language models, and so her mitigation was often to isolate a particular word and then to figure out what she could do with it. Following are notes from three months later:

C	I looked everywhere. I didn't find the key.
I	**The cave is locked. I locked it.**
C	I don't have anything to use.
I	**Now I'm the nice crab.**
C	Crab, I can't get into the cave. It's locked.
I	**I don't have anything.**

It is interesting to see how Izzy changed places with the clinician so she could practice using the word "anything" herself. As can also be seen from this sample, Izzy could now generate grammar that she could call her own and had enough flexible language to emerge into the world of story-telling like she had imagined back when "Whoosh!" was her only stage direction. As time went on, Izzy only got better, and by the time she was five years old, Izzy had taken part in many novel stories that were not contaminated by learned scripts. One year into language therapy, she had enough flexibility to even tell some her old favorites in new ways. Such was the case with this story about her perennial favorite, mermaids:

I	**Pretend I'm Ursula and I live right here inside the cave.** (crawling under the trampoline)

C	Okay!
I	**Watch out for Ursula!**
C	Where is she?
I	**Pretend you talked loud and Ursula was awake.**
C	And Ursula heard me?
I	**And Ursula heard you.**
C	What about this cave—
I	**I woke up in the morning.**
C	Ursula, I want my magic wand back.
I	**I'm sitting on top of it.**
C	It's mine.
I	**It's not yours. It's mine.**
C	You stole it from me.
I	**You can't have it now.**
C	But I want it back.
I	**You can't have it.**
C	I'll go find something to trade for it. What do you want?
I	**I don't want you to trade for it.**
C	You don't want to trade?
I	**I'm gonna pretend I put a spell on it and change my mind. I don't want to sleep again. You have to say that.**
C	If you have the magic wand, you'll put a spell on me. I don't wanna sleep.
I	**Pretend you change your mind. You don't want to sleep. Say that.**

Obviously, our little story-teller was also the narrator and director, all roles she relished. As the next year of her therapy went on, her cast grew so that each person had a particular role, and Izzy didn't have to jump back and forth. A year later, by the time she was six, Izzy could create a story, hold the plot in her mind, use most of the language it required, and begin to show the flexibility needed to create with other people. Following is one short segment of one long story. As always, clinicians took their conversational turns, although they are not included here:

> **Bzzzzzz.**
> **Pretend I got the honey back!**
> **The bee who stings you because you're trying to take our honey and take it to your house.**
> **I'll bring some honey and put it in a honey jar for you and your mom to eat.**
> **And pretend I give you the orange sweater as honey.**
> **It's because I sell this honey for people.**
> **I make this honey for people.**
> **Here you go, here's your honey.** (Inviting a second clinician into the play)

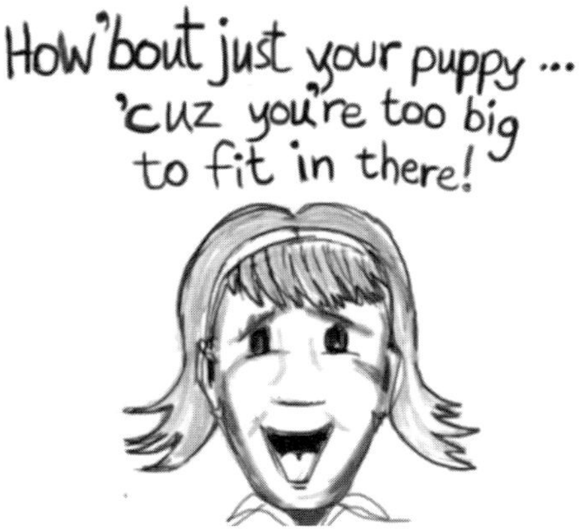

Want to join my beehive to eat your honey and you can wear this sweater in case you get cold?
Help me.
Make sure you get yellow and white dandelions.
Get yellow dandelions.
I think, I think, I think you could have a sleepover at my hive tonight.
And then not sting you because your puppy tries to steal it.
I sell it for people; you have to get some money; you can't just buy it; you have to get some money.
Just pretend.
Gimme 3 quarters. (Inviting a third clinician into the play)
Cuz it's 75 cents.
You get a big jar.
I filled it with honey just for you and your puppy because I know you're hungry and you can eat at my hive and have a sleepover and for you and your puppy.
How 'bout just your puppy 'cuz you're too big to fit in there.

Izzy went on to become a flourishing linguist and kindergarten-level playwright. During the time between age 6 and age 7, when she was ready to be dismissed from therapy, her goals shifted more and more to social interaction and the remaining regulation challenges she still faced. This tiny little director with a huge heart moved on to a new school venue which never suspected her earlier diagnosis.

Andrew had mitigated long before anyone could understand him

Andrew's story is quite different and quite short, because he was not language-delayed when we met him. We didn't realize it, however, and his story is a good reminder that a minimally-speaking child might already be at Stage 4 or higher in language competence. We met Andrew at when he was two years old, and at that time, it was impossible to know what his language development level was. Andrew was vocal, but his vowels, his intonation, and his timing was all undifferentiated. We suspected Andrew was verbal, but it was not until he was two and a half that he was able to begin demonstrating his intelligence and his language skills. It took some folks who really knew Andrew well to recognize the signs, but by the time he was three and a half, his parents and loving professionals recognized Andrew's genius and his mastery of language to at least NLA 4. Because of his severe apraxia of speech and whole body dyspraxia, it took every fiber of his physical being to demonstrate his understanding of language, but as a team, his friends "got it."

Andrew's dyspraxia was much more challenging than was Jake's, whose story is told in Chapter 9. Andrew worked at it as hard as any child we have ever known, but over the years, Andrew had to pick and choose which sentence patterns he wanted to practice in order to make them intelligible. Andrew wisely selected a handful of intonational patterns, using his musical ability to perfect the tone changes in them. His vowels became impeccable, and he judiciously worked on consonants that did not constrict his airflow and create unnecessary stops and starts of his voice. Andrew also became a rapid typist, and his keyboarding skills allowed him to reveal his growing command of the language that became exquisite.

Andrew's story has so much to teach us. So many of our kids are challenged by apraxia of speech and body dyspraxia and are often misunderstood as not having language competence—sometimes as not having language at all. Because 40% of our kids are dyspraxic, we need to remember that speech is not language and language is not speech.

Speech is not language; language is not speech.

Speech is a set of motor skills and is not necessary for language: receptive, internal, or expressive. Understanding language is competence in processing and is applied with both listening and reading (visually or through another modality like Braille). Internal language means thinking with language. Expressive language is different still and can occur through a variety of modalities: signing, typing, accessing alternative means of communication, or speech.

Andrew had all forms of language in spades. Expressing it through two-finger typing became easier and easier. But expressing it through speech was an enormous challenge Andrew always kept working on. Over time, Andrew became a fluent keyboarder and excelled in written language when his speech skills could not keep up with his oral language. Andrew zipped through school with an idea in his head: he had always wanted to be a filmmaker, and with his creativity and drive, Andrew was developing the technological competence to realize his dreams.

Russel just loved letters

Now, let's turn to Russel, whose story is much more complicated than Josh's or Izzy's and was the subject of a series of columns in the *Autism Asperger's Digest* ("Finding the Words ... When They're Pictures!" 2006). Much can be learned from Russel, not because he is typical, but because he is not. Like your child, Russel was his own person, and his fledgling sense of language needed to be his own to matter to him.

When we first met him at age two and a half, Russel preferred his modalities pure: the purely visual or the purely musical, but not mixed. Russel had a sense of the gestalt, however, in his appreciation of story: that is, a story with cadence but no words. It appeared clear that Russel's journey would be a longer one, as his peaceful little soul was not about to be hurried. One could try; but it wouldn't work. Thus, his story begins here, in this preschool chapter, and continues in Chapter 12, when Russel entered elementary school. Everything happened in due course: Russel developed good language skills and, throughout his childhood, managed to weave all the really important events into vignettes, the telling of each accompanied by a theme, a rhyme, and a twinkle in his eye.

But all that took time. Between the ages of two and a half and three, Russel appreciated patterns, logic, completeness, rhythm, and the visual. And Russel was very exacting. He didn't like sound with his visuals, and the visuals of the alphabet were what he loved the most. His preferred "sound" was silence, punctuated by quiet speech delivered in a cadence and gentleness that matched his auditory temperament. The "key phrases" of his life consisted of the predictable rhythm of poetry, into which almost any words could be placed.

By age three, Russel had an assortment of communicative language. He used some gestalt language meaningfully, such as: **"I wanna pick you up"** (meaning "I want to be picked up"), **"Shall we erase it?"** (meaning "I want to erase it"), a small assortment of mitigations, such as "Should we" and "How 'bout," and many Stage 3 single words and two word combinations, such as **"Pen," "Buckwheat," "Circle," "Experiment," "Root beer," "No magic door," "No magic key a duck," "And purple forests," "Up to forest," "Ben and Jen Juicy Juice," "Daddy Juicy Juice."** He also had some Stage 4 beginning sentences, such as: **"Grass is outside," "Marie's not home," "I want some mango honey," "It's buckwheat," "Mommy drink Juicy Juice."** But Russel was not a strong candidate for the kind of language work Josh or Izzy craved. For a long time, the only thing Russel wanted to mitigate was the alphabet, but even that was in his own way, with his own timing.

So, life in his slow, gentle lane meant thinking "outside the textbook" that Dylan had helped create. Russel's own story book had more chapters, and there were several that needed to be written before the one about language. The *Digest* article included those details, because they offer a template for other children who aren't really interested in language yet. These were the "chapters" we wrote for Russel:

> Chapter 1 – Things that delight Russel
> Chapter 2 – Delightful referents he shares with others
> Chapter 3 – Sound tracks of these delightful referents
> Chapter 4 – Language of these delightful referents

From the time Russel was two and a half, his family and I could fill in the first entries:

> Chapter 1 – Russel's delights: things that visually move, like automatic doors, cars going down the street; things that fit well, like shape cubes, boxes with well-matched lids; sticky-sweet desserts; his father's music, but at a distance
>
> Chapter 2 – Referents Russel shares with his family: looking at the night sky; watching trees swaying in the breeze; going through the "magic" doors at a local drug store; sharing books turned page-by-page; playing with letters of the alphabet; hearing favorite poems; sharing sticky-sweet desserts

And except for the sticky-sweet desserts, the letters of the alphabet were Russel's favorite things. That other people also liked them ignited Russel's sense of fun, and his visual pastime became his passion. He loved putting the letters into alphabetic order and delighted in seeing key words in his visual environment. The lighted "Exit" signs were his favorite, especially if they pointed the way to "magic doors."

Russel was quite OK with us saying the names of the letters, slowly and gently, as he put them into order. We were careful to say each name softly, with gently-rising inflection, just after the letter was set in place, so the visual experience was not altered. It was tempting to go faster, or to "teach" him in our way, but our little probes were effectively shut out and didn't work. To honor Russel's chosen experience, however, we could introduce the letter names in such a way as to create a sound track he liked, one he would come to appreciate as his Chapter 3. If we showed him that sound could enhance his experience, rather than detract from it, we hoped it would become the foundation for a successful language experience when Russel was ready for Chapter 4.

Once he trusted that people would not break the "rhythm," Russel began to love our letter naming. He didn't like the ABC song, and he didn't like rapid or non-melodic speech. Russel's pleasure was maintained only if the timing of our words was predictable. For six months, Russel had fun with sound and loved the social interaction we provided around his letters. Slowly and respectfully, as we created an atmosphere of fun, we were preparing for the next chapter, when language beyond A-Z would also be fun.

Russel turns three

As quietly as it had begun, when he was three years old, Chapter 3 came to a close. Other letter orders besides ABC emerged as the words Russel liked to spell. "Boston," "Turkey," "Exit," "Stop," and "Emergency" entered Russel's realm of the visually-intriguing. And the grammar we gently introduced to Russel also referred to the visual present, the existence of the letter. In a sense, Russel had mitigated individual "words" from the gestalt of the alphabet and had re-sorted them into spelling words. We wanted our first grammatical models (his Chapter 4) to fit in just as gently. I also wanted them to be grammatically easy-to-mitigate and to have the same common denominators Russel had already isolated: the letter names. So, "It's an A," "I got a B," "We found a C" seemed like ringers.

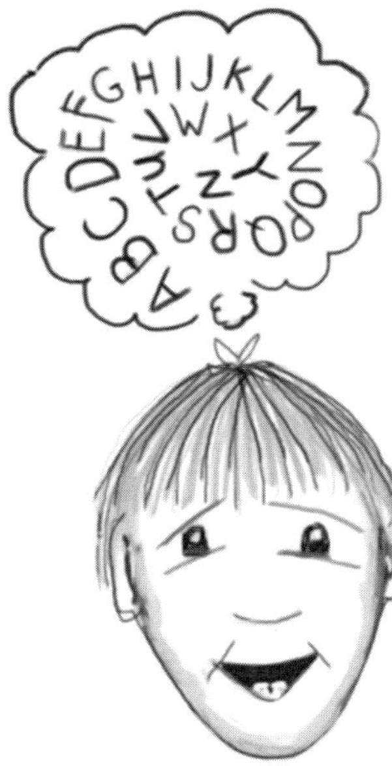

Once I gave him the "I got a A" sentence, Russel quickly proceeded to produce all the combinations of "I got a ..." all the way to "I got a Z." Realizing that Russel was actually doing a "mix and match" with our first grammar models just like he was recombining the letters of the alphabet, I decided that the next gentle step would be to make sure he had every opportunity to mix and match all of his favorite concepts: colors, letters, and spelling words.

Yes, it was with his own vocabulary and the grammatical forms he found pleasant, but by the time he was three and a half, Russel had moved solidly into using beginning generative grammar. Many of Russel's sentences communicated; many did not, at least in a conventional way. Following is a small composite of both types:

> **They're puffy clouds. They're like a blanket.**
> **Are you do castle bangs?**
> **It erased. It's flappy.**

An interesting recommendation came from his progress report at the time: "Consider Russel's learning style and his own rhythm in interactions with him. He is auditorily adept, so he will apply the first language he hears in conjunction with whatever *he is focused on.* Make sure the first language you use in a situation is the best language for him to use later, because he will remember it! The best pace for Russel's language processing is the one he himself uses. Because he is now producing language at about 4.5 utterances per minute, his own slow, sing-song pattern is ideal for language modeling."

By the time he was four years old, Russel began playing with language as if to practice it. He would produce a series of utterances in a manner that continued over the years, even as the sentence patterns became more complex. At age four, a series might sound like these: **"Look at that; Look at that Etch-a-Sketch; It's a Etch-a-Sketch,"** and **"Marge Blanc forgot; I forgot; You forgot."** Russel's oral practice extended to original words as well. Starting with "moniker," Russel variously referred to people this way: **"Mom-a-ker; Dad-a-ker; Marge-a-ker".**

When Russel was four and a half, his emerging sense of dialogue was a common subject of practice. He would suggest a favorite topic, such as a "T," and say, **"Here's one—would you like a 'T'?"** By his response, or lack of response, to what his partner said, it became clear how much of a "turn" the partner could take without upsetting the dialogue Russel had in mind. It was as if the story was already written in his head, and life was the stage on which it would play out. And his partners were challenged to remember all the stories Russel had ever heard, read, or told them, because **he** would.

Also at this time, Russel was becoming inventive in naming and describing things, using decidedly visual referents. Trying to ask for a particular toy, Russel asked, **"Let's go get your—Marge Blanc's rainbow toy."** He continued, **"It's a fizzy something."**

Russel turns five

By the time Russel was five, he was spelling in earnest with just a little help. His language reflected his pride: **'Boston' down there spells BOSTON and 'Stop' up there spells STOP and 'Exit' up there spells EXIT."** Regardless of the grammatical accuracy, the use of sentence structure was wonderful. Russel still had some of his old gestalts and mitigations, but his own generative language was catching up with them, as in: **"Should we do some spelling?; We doing some spelling; Let's do some spelling."**

By the time he was five and a half, Russel was telling jokes of this type: **"Wanna eat the rug?" "Wanna eat the cushion?"** And his grammar was coming along nicely. Russel clearly preferred his own generative grammar to gestalts, even if he didn't know how to fully form a construction: **"I'll show you—you eat"** (meaning: 'I'll show you what you can eat') He practiced conjunctions over and over again, but always with the ultimate joke in mind (often an invented word, using "self-generated" spelling): **"We watched the Teletubies for a long time—but then the show was over"**; **"We watched the exit signs, but then**

the loge is over—they're gone."

By the time Russel was six and beginning kindergarten, he had become a fledgling conversationalist and story-teller. It was clear that multi-sentence accomplishments required considerable concentration, absolutely silent surroundings, and an adoring audience. When something interfered, grammar quickly broke down, as in the following dialogue:

R	**Take the markers and go out—**
C	Outside?
R	**No outside.**
R	**Go out.**
C	Go out?
R	**Out to the front.**

On the other hand, sometimes everything went right, such as when Russel dropped a set of colored sticks, prompting him to pretend we were having a "barbeque" and then to get some real food to add to the party:

R	**Barbecue.**
C	We're having a cook-out.
R	**Should we—**
C	Absolutely.
R	**Wanna eat the hotdog.**
C	Sure, we can have hotdogs.
R	**Cheese.**
C	Oh, hot dogs and cheese.
R	**Wanna eat the hot dog?**
C	We sure can.
R	**Wanna go in.**
C	We could get some real food inside.
R	**Wanna get out.** (meaning "stay outside")
C	We can stay outside.
R	**Wanna go get some hot dogs.**
C	And bring them outside!

Russel was making good language progress, but he was far from matching his linguistic potential. Russel was a communicator, more selective than any of the preschool children we have highlighted so far, but a communicator in the realms that mattered to him.

As Russel moved into the elementary grades, we continued to work with him, and we will pick up on his continuing story in Chapter 12. For now, however, let's pause and summarize what we have come to understand about the NLA process for preschoolers.

Summary

Natural language development is built into our kids' fabrics, waiting for the right cognitive maturity and self-regulation to unfold. We need to be there at the right time so we can help make it happen.

The preschool years are by far the most conducive time to begin language development and to use the principles of NLA to support it. Natural language development is built into our kids' fabrics, waiting for the right cognitive maturity and sense of self-regulation to unfold. It is up to us to be there at the right time so we can help the process unfold, either in a "textbook" manner like Dylan experienced, or in one of the myriad chapter-book ways illustrated by Jake, Josh, Izzy, Andrew, and Russel.

NLA offers us a textbook progression to keep in our minds, but each of our kids is unique and special. Because each of them is an individual, our set-up, materials, and technique need to be individualized. Being a gestalt language processor does not suggest which language gestalts an individual child is interested in any more than being an analytic language processor suggests which vocabulary an individual child is interested in. Clearly, Dylan's story could not have been superimposed on Russel's, and we would have ended up ignoring Russel's own style and intentions had we tried to do so. Mixing basketball games in with alphabet sorting doesn't work for avid spellers. And teaching *Cars* vocabulary is anathma to a young mermaid girl. It's what any of us cares about that creates our first successful language experiences and our early language.

There are plenty of commonalities in our kids' journeys, of course. The capacity to develop a system of grammar to talk about Lightning McQueen or barbecues is part of our humanity, what all of us in our language community share. Each human community tacitly "agrees to" a set of rules about how its particular language fits together. The resulting code, the grammar, is a tool for the individuals within that language community to use for their own self-expression. What we do with that grammar is our own: our personal thoughts, feelings, insights, and "takes" on life. Our language then becomes our way of communicating ourselves to others.

Real communication is sharing what we care about with people we care about.

So, beneath our communication and powering our communication are our communicative intentions. Authentic communication is sharing what we care about with people we care about. Outside of communicative intentions, language is like a "clanging cymbal" without a heart and soul; it says nothing. We can teach a certain amount of language outside those intentions, but we end up with a set of skills, sometimes just an assortment of "splinter skills" with limited application. To our dismay, we find that these skills never lead to language development and never even generalize—because they are not a developmental language system. Isolated skills or verbal behaviors are just that; they never become a flexible system, the generative tool we had hoped for.

Language can certainly exist outside of communication, but why would we want it to? And why would we want to teach it this way to our children? Far better to start with each individual child, with his or her hopes and joys, and build something from the inside out: something kids will love, and use, and call their own. In the next chapter, we will take that inside-out approach and offer some specific ideas as strategies to use with our preschoolers.

Chapter 11
Preschool Strategies and Considerations

We know the value of early intervention, but we also know it needs to be the right intervention if it is going to lead to the development of flexible language systems for our children. This chapter will present the general principles that best support natural language acquisition in young children. It is based on the general linguistic process of NLA and supplemented by what we know about the individuality of young children.

Naturalistic means that we begin with children's authentic experiences of life, the ones where kids feel safe and happy.

Appropriate preschool intervention has four key ingredients. It is naturalistic, interactive, personal, and supported. All four ingredients offer us descriptors of where to begin.

Interactive means that we begin with our kids' joyfulness and share that joy with them.

The first ingredient—naturalistic—means that we begin with children's authentic experiences of life, the ones where kids feel safe and happy. We take special notice of when kids are happiest, share those times, and gradually superimpose sound and language on them. We don't approach language out of this context any more than we would with any child. Not to belabor the point more than is warranted, but our kids have the capacity to develop natural language, and they do develop natural language—in natural environments—naturally.

The second ingredient—interactive—means that we begin with our kids' joyfulness and share that joy with them. It is this sharing of joy that is the heart of interaction; it is the dance of reciprocity that underlies non-verbal conversation and, ultimately, verbal conversation. Don't wait for a child to initiate sharing; when we share in our children's joy, we establish the interaction.

Personal means that we begin wih communicative attempts that come from inside our kids, and are intentions they want to share.

The third ingredient—personal—means that each of our children's early communicative attempts starts from inside them. Communication bubbles out from within. It is personal, meaningful, and comes from a desire to share. Person-to-person sharing precedes communication, and shared joy leads to continuing that shared joy, which leads to our kids' first communicative intentions. Later, we will talk more about the development of communicative intents; for now, it is enough to know that communication is personally motivated.

Supported means that our kids need to find places of safety and joy for the first three ingredients to matter.

The fourth ingredient—supported—means that our kids need to find places of safety and joy for the first three ingredients to matter. Without being regulated enough to feel safe, our kids are not in a place where personal communication, or language development, is even on the radar. We have lots of resources available to us to help our kids regulate, and finding the right formula for your child—the right "sensory diet"—is the support that will make the difference. During times of optimal self-regulation, natural joy is possible, sharing joy is possible, and natural language opportunities are possible.

Principles of NLA for preschoolers

Beyond these four overarching ingredients, some principles for introducing NLA to preschool-aged children are important to think about before you start. It is a good idea to plan how you think you might include these principles and practice some by yourself or with a partner. Here are the main principles:

1. Gestalt language processors need gestalts

Successful language development for our kids depends on there being natural language gestalts in their environments. The process begins when kids are able to tolerate auditory input and they selectively tune into the gestalts around them. Depending on their age, tolerance, and propensities, these might be songs, jingles, movie lines, environmental sounds, the hum of conversation, or the drone of life around them. Our kids will hear whatever parts of these things they are drawn to, but when we build intentional sound gestalts into their lives, we increase the chances they will extract what we hope for once they're ready: language.

This principle means paying attention to sounds your child tolerates and likes—and planning to include similar sounds as a part of your natural interactions. At first, the sound is just a back-drop but, more and more, it can assume a greater focus until there are some predictable melodies, tone patterns, rhymes or jingles that are a part of the shared joy. All these auditory gestalts then lead naturally to language gestalts whenever a child is ready.

2. Natural language development needs natural language

Language is part of a natural environment, and that's where it should remain. We know that because "play is the child's work," language should be in the context of fun and play. As you progress in the auditory environment you plan for your child, natural kid language is what you want. If expressions like, "Yea!!" and "Whoooa!" or "Wowowowowow!!" appeal to your child, good; if other sounds like "Vroom!" are more his speed, fine also. Your child's loves and passions—and his auditory system—drive your selections.

3. Kids need to feel good to care about communicating

Regulation matters to all kids, and because our kids have greater regulation challenges, they need greater regulation solutions. If your child is receiving PT and/or OT services, regulation is probably something you understand, and can support. In case you haven't heard this way of describing autism from an "arousal" or "alertness" perspective before, I will share it with you. It was shared with me by an OT long ago, and I have found it so useful in understanding the ebbs and flows of our kids' days. "All kids have a range of arousal or alertness that works for them," I was told, "and this helps them go though their days with minimal meltdowns. But with autism, that optimal range is pencil-thin, and kids move through it too fast for us to use it to their advantage. They might go from under-alert to over-alert in a matter of minutes, passing through the optimal range for just a few seconds. Part of treatment is increasing the size of that optimal range so kids can actually do something productive, learn something productive, during it." In the classic educational vernacular, it is the "teachable moment," which may be fleeting for our kids. But just knowing what it is helps us recognize it, support it, extend it, and, finally, use it to our kids' advantage.

All kids have a range of arousal or alertness that works for them. With autism, that range is pencil-thin, and kids move through it too fast for us to use it to their advantage.

4. Individual kids need to be approached as individuals

There is no "one size fits all" to NLA, any more than there is a "one size fits all" to language development off the spectrum. The only "one" is the system of grammar that all kids in our culture aim towards. But we all build our own messages, our own style, in our own way.

Ways of presenting language are as varied as our kids and the families they come from. The ingredients may be the same in principle: naturalistic, interactive, personal, and supported, but they all imply that the individual is at the heart of the process. So your living room won't look—or sound—like anyone else's, nor should it. Imagine the silence of Russel's alphabet floor compared with the engine roar of Josh's race track.

5. Kids need to interact with people who care about them

This might seem to go without saying, but even as we do our best to make sure our autism programs are delivered by trained, caring people, nothing can replace a true family, extended family, and family-chosen circle of interactants for our kids. We turn to professionals as coaches and partners, but it all comes back to real relationships that nourish communication and the language that communication will eventually depend on. Our best advice is to partner with an SLP who can help you along the way. A long-term relationship with that person means that you will have widened the circle you create around your child and means that, together, you can continue to develop the relationships and interactions that will support your child for years to come.

6. Kids need to have their communicative attempts acknowledged

Our kids' first communicative attempts are notoriously difficult to detect. Our kids are motor-challenged and typically lack the body proximity, facial expression, and vocal control to make their early communicative attempts clear. Our job is to bend over backwards to notice the subtle clues and to acknowledge our kids when there is no "writing on the wall."

Our job is to notice the subtle clues and to acknowledge our kids when there is no "writing on the wall."

It is extremely difficult for any parent to be a good observer of his own child at first—that is, until he can stand back far enough to simply watch and listen.

One practical way to do that is to make some short movies of your child when he is with you and perhaps others in your family. From the vantage point of an observer rather than an interactant, it is easier to spot glimmers of emotion, shifts of eye gaze, subtle changes in body orientation, and jagged reaching that signal intention. During the interactions themselves, such fleeting moments are often difficult to notice, but watching them over and over on a movie really helps bring them into focus. Having stepped out of the dyad long enough to observe, you will develop a better sense of the fleeting clues that are easy to miss in the brief moments they occur.

Once you return to the dyad, then, you will feel much more confident about doing these things:

1. Attribute meaning to your child's actions. This is hard to to do until you get started. Until then, you may feel foolish assuming your child had something in mind when he moved this way or that. But once you get started, that all changes, because kids learn that you are watching for signs and that their actions matter. You are not likely to see dramatic changes in your child right away, but then you add the next element.
2. Give your child the benefit of the doubt. How many stories have we now read of older ASD kids who learned to type and could finally let their parents know they are smarter than they appeared using conventional standards? By presuming intelligence, you can give your child a head start on communicating themselves to the world. We often fear "wishful thinking" and attributing more intelligence to our children than they demonstrate. So what? My clinical experience convinces me that all kids appreciate our admiration, and kids with true cognitive challenges do many, many smart things. These kids feel smart if we tell them they are. Presume the best; your child will achieve.

By presuming intelligence, we give our kids a chance to share themselves with the world.

7. Kids need to have their language development progress acknowledged

The ideal environment would have everyone on the same page, and no one working at cross-purposes with anyone else.

When we understand how important language gestalts are, we can make sure others in a child's environment understand this as well. The ideal environment would have everyone on the same page and no one working at cross-purposes with anyone else. When kids are processing gestalts, they process all sound, all language, as gestalts. They have no choice.

But a common situation is this: kids are receiving services from more than one provider and each provider takes a different approach—a different approach to autism, yes, but even a different approach to language development. Let's follow two different scenarios:

First, if an SLP is approaching language development from an NLA perspective, that's good. But what if another provider is approaching language as a behavior and feels that single words should be taught? We know that if a child is at Stage 3, those single words will be appropriately processed as single words. But if a child is at Stage 1, those same single words will be processed as gestalts. If so, the child can learn them, but they are actually a detriment to true language development. This common mismatch of language input can stymie or stop development until either the providers can coordinate their input or the child's SLP is given a free hand until the child has moved past Stage 1.

The second scenario can be even more problematic. What if no one really knows if a child is processing language at all? What if a child seems to have so little understandable speech that we think of him as "non-verbal"—not just expressively, but receptively? This is an all-too-common scenario, with kids being mis-labeled as "non-verbal," with their communicative attempts falling on deaf ears. We hate to think of ourselves this way, but adults seem to need "evidence" that kids are talking to really believe it. And evidence with our kids often only comes years later, after kids' speech is finally clear enough that parents realize their children were talking for years.

Adults seem to need 'evidence' that kids are talking to believe it. And evidence often only comes years later, after kids' speech is clear enough that parents realize their children were talking for years.

We have to remember that our motor-impaired gestalt kids are trying to say some pretty long lines of song and prose, things that are much more difficult than "ball" or "bottle" or the words that parents hear their analytic kids say. For many of our kids, putting together an intonational contour with or without a few vowel sounds is a big enough feat. Making it intelligible is simply impossible for some years to come.

If this is the case with your child, you will likely be enlisting an SLP and an OT to help you think through your child's speech development to make sure you're supporting it in the best ways possible. But if one of your service providers is not on board with you and feels that only intelligible, non-echoed utterances are of value, your child is the one who suffers. Consider, for example, the intervention study in *Pivotal Response Treatment for Autism* (Koegel and Koegel, 2006). When the authors surveyed parents about the "expressive words" used by their ASD children under the age of three, both echoed language and unintelligible language was excluded from the utterance count. The results of the survey were that these children "used no or very few expressive words." Then PRT was instituted and "considerable progress" was made. Typical numbers of words "evoked" in 10 minutes jumped from an average of 16 to more than 200.

Now let's read the fine print and then between the lines. Many ASD kids under the age of three would likely be echolaic and unintelligible. So by Koegel and Koegel's standards they would have "no to very few expressive words." If the PRT program taught a child to make a request and the child repeated that request 200 times in 10 minutes, he certainly has learned a powerful skill. But learning a small handful of words this way fails to translate into language development. As a point of illustration, the book uses a case example of a four-and-a-half-year-old boy, "nonverbal" at the start of the program, who learns an expressive repertoire of 35 words and even a spontaneous sentence, "I want more sauce" (Koegel and Koegel, 2006, p. 159). In the vernacular of NLA, however, he has not developed beyond Stage 1.

The experience in our clinic is that kids are dealt a double whammy here, as some of those well-trained, well-practiced requests, usually the first one(s), become locked in for the duration of childhood. Some are benign and don't get in the way of language development ("Ready, set, go"), but others interfere in

Learned gestalts like single words and scripted requests don't break down naturally; kids end up with unmitigable language and little else to work with.

a significant way. Learned gestalts like single words and scripted requests don't break down naturally, and kids end up with unmitigable language and little else to work with. In our clinic, we frequently see kids whose language is like that cited in the case example above. It is at such a point that many parents seek out SLPs. They describe their kids as having "some functional speech" but that generalization is uneven and progress has stopped. As they enter elementary school, such children often are introduced to NLA for the first time. These are the kids we will follow in the next section.

Preschool kids: a review

Before we move on from our preschool-aged kids, let's review what we have learned. First, we have identified four key ingredients of a productive language environment:

1. Our kids need a naturalistic environment in which they feel safe and happy.
2. Our kids' environments must be interactive ones, where we share joy with our children.
3. Our kids' first communicative attempts must be personal to them and must come from them, inside.
4. Our kids need to be appropriately supported in the individual ways they require to be regulated and feel safe and happy.

We have also identified seven principles of preschool language development programs. They are:

1. We need to provide appropriate, mitigable sound and language gestalts for our gestalt kids to hear and process.
2. We need to use natural, kid-sounding language to make their mitigation tasks easier.
3. We need to help our kids feel good, because we want them to feel good about communicating.
4. We need to approach each of our kids as an individual: with materials, activities, and sounds they are drawn to.
5. We need to provide our kids with play and communication partners who truly care about them.
6. We need to make sure that our kids' communicative attempts are fully acknowledged.
7. We need to ensure that the people around our kids understand the natural language development process we want them to experience.

We have many things going for us as we embark on our preschool child's language development journey:

- We know our child has the potential to have fun and be playful.
- We know our child's language exposure is largely in our hands.
- We realize we have the opportunity to set up our child's environment the way we want, to his or her best advantage.

- Once we tackle how to support our child's health, safety, and self-regulation, we know we have the opportunity for shared joy to become the core of her language development program.
- We appreciate that our child is a unique individual and that his progress will not look like anyone else's.
- We realize that our child has her whole childhood to develop grammar and that it doesn't need to be complete by the time she is school-aged.
- Finally, we will learn later in this journey that grammar is just one part of language and that our child has her whole life to learn other parts of language and to extend its use in myriad ways.

In summary, our kids have many, many productive years of development ahead of them. Our next topic will be the elementary years, which are a rich time for language development.

section 4

Elementary School Kids

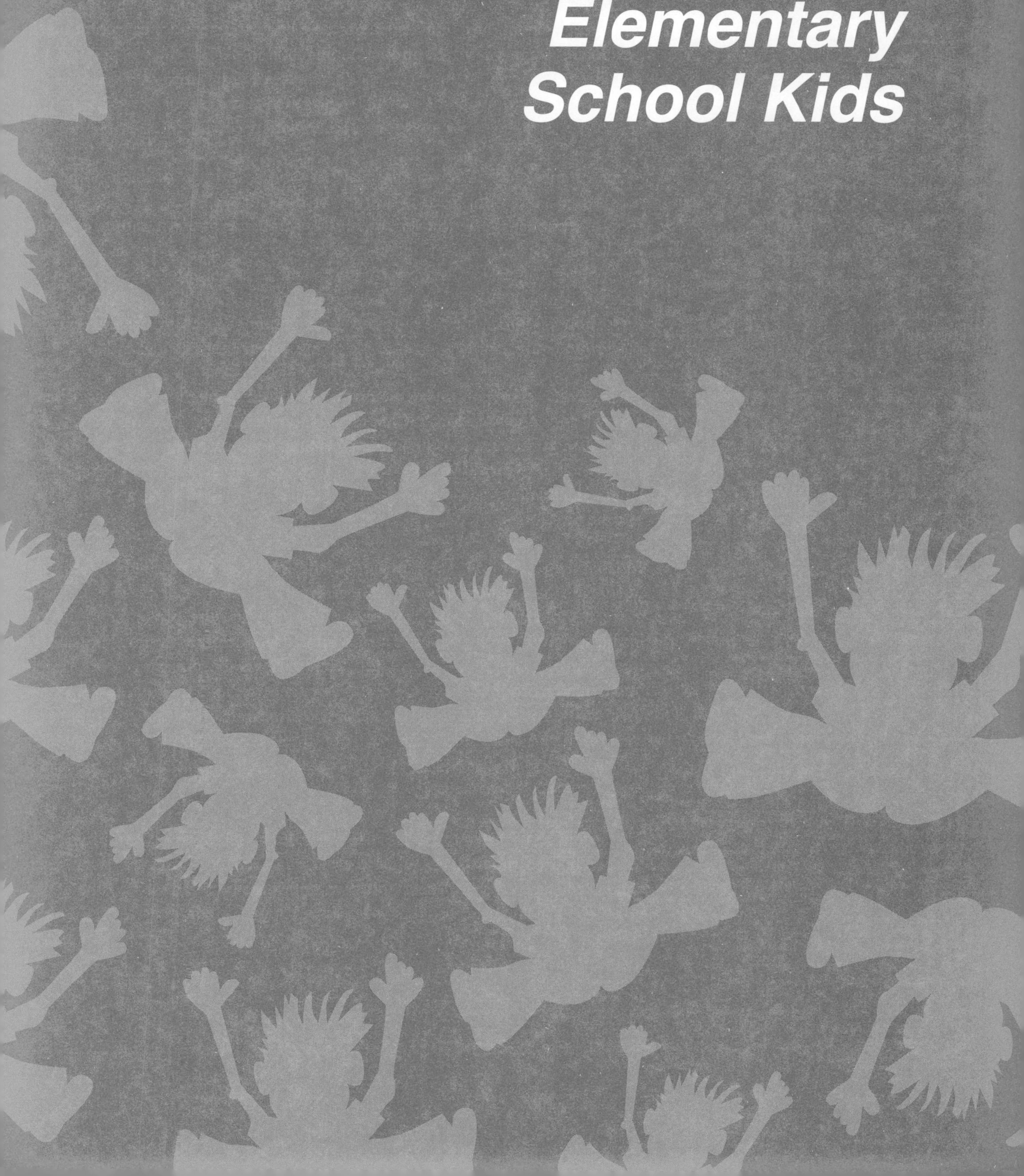

Introduction

Our kids can continue to develop their language systems throughout childhood.

The child who has successfully begun the NLA process before he enters school and receives continued understanding and linguistic support can continue to develop his language system throughout his childhood and achieve a grammatical system to the level of his potential. The school years are not as easy as the preschool ones for planning playful language experiences, but our kids' growing sense of self-regulation allows for a greater variety of activities.

Some of these activities can take place at school, but it is often at home that kids' language development is best targeted. With each year, there is less free time at school, less physical activity, and less-frequent time for natural language modeling. The language of the classroom becomes more didactic, with more "school language" and less opportunity to talk while playing. Families are in the position, then, of becoming more creative with after-school time, transforming their homes into little playgrounds and finding local gyms and outside playgrounds for their language-development opportunities to take place.

Such was the case with Dylan, whom we followed through his preschool years and will continue to follow in Chapter 12 as an elementary student. We will also look again at Russel and his continuing language development journey through the elementary years. Both boys were self-generating language by the time they entered elementary school, and both were able to achieve a full grammar system as time went on.

The sheer amount of gestalt language amassed by older children makes their first mitigation a highly complicated process.

In Chapter 13, we will take a new road and introduce some children who had not begun NLA intervention until elementary school. Their process is much more complicated for many reasons. First, there are the constraints inherent in the structure of the school day and limited opportunity to hear appropriate mitigable language models. Secondly, children have been exposed to a largely uncharted territory of language gestalts by then, without a rudder to help steer their way through. If they have managed to mitigate some, they have a good start on the process. But if they have not, the sheer amount of gestalt language amassed by these older children makes their first mitigation a highly complicated process.

The stories in Chapter 13 are less like a textbook and much more idiosyncratic to the children themselves. While the stages of NLA remain the same, each child's language encyclopedia is his own and must be addressed by the adults in his life for linguistic progress to occur. A lot of credit goes to these older children, and a lot of credit goes to their parents who believe in them and in their linguistic futures.

Chapter 12
Our Preschool Kids Grow Up: Continuing the NLA Process in Elementary School

Returning to Dylan's story: development of grammar

After Dylan had been in therapy for a little over a year, he started kindergarten. He had been at Stage 4 for a few months and was starting to use his own generative grammar. Dylan still used some short gestalts and some mitigated utterances, but it was obvious which utterances were constructed from scratch. These were the ones with grammar errors that made them sound imperfect. Following are some of Dylan's beginning grammatical utterances which help paint a picture of what Dylan sounded like when he used the grammar he had available to him.

"I got magic!"

I slam it.
Door's lock.
You go in there, Mom.
I want move mattress.
I got magic!
Go get a magic.

Dylan's sentences didn't sound like what we expect of children entering kindergarten, but they gave Dylan some flexibility with his self-expression. And knowing where Dylan had come from, his fledgling grammar represented real progress. As we continue to trace his language development, we will look first at the building blocks Dylan had to work with and then at a rationale for what to do with them.

Next steps into grammar

"Some magic?"

Dylan worked at language in earnest. His Stage 3 concept combinations continued to expand, each one providing a place to add grammar. Following are a few examples from the session cited above:

It two books.
Red and blue.
My—me.
All done balloon.
Some magic?

Such utterances were a nice training ground for further development of grammar. You will recall from Chapter 5 how beginning grammar naturally emerges from two-word phrases, and how it then evolves into higher level grammar. You looked at grammatical development as a series of levels, each level more developmentally sophisticated than the one before it. You learned that treatment of developmental grammar targets structures that naturally develop all at the same time. Knowing this gives you permission to choose from among several developmentally-appropriate targets, depending on the interests and activities of your child.

With analytic kids, an advanced construction they're not ready for will just wash over them. But gestalt processors will probably learn it as a gestalt.

In Chapter 5, you also were introduced to a general process for targeting grammar in your play and conversation with your child. Now, as we look at school-aged children who are ready for more sophisticated developmental grammar, we need to re-emphasize how much the developmental order of language targets matters. With little analytical kids, if we use an advanced construction that they're not ready for, it will just wash over them. But with our little gestalt processors, they will probably learn it as a gestalt. While this is not necessarily bad, it can slow down their true language progress. If it's a catchy phrase and they repeat it, they may remember it and then just have one more phrase or sentence to break down. As we cautioned in the Preschool Section, we want to make doubly sure we don't interfere with the developmental stage our kids are working on, and the surest way of interfering is to inadvertently model a gestalt sentence after they've progressed through Stage 2.

So how much do you need to know about grammar in order to help your child? You don't need to become a grammar specialist and diagram sentences like you did in English class. But you do need to develop a working sense of the general order of grammar development. The best way to do this is to take one level and practice it. Talk to yourself a lot when you're alone, such as in your car or when you're taking a walk. Try out lots of sentences at DSS Level 1 until you can sound like a child again. The entire DSS chart is Appendix D, but for quick access, just write the following abbreviated DSS "cheat sheet" on a set of post-it notes to carry with you and practice for a few minutes as often as you can.

Table 18: Highlights of Developmental Sentence Scoring Levels
1. It, that, I, my, mine, you, your, simple verbs, not, Is it?
2. He, she, verb+s, verb+ed, gonna, gotta, let's, what, where
3. We, they, those, more, some, and, to+verb
4. Some, more, can+verb, can't+verb, don't+verb
5. But, so, or, if, when, how
6. Wh pronouns (I know what to do), could, would, because
7. Why, everybody, first, last, passive voice (has gotten)
8. Which, embedded clauses (I got soaked when it rained)

Now think about how a child sounds at the first level. This is your target for how you will sound. Try out all kinds of phrases and sentences, some that are correct, and an equal number that are not. At Level 1, a child only has so many constructions to work with, so role play it like that child.

> That's blue.
> I want it.
> It's not mine.
> Is it yours?
> It's falling.
> I fall down.
> I not want it.
> You want blue ball?
> That ball mine.
> Not getting it!
> Not take it!

A child working at Level 2 will also have the constructions at Level 1 available to her and can construct many more types of sentences. Your practice will include grammar like the following: sometimes correct, sometimes not. Your task is to internalize the process kids are working with, so use the following as an example:

> He's climbing a hill.
> She's gonna get that book.
> You're gonna go now?
> Let's go to school.
> What's his name?
> Where's he's going now?
> He's gots hers ball.
> I gotted a new bike
> I not had it, not eated it.
> I'm gotta get out!

As you read these sentences, notice how many constructions are not a part of a child's generative repertoire by Level 2. So many constructions that make up typical gestalts aren't constructible yet, and visibly missing are words like "don't," and "can't." Our kids will tend to say sentences with useful words like this, but at this point in their development, they will be gestalts or mitigations and not self-generated. Also be aware that while we may be tempted to teach our kids polite forms like "Can I … ?" this construction doesn't appear for several more levels, and if it is learned, it is learned as a gestalt.

While we may be tempted to teach our kids polite forms like "Can I … ?" this construction doesn't naturally develop until later, so if it is learned, it is learned as a gestalt.

After you become familiar with how it feels and sounds to talk like Level 1 and then Level 2, continue up to at least Level 3, which will give you a complete beginning grammar. After your child has moved on to higher-level grammar, you can practice the next levels, but you will have plenty of time for that later. By then, you may want to hand over the lion's share of this practice work to your child's SLP.

Continuing Dylan's story

"I gonna running."

Now it's time to pick up Dylan's story again and join him a few months into kindergarten, when he was producing a preponderance of grammatical constructions. Again, he continued to use some nice two-word constructions, as would be typical of any language-developing child, and experimented with a few higher-level grammatical constructions. Following is a short snippet of his language, illustrating its variety.

> **I gonna running.**
> **Don't move!**
> **I rolling.**
> **Scary monster.**
> **I can fall.**
> **I get a pillow.**
> **Mommy, no out.**
> **I don't like it.**
> **Whoa, I'm gonna get bounce.**
> **Hey, can't falling.**

"What you going?"

We now jump ahead to the next summer, after his kindergarten year, following some months when Dylan experimented with his new grammar in all aspects of real life. By then, his grammar served as a tool for functional language, and his social interactions were blossoming. Dylan's language was solidly based on NLA 4 (DSS levels 1–3), with healthy experimentation at higher levels of grammar. His grammar was sometimes correct, sometimes not, but it allowed him great expressive flexibility. Following are some examples from a single session:

> **Yikes, she's got hurt.**
> **Curious George is—climb tree.**
> **You get the rhino.**
> **I'll teach him on a rope.**
> **What you going?**
> **I take him map.**
> **I gotta fix.**
> **Oh, the ship and the house.**
> **Where did the ladder go?**
> **Tigger, are you promise?**

By the time of this language sample, Dylan was 6 and a half years old and was viewed as "language delayed," rather than "echolalic." He was producing a nice variety of original sentences in near non-stop dialogue and used language gestalts sparingly. Dylan still loved to quote from his favorite videos, but this was usually to research an idea or to find a subject he wanted to understand. Quoting from *The Lion King* meant that Dylan was a gestalt thinker, and he looked to whole stories, whole ideas, and whole patterns as his prime source of meaning. He liked reciting whole lines from a variety of sources, but, unlike a few years before, Dylan usually mitigated these gestalts quickly, found what he wanted from them, and used these extractions in his own unique ways.

Dylan's dismissal from therapy

"I don't want to balloons—I don't want to blow a bubble."

Dylan continued his steady language progress for another half year, and at the time of his dismissal, he was speaking with far greater accuracy and was regularly reformulating sentences to make them more understandable to his listeners. Dylan was dismissed from our clinic because he was able to flourish with continued therapy in public school.

A few examples of Dylan's sentences at age seven give a nice picture of a boy who could act out stories with toys and with his peers and who could also begin to advocate for himself:

> **We got it—we got the treasure, Pooh.**
> **Pull—let's pull—let's pull the rope!**
> **Oh, Tigger, you got to get the anchor.**
> **What's this? A star!**
> **I don't want to, Marge—I don't want to balloons—I don't want to blow a bubble.**

While Dylan's story was far from complete at age seven, he was clearly progressing as a generative language user. Dylan was later able to catch up with his peers, who, by third and fourth grades, were just beginning to learn about story construction, the moral of a story, and the meaning of metaphor. Dylan had understood stories from the time he was immersed in them at age four, so it made sense that once he had grammar, he could catch up with other kids at that time.

As we now close this chapter of Dylan's story, we will recap his language accomplishments between the ages of four and seven. As a preschooler, Dylan successfully moved from using language gestalts (NLA 1), to mitigating them and recombining them (NLA 2), to isolating single words and combining them into original phrases (NLA 3), then to beginning to develop simple sentences (NLA 4). Once he moved into elementary school, Dylan solidified his simple sentences and continued to develop a variety of verb tenses and phrase relationships (NLA 5), then began forming complex sentences with more advanced verbs and conjunctions (NLA 6).

As well as Dylan's language continued to develop after we dismissed him, he remained challenged by sensory input. In later elementary school, he was able to ask his peers to help him when he faced sensory overload. His own written story was published in *Walk Awhile in my Autism* (McGinnity and Negri, 2005), and his insights will be helpful when we grapple with some of the challenges of our older elementary school students.

And now back to Russel

But for now, we return to Russel, the boy who loved the alphabet, whom we met as a preschooler. You will recall that Russel's beginning steps with language were not out of a textbook, because he didn't take to language in the same way as Dylan. Rather, he spent his preschool years playing with sounds in a style and a pentameter that was all his own.

As a kindergartener, Russel began to use language more and more, especially if the environment was gentle and conducive to his style. He was fortunate that his kindergarten was in the same University school as his preschool, so his gentle environment continued until he was seven.

When Russel was six and a half, his language reflected both his first love, thinking about the alphabet, and his second love, studying it in a predictable format. A dialogue could take place if his partner agreed to play his or her limited role "to a T":

R	**What letter comes after A?**
C	B
R	**What letter comes after B?**
C	C

His grammar and word order struggled to keep up, as in the following dialogue:

R	**What does A make a sound?**
C	"aa"
R	**What does B make a sound?**
C	"buh"

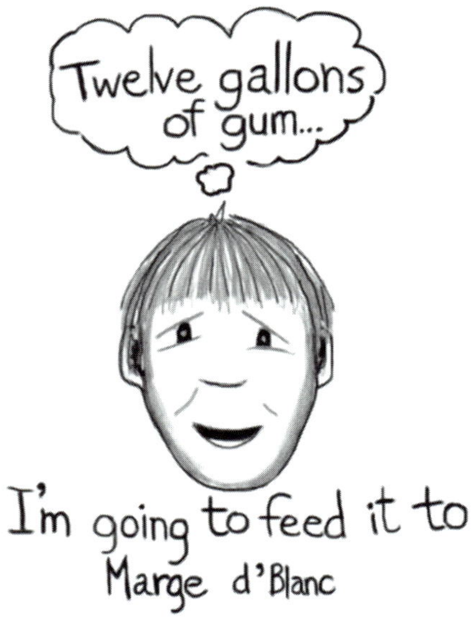

By the time Russel was seven and in first grade in public school, he had managed to integrate auditory input enough to use predictable words in his original, toneless songs. Using 'closed sets' like the alphabet and numbers, Russel created a continuous scat-like chant for up to 15 minutes at a time. For this, Russel used his tongue, throat, and nostrils, both inhaling and exhaling, to sing a rendition of the numbers 1-150. Clearly, Russel loved the unconventional creations of his stories and songs more than he enjoyed the conventional ways that people tended to approach communication. But in the company of those who loved and appreciated him, Russel communicated his enjoyment of song and entertainment with rewarding comments that bubbled up from inside. **"This is fun!"** he would announce.

Russel also communicated in other entertaining, albeit idiosyncratic, ways such as when he decided to feed his SLP friend **"twelve gallons of gum."** Using a nice mix of grammar, Russel accompanied his feeding frenzy with comments such as:

I'm gonna feed it to Marge d'Blanc.
We need more gum.
I think we need more gum.
Put the gum in Marge d'Blanc's mouth.
Do you wanna eat them up?

Moving on to candy, Russel continued:

I'm gonna feed Marge d'Blanc these coconuts.
All I want is my good old white mint.
Can I have my white mint?
I—that mint I love.
Can I have my white mint—yeah!

As this sequence of events illustrates, even the unconventional can be constructed with conventional grammar!

Russel's progress during elementary school continued in his slow and gentle way, and while a complete rendering would create a delightful story, the general message can be more simply conveyed. Suffice it to say that Russel made steady progress in grammar, in vocabulary, in story, in song, in joke-telling, in conversation, in social interaction, and in self-advocacy throughout his elementary school years. Russel wasn't quite finished developing a full grammar system then, but he added the higher reaches of NLA 6 in middle school. Once he could use all manner of embedded clauses in a flexible manner to convey all the contingencies of time and space, his grammar was finally declared complete.

It is not unique for our kids to have more than one language challenge, but developing a profile can take time.

All along the way, Russel spent concentrated time practicing and, in this way, learned to overcome the concomitant language challenge he faced: word finding, or more accurately, language retrieval. It is not unique for our kids to have more than one language challenge, of course, but developing an accurate profile of challenges can take time. Russel discovered for himself that he could work on grammar or vocabulary, but not both at the same time. He chose to practice grammar using a predictable set of vocabulary words, and vice versa. Following is a short segment of one such practice routine later in elementary school that illustrates how Russel used a few sentence patterns to practice retrieving the names of songs:

Push the "R"—That's Yankee Doodle.
Push the "S"—This is called She'll be Coming Round the Mountain.
Push the "B"—That's Pop Goes the Weasel.
Push the "Z"—This is 509; it's instrumental; it doesn't have any words to it.

The next segment shows Russel using limited vocabulary so he could practice the advanced conjunction he was working to perfect:

After the milk chocolate M+M's, we're gonna have some peanut M+M's.
After the peanut M+M's, we're gonna go.

Russel later put the last sentence into a dialogue:

R	**It looks like an E.**
C	It does look like an E.
R	**The M looks like an E.**
C	All those M's look like E's.
R	**It says M; tip it on its side and it looks like an E.**
C	It's quite cute looking like an E.
R	**After the M+M's, we're gonna go.**

Following are a few more vignettes, offered as illustrations of the individual styles of communication kids develop along with their grammar. Russel was always working on all aspects of language, with each nuance of grammar quickly applied to his poetry and prose. The first shows how Russel used the polite forms of grammar to protest his friend taking notes during our play time:

M is for Marge writing a note. Oh, you gotta stop, Marge!

The second is a dialogue that starts with Russel directing his friend to research something and ends by communicating his resignation again, very politely:

R	**What's that green thing down there?**
C	I can go look.
R	**I can't.**
C	That's OK; I'll take a look.
R	**What's that green thing?**
C	Is it lower down? I can't see it.
R	**Lower down. Pick it up and show it to me.**
C	I still can't see it.
R	**Should Marge come back up?**

Like Dylan, Russel experienced continuing challenges with sensory input, particularly auditory. Even his usual polite language shifted to a more pragmatic plea when things got rough:

C	I looked everywhere and I can't find any money for snacks.
R	**Stop being so—sick of it!**

And another instance:

R	**Oh, it won't work.**
C	It will work; we j—
R	**Stop the questions!**

In summary, Russel's story nicely illustrates the long-term potential of continued grammar development in our kids. Although we have long thought that grammar development would end at age six or seven, kids like Russel demonstrate that grammar delays are met with surprising windows of potential for more development. Russel's story is just one of many, but its uniqueness demonstrates how one size never fits all. More accurately, one size never really fits anyone. Russel's story is his own, just as your child's story is her own.

One size never really fits anyone.

The lessons learned from Russel have applications for all the children whose journeys into full grammar continue through the elementary years. Here are some of them.

First of all, the very principles we know are important to preschoolers are equally important to school-aged kids. Kids need natural, meaningful language environments to share with people who care about them. Kids need to feel safe, happy, and regulated to be free to communicate what is important to them. What makes one environment work for one child is not what makes another environment work for another child.

Secondly, communication still comes from the inside out. Even when we do everything we can to support a child maximally, kids make their own progress in their own way in their own time. Russel's story amply illustrates this principle. Hurrying things just causes the dyad of you and your child to split apart, and that doesn't serve anyone's purposes.

Even when we do everything we can to support a child, kids make their own progress in their own way in their own time.

Third, grammar is just a tool. What each of us does with this useful, flexible tool is what matters. Each of us has our own thoughts to convey and own style to create. Grammar is important, but grammar is as grammar does. Each of our children has a world to paint, in his or her own unique way.

Finally, using language is one way kids learn to support their own regulation, advocate for themselves, and help themselves stay safe. Russel had a myriad of ways to help make the auditory environment work for him. It takes a little experience and maturity for kids to get to this point, but starting in the elementary years, these skills start to develop. We will see them develop even farther in middle and high school, which is a good reminder that even when grammar development ends, pragmatic language continues to broaden and deepen all our lives.

Using language is one way kids support their own regulation, advocate for themselves, and help themselves stay safe.

We now turn to those children who did not begin the NLA process until their elementary school years. Besides Bevin, whom you know from earlier in the book, you will meet Joey and Kyle, who represent two very different profiles of elementary-aged children

Chapter 13
Starting the Process at the Elementary Age

Starting the NLA process once a child is older presents a different slant to the picture we have of Dylan, Russel, and their young cohorts. Preschoolers have plenty of time and freedom to play and learn about their world, and plenty of time for language to develop. By the time Dylan and Russel started elementary school, they were generating most of their own grammar, and this made their lives infinitely easier than it is for those echolalic kids who begin the process later.

The same language development process works for elementary-aged students.

The most important thing to know, however, is that the same language development process works for elementary-aged students. Depending on the age when they begin and how much they have already begun to mitigate on their own, children who start NLA at age five, six, or seven can make good progress that looks similar to that of preschoolers.

Please also know that even kids who start NLA when they are older than seven can make good progress too, depending on how much mitigating they have already accomplished. Eight-year-old Kal was such a child, and we will outline his process in this chapter. Older kids may not make it all the way to a complete grammar, but they can develop a useful one with which to share, communicate, and create in ways that were previously impossible. Nine-year-old Joey was a child like this, and we will turn to his story after Kal's, in order to show what another picture of progress looks like.

The biggest challenge for older kids is dealing with the large number of language gestalts in their brains, particularly when they have no method for breaking them down.

The chapter then returns to Bevin, ten years old when he began, in order to follow the development process over time. Besides the expected challenges of finding time during the busy day to work on language, the biggest challenge for older kids is dealing with the huge number of language gestalts in their brains, particularly when they have no method for breaking them down. When they were young, these kids were seen as simply echolalic, but now they seem intractably echolalic. Echolalia was a good sign, and it still is, but the longer kids remain echolalic without mitigating, the harder it is to take the leap into mitigation and beyond.

The longer kids remain echolalic without mitigating, the harder it is to take the leap into mitigation and beyond.

So, the first rule of starting in elementary school is simply this: start. Start now! Kids still have a chance, and until we start with them, we will never know how far they can go. Sadly, one hurdle to starting is often that the system seems to have given up on our elementary-aged kids developing natural language. Going on the mistaken notion that their critical learning period for grammar has passed, goals for these kids have become simply functional. Without explicitly saying so, the language goals for older kids suggest we have given up on their ability to develop flexible linguistic systems. Instead, the goal statements focus on teaching kids to use functional phrases and sentences or to access them with AAC.

Let's look at a few scenarios that illustrate this point. In my own twenty years as a public school SLP, I have read countless IEP goal statements like this: Johnny will state his wants and needs in 6/10 opportunities by saying, "I want x, please," when given three options. This IEP might go on to state several other practical language skills that, beyond a doubt, would help Johnny in the classroom, but fail to recognize Johnny's potential to develop a useful linguistic system.

The next year in Johnny's life, a particular goal might have become accomplished at a particular criteria, so the new criteria of success might be 8/10 opportunities instead of 6. Do we ever stop to think about why such goals take so long to generalize? Do folks have the background to recognize that a sentence such as, "I want chips, please" is a gestalt, quickly learned when a child asks for and receives chips? But, if chips are not available, or if the child really wants water, the gestalt isn't spot-on, and the child has no developmental template for mitigating it and saying, "I want water, please." This second request is viewed as "generalizing," and we come away from the experience thinking that the child cannot.

If a child learns "I want chips, please," as a gestalt, he has no developmental template for mitigation and flexible use.

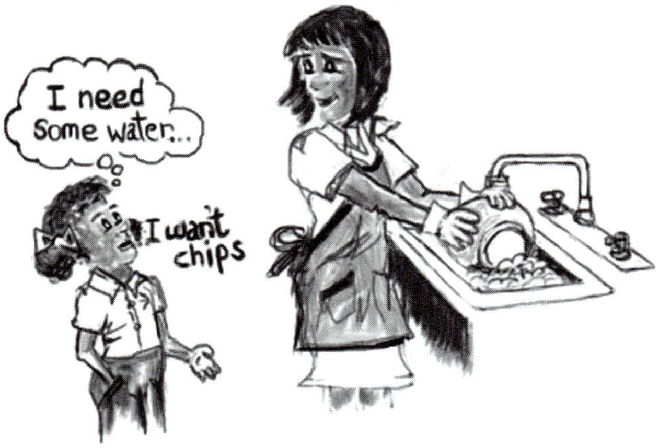

So, a goal statement the next year might be: Johnny will produce the following requests when given a choice of chips, water, and paint: "I want chips, please; I want water, please; and I want paint, please" in 5/10 opportunities when one of them is available.

In hypothetical Johnny's life then, such language learning may well continue for his entire elementary school career, and by fourth or fifth grades, well-meaning folks might decide that his now-well-ingrained "I want ..." statement sounds too demanding, and that he should be taught, "Can I have...?" instead. So, his next set of IEP goals say, "Johnny will request one of five items using the question, "Can I have x, please?" in 7–10 opportunities. Our good intentions made Johnny sound more polite, but have effectively kept him at NLA 1, and his linguistic development was stalled.

The first rule of starting NLA in the elementary grades is: start now! You can then watch your child get unstuck.

This is why the first rule of starting NLA in elementary school is this: start. Start now. Start with a real language development system, and get Johnny unstuck!

And this is what we did with Kal and Joey. Kal sounded generative but odd. His utterances had a script-like redundancy to them that was hard to figure out until we applied NLA to it to see where he was operating. Joey, on the other hand, did not sound generative at all, and he wasn't. He had some firmly-entrenched NLA 1 and 2 utterances, but he was eager to communicate. This is how we began with each boy.

Kal's story

Kal's family wanted our opinion on their boy's language. At eight years old, Kal talked fairly well and essentially non-stop, but there was something odd that no one could quite put their finger on. A few minutes of one of Kal's first language samples is included here. It is divided into segments so we can comment along the way, but in real life, it was continuous. The first segment begins with Kal stuck in an inner tube and seemingly suggesting moving it to a different place even though he was inside:

K	**I'm stuck.**
C	Oh no.
K	**Hey, wanna move over the tube?**
K	**We'll go bring the tube up here.**
C	It's pretty big, but we can do it together.
K	**I think we shouldn't.**
C	Why?
K	**I dunno!**
C	Because now you are sleeping in the tube.

All these comments went by so quickly that they were difficult to analyze. But once transcribed, some of the loopholes in Kal's grammar become more apparent. Note that Kal seemed to be formulating his idea the way he wanted, but then he seemingly changed his mind and could not explain why.

Kal quickly continued with an invitation to go to a movie, commented on some seemingly conflicting ideas about having a cell phone, and then seemed to uninvite himself from the movie. Again, he appeared to be changing his mind often.

K	**How about we go to a movie me, princess Kar—princess Kal, but I have a pink pull-up.**
C	You're funny!
K	**How about The Big Moose who ate New York?**
C	Let's go see it with Princess Kal?
K	**How about Princess Polly?**

C	Princess Polly, Princess Kal, we can all go. Can Chloe come?
K	**Uh huh.**
C	Sounds like a good time to me.
K	**How about we go to Newman's Island?**
C	Ok.
K	**Mmm-hmm.**
K	**I don't leave a message on my cellphone.**
K	**But I don't need a cellphone.**
C	Nah—
K	**If I went to the mall and got a cellphone, I'd keep it.**
C	Yeah?
K	**Yeah, I'd call you that we can go to Newman's Island.**
C	That's a good reason for a phone—
K	**I can't go to the movies with you.**
K	**If I finish cleaning my house, soon as I get rid of the nasty old Perky.**
C	You have a lot to do first before we can go?
K	**Yeah.**
C	You gotta clean before we can go.
K	**Yeah, but I don't, we don't have time. Sorry.**
C	Yep this weekend is busy for both of us.
K	**I'm going to Three Wolves Lodge.**

Once we were able to look closely at Kal's use of language, we could identify places where it was just as stuck as Kal was in the inner tube. He had lots of generative grammar, to be sure, but rarely constructed from scratch. Rather than constructing from isolated single words (NLA 3), Kal had numerous remnant mitigated phrases (NLA 2), which limited the flexibility of his final constructions. Following are a few examples of how Kal's sentences could be analyzed:

Hey, wanna move over the tube?
We'll go bring the tube up here.
I can't go to the movies with you.

While these undivided units seem rather benign, consider next how much more flexibly Kal constructed sentences when they were completely from scratch. The number was limited, but they suggested what Kal could do once he'd spent some more time getting unstuck from his NLA 2 phrases:

It's a scary movie.
Hey, I found a drumstick.
Yeah, I like it.
I found Shrek.
That's a party hat!
And they hit.

The constructions above used simple grammar and worked well for Kal. Using higher level grammar was troublesome to him, however, and tended to paint him into corners he couldn't get out of. A few examples:

> **I'm so tired because I just sleep good.**
> **Because I couldn't have a good night's sleep.**
> **How 'bout we go to a movie, me Prices Kar—Princess Kal, but I have a pink pull-up.**
> **What if you ate an Oreo with toothpaste on it—and I have then been to the principal's office.**
> **If I went to the mall and got a cell phone, I'd keep it.**
> **Yeah, I'd call you that we can go to Newman's Island.**

Kal's therapy plan

We began by helping Kal get himself unstuck. It seemed likely that Kal had simply moved into grammar before he'd finished Stages 2 and 3, and the results were often perplexing to everyone. Kal was so verbal that the process had probably just moved too quickly. To begin, we targeted pronouns + simple verb, and let Kal hear sets of them in the course of the active play he loved. Here's an example of the dialogue:

C	Hey, let's get up on top.
K	**I can't!**
C	I'll help you get up there.
K	**I gotta fly off there so the monsters come—take that!**
C	I wanna help you! I can reach you from here.
K	**Aaaaa! Take that.**
C	I'm reaching so hard! Take my hand.
K	**Noooo—you can't catch me.**
C	I don't wanna catch you; I wanna save you.
K	**Oh, thanks, Jessi.**
C	You're welcome. Hey, let's jump!
K	**Nooo—never—I'm landing under the ocean.**
C	I'm coming in with you.
K	**Nooo—don't jump on me.**
C	I'm not; I'm very careful; See me coming?
K	**Oh, ok. Hey, watch out!**
C	What's wrong? Are you stuck?
K	**I'm not stuck; I'm just drowning.**
C	Don't worry; I got a branch for you. Here, reach!
K	**I can't reach; It's supposed to be short.**
C	I got a longer one: here! Hold it really tight.

The clinician had a fun but mentally-challenging job to do: She had to keep beginning grammar in her mind, and rather than teach it per se, she had to put it into similar sentences for Kal to discover and mitigate on his own. Sometimes

Jessi, his clinician, presented things in more logical groups, like the following:

> (1) I see it! It's tall; it's blue; it's got wings; and it's coming to get us.
> (2) She got me; She's coming to get you; She's my favorite monster.

It all made sense to Kal, and he started to get unstuck.

Kal's progress after four months

Kal made rapid progress, as reported after four months of therapy. His Progress Report is quoted verbatim in the next seven paragraphs, and the rest of this section details how Kal and Jessi structured each of their hour sessions together:

> When Kal starts each session, he typically relies on combining his longer Stage 2 utterances into pragmatically relevant sentences to initiate his favorite games with the clinician. For example, Kal will introduce his idea to play 'Rapids' by accessing his Stage 2 phrases such as **"Let's see if Periwinkle and Magenta Drew can go down the rapids,"** or **"Maybe the dragon can go down the rapids,"** or **"Should we play Alligator?"**
>
> Usually, Kal uses a wide variety of Stage 2 phrases for the first 15 minutes of a session before he begins to modify his longer utterances. During this 'warm-up period,' the clinician models further mitigations of Kal's Stage 2 phrases, as well as ... recombinations of the mitigated utterances. Kal is very astute at integrating these mitigated phrases into the relevant context while the clinician and Kal are engaged in play. For example, during a game of "Rapids," Kal and the clinician maintained a scenario for approximately 5 minutes:
>
> | | |
> |---|---|
> | **K** | **Magenta, grab the trees and climb up.** |
> | C | Grab it! |
> | **K** | **Grab it the trees!** |
> | **K** | **Magenta, grab the trees! Grab!** |
> | C | Climb high! High trees! |
> | **K** | **Climb! Climb and grab the high trees!** |
> | C | Climb higher! Higher! |
> | **K** | **Grab! Higher! Higher!** |
> | **K** | **I climb! Grab the trees! I can't grab! Help! Help! Do something!** |
>
> During this example, Kal successfully took feedback from the clinician to break down some of his Stage 2 phrases and create new combinations. For instance, Kal was able to isolate 'climb' from his initial Stage 2 phrase "climb up" and use it in different combinations such as **"climb and grab ..."** and **"I climb,"** as

"I'm afraid I'm stuck."

"I'm afraid of I'm stuck."

"I'm stuck."

well as **"Climb!"** in isolation.

As the session progressed, Kal becomes more fluent in further mitigating his Stage 2 phrases and using each part in relevant contexts (e.g., in a game of 'Rapids') as well as carrying mitigations over to other, similar games (e.g., playing "Monster"). For example, on another day Kal came into the clinic using many longer Stage 2 sentences:

I can't quite climb.
I'm afraid I'm stuck.
I might get stuck.

However, after about 15 minutes of engaging in a shared activity, Kal began to mitigate his Stage 2 phrases:

I'm afraid of I'm stuck.
You're scared in the movie.

By the end of the hour, Kal was able to further mitigate his Stage 2 utterances into two-part phrases, which demonstrated the productive use of "I'm ..." in a nice variety of short sentences that show how Kal is successfully mastering Stage 2, allowing him to move into Stage 3 word-isolation and Stage 4 grammatical development:

I'm stuck.
I'm scared.
I'm climbing.

Overall, Kal has made significant progress in his grammatical development, with each successive session requiring a shorter "warm-up period" before Kal begins to mitigate his own Stage 2 phrases, recombine his shorter mitigations into different sentences, and increase his use of single words combinations in relevant contexts (Stages 3 and 4). With the help of the clinician's continued consistent modeling, as well as that of Kal's family and school personnel, it is anticipated that Kal will continue making significant gains in developing his generative grammar skills through further mitigation of Stage 2 phrases, isolating more Stage 3 single words, and using these words in Stage 3 combinations and Stage 4 grammatical sentences.

Kal after eight months

Indeed, after four more months, Kal had not only moved successfully through NLA 2 and 3 and solidly into beginning grammar, he was able to use his new-found skills to engage in pretend play and create imaginative stories. Included here are two excerpted paragraphs from his Progress Report after another four months had gone by:

> Kal has expanded his play games, such as 'Jessi eating monster' and 'crocodile,' to include action figures as additional characters, role-playing characters' voices, and describing the action of the play. As Kal becomes more fluent with mitigating language gestalts, his stories are becoming richer in detail and variety. Kal is able to tell what is happening in real-time and is also able to talk about an event that is going to happen as well as retell an event that has already occurred. Kal demonstrated this when he narrated what was going to happen, what happened during the story, and then retold the event later back in the play rooms:
>
> (heading down the hall to the elevator, on the way to the 'salmon run')
>
> **K** **Let's go to the salmon run.**
> **K** **We just have to go up to the third** (floor).
> **K** **We have to get to the highest level.**
> C How many salmon are at the salmon run?
> **K** **Two—two salmon hahaha.**
>
> (K and C sat in hallway waiting for it to start)
>
> **K** **I can't wait to see the salmon run!**
> **K** **The glacier passed the bathroom, and the rhino is in the salmon run.**
> **K** **The rhino won.**
> **K** **The salmon run's over. Let's get on our hot chocolate.**
>
> (back in the play room)
>
> **K** **We watched the salmon run.**
> **K** **The rhino won and the glacier passed away to the first floor.**
>
> This sequence of events illustrates Kyle's use of space as a support to creating a timeline for his story. Kyle was able to talk about going to the salmon run as he and the clinician headed towards the elevator; Kyle was able to narrate the action sequence of the salmon run as we sat in the hallway watching it happen; finally, when the clinician and Kyle were back in the play rooms, Kyle was able to talk about what we had just observed. By moving through different spaces, Kyle was able to build a framework to flow through his story in a logical, cohesive sequence.

During the next half year, Kal was able to develop grammar in earnest. No longer hampered by the gestalts and mitigated phrases of a year ago, Kal was able to try out the grammar he had found so confounding in his first language sample. The following four paragraphs are taken from his Progress Report approximately a year into therapy:

When the clinician arrived at Kal's house, he was finishing the final scenes of the movie *Jurassic Park: The Lost World.* Kal informed Jessi that, **"When the movie's over, I'm gonna ask what was your favorite part."** After the movie, Kal discovered what Jessi's favorite parts of the movie were, but also offered what his own highlight of the movie was:

I liked the part where the man was running away from the baby dinosaurs and he slipped in the puddle and got splashed and he got bit 4 times.

The above example is wonderful for illustrating Kal's increasing narrative abilities using his own generative grammar to retell a scene from a movie. Kal was able to offer a short narrative such as the above example for not just one, but at least three different scenes from the movie.

After the movie, there was a preview for a Jurassic Park themed amusement park ride at Universal Studios. Kal, who is very interested in theme parks of many types, had the following conversation with Jessi:

"Hey, what is scary about—um—Terminator 2-3D?"

K	**This Lost World is trying to be more scary than 90 Jurassic Parks.**
C	The Lost World is much scarier than Jurassic Park! Like 90 times as scary!
K	**How would we have Universal Studios Jurassic Park, The Ride in our backyard?**
K	(asking another question regarding building in the backyard)
K	**Wish we could build in our backyard!**
C	Wow, Kal! That would be so cool to have that ride in your backyard!
K	**It would be warmer and warmer, heavy.**
C	You are right, it will have to be warmer outside and the ride and dinosaurs would be very heavy!
K	**How are we gonna find a Jurassic Park, the Ride in our backyard?**
C	I don't know where to find dinosaurs.
K	**Hey, what is scary about—um—Terminator 2–3D?**
C	That they look like robots?

K	**Let's play Terminator 2–3D.**
C	We could build robots that look like dinosaurs!
K	**Jurassic Park, the Ride has to be scary.**
C	Right, as scary as The Lost World. It looked scary on the movie.
K	**Jessi, many kids have been to Jurassic Park, the Ride, Universal Studios.**
C	That's right. It wasn't too scary for some kids, but we could make the ride less scary for all kids.
K	**Let's play the game.** (referring to an arcade-style game Kal turned on in his basement)
K	**We should make an arcade down here.**

In this sample, Kal maintained nice cohesion with his topic and his partner's input. It did not represent perfection, but showed how well Kal had made his new language skills his own. Four months after this sample, Kal was ready to be dismissed from therapy. He had moved on from narration to social interaction with his siblings, self-advocacy at school, and explaining new games to all his playmates. His family was able to maintain language work at home with the built-in social network his siblings provided. Kal was not only unstuck but leading the way with his linguistic flexibility.

We now turn to Joey's story, as it represents a very different picture from Kal's. That Joey was older was one factor, but Joey had done little mitigating on his own, and so presented a linguistic picture of a NLA 1 language user with a sprinkling of the other levels here and there.

Joey's story

We first met Joey when he was nine years old, after he had recently moved to Madison. An SLP report from a year earlier noted that Joey could identify vocabulary words such as 'jungle,' 'happy,' and 'melting,' could label nouns such as 'sofa,' 'penguin,' and 'tiger,' and that his most challenged area was expressive communication, although he was seen as "an intentional communicator" who combined "gaze and gestures to indicate intent." Joey was observed to combine 3–4 words to request ("I want xx") but was seen as primarily using "perseverative delayed echolalia," for example saying, **"Welcome to my world"** 15 times in two minutes.

Joey's first session was at home, where his spontaneous language was recorded and later transcribed. Joey's speech was difficult to understand: rapid, under-articulated, and poorly timed with his body and his communication partners. It took us a while to understand him well enough to inventory his language and determine his development levels, but his assessment report noted many useful gestalts, some mitigations, and a few isolated single words. Following are a few examples of Joey's most useful language at NLA 1 and 2:

NLA 1	**Where am I going?** **You must be kidding.** **Come on!** **Just disgusting!** **Be careful.** **Very fascinating, I'd say.**
NLA 2	**Can you?** **Where's Bianca?** **It's Bianca.** **It's yellow.** **Hey, comin' on!** **Gotta get.** **Gotta go.** **Gets out.** **We got.** **What's you got?**

Our report noted that while Joey had successfully negotiated the steps to NLA 2 mitigation and even NLA 3 single words, the resulting language had "limited breadth of application and what seems like 'tentative' confidence." Indeed, Joey was the most animated when he could deliver heart-felt but less-flexible lines like these:

One night, a long time ago—stars shining on ice.
I'm lost at sea without a friend—who will rescue me?

We were thrilled that Joey had successfully negotiated some mitigation on his own, but realized those shorter phrases and sentences seemed truncated to him, and less communicative. Our second job was to help Joey understand what he had accomplished through mitigation. We wanted him to know that he would be able to communicate through his mix of short phrases, and that we would understand the emotion beneath them, even though they didn't sound like movie language. Our efforts were rewarded with dialogues such as the following, in which Joey played with phraseology that helped him move into NLA 2 with confidence:

C	It's a little hard. (referring to climbing a steep slide)
J	**You're telling truth.**
C	You're telling truth!
J	**You got truth.**
C	You got truth!
J	**You got truth.**
C	I like those challenges—a little hard but not too hard.
J	**You—telling truth!**
C	It's the truth. We're telling the truth.

In another linguistically-similar exchange, Joey played out his role in *The Rescuers* with his clinician friend, "Bianca," as a second clinician "narrated" with him. We did this so Joey could see that dramatic scenes could be acted with simple language:

J	**Bianca!**
C	What?
J	**Where's Bianca?**
C	Oh, where's Bianca—you—you—
J	**It's Bianca; it's Bianca!**
C	Yes, it is.
J	**It's Bianca!**
C2	Here I am!

Having communication partners who were attentive to movie language was something new to Joey, but as the first months went on, Joey became more comfortable with this and relished purposeful glosses of his language and opportunties for multi-part conversations. In turn, his mitigation increased, and after three months, Joey produced more useful NLA 2 combinations and NLA 3 isolated words such as the following:

"Want a Fozzie."

Want a Fozzie.
Want a Kermit.
I get stuck.
Stop pulling.
They're scare.
Get the heavy.
Climbing.
Heavy.
Go.
Ouch.
Up.
Can.
Water.
Cows.
Lie down.
Good. Go get.
Get out, out.
Gets out.

Sprinkled in with these short language chunks, Joey always used beautiful gestalts as well, and these remained the comments that seemed to resonate the best with him. They ranged the gamut of emotion, and included comments such as:

What a nightmare.
Find your way home.
This is the way home.

Joey after six months

Joey made gradual steady progress, the most significant being that he was satisfied with his simpler language. He knew that his play partners weren't fooled by its mundane quality, and he still believed that his internal world was one of starry nights and brave rescues by friends. Joey talked as he moved in the clinic space, and this seemed to anchor his new language to his body. Following are a few of his flexible utterances, primarily NLA 2. Joey had not separated "I" from a handful of verbs he commonly said with "I," nor had he isolated the other pronouns. Even though Joey could use some verbs in more than one way, they did not appear completely independent of their original contexts. In the following, the slash marks signify Joey's mix and match of phraseology:

"See—I wanna see."

See—I wanna/see.
Want/the bear.
Did you/got it?
Go get/Fozzy.
He's/lost.
He's/getting away.
Enjoy—let's/enjoy.
Let's/go.
Just same—that's/just same.
It's/locked.
It's/easy.
It's/heavy.
It's/rusty.

Joey after nine months

After nine months, Joey was relishing the regular conversational exchanges with his play partners and grew more confident in using his semi-flexible language along with his body moving in space. Joey had not isolated many pronouns yet, so these comments were usually semi-original:

It's about this.
It's about China.
It's gone.

Joey was beginning to isolate "I" and "my," however, and these helped him communicate more specifically:

I fight Big Bird.
Help my neck.

More often, however, Joey used pronouns within short phrases, and his flexibility was tied to them. Following is a wonderful set of comments Joey made while listening to the story, "The Mixed up Chameleon." Joey communicated beautifully about himself, in spite of the limited flexibility of NLA 2:

I wish I could like a fox.
Smart like a fox.
I wish to shell like a turtle.

J	**I wish I can be.**
C	I wish I can be—happy.
C	I wish I can be—
J	**I wish I can be myself.**

Joey after a year

During the next three months, Joey became more facile at using his newly-isolated pronoun, "I," as in the following sentences:

"I silly."

I do that.
I not through yet.
I not doing it.
I silly.

Other "I" sentences were obviously single units of language, however, NLA 1 or 2:

I can't.
I love doing that.
I can explain.
I am a dog—you're a wolf.
I'll be blue—you be yellow.
I know where we're going.
Only I could.

With grammar now emerging, however, it became less important which was which:

J	**Come on!**
C	I'm coming!
J	**I like it!**
C	Me too!
J	**Do you—**
C	Do you like it?
J	**I do!**

As the above utterances clearly show, Joey was coming into himself as a communicator, able to express himself from his own perspective, and establish conversational exchanges through the use of "I" to refer to himself. Joey's intonation had become more natural-sounding as well; his rate had slowed, his timing matched his body and his partner, and his speech clarity had improved markedly. One of Joey's themes throughout the year had been his wistful desire to become a "real boy," à la Pinocchio. He now knew he was one, expressed pride in himself, and, in three months, had not returned to the Pinocchio reference to reexamine the question.

Joey after a year and a half

Joey spent another half year with us before moving back to his home state. During that time, he shared life with his clinical friends, and although he continued to isolate more words at NLA 3 and develop beginning grammar at NLA 4, the main emphasis of our time together was exploring life themes of Joey's real interest.

*"I tired.
I'm very happy."*

As the day of Joey's move came closer, he talked more and more about how much Bianca and her crew had meant to him and how much he would miss us. On one of these days, Joey cheerfully trudged up to our upper loft, laughing and declaring these things:

> **Happy Wednesday!**
> **I tired.**
> **I'm very happy.**
> **Happy as can be.**
> **Happy day, happy day.**

After a story about a "happy wind," however, Joey said his good-byes, announcing, **"I must be going."** Joey had a way to juxtaposing emotions with his words, as in the following:

> **It's not fair—it's just goodbye.**
> **But hurray!**
>
> **Everything changed. It was delighted.**
>
> **Hey, look out Percy! That's no time for teasing.**
> **And he got stuck. Something broke.**
> **Do you know what it is? Something borrowed,**
> **something blue. You'll find out.**
> **Stuck. Henry began crying and—stuck.**
>
> **Either way, it sure is a shame. Tally ho!**
> **I've done it; well done.**

We were unable to watch Joey continue his journey after this, but we could say with great pride, "Well done!" Joey was such a strong communicator that his fledgling grammar was starting to add the flexibility his communication had lacked. We could even add, "Tally ho!"

It is our intention in this book to follow an older student's story over time, however, so we now return to Bevin, whose journey takes us many places and teaches us as it illustrates. The first lesson from Bevin's story is how challenging mitigation is for a ten-year-old and how little credit you receive for all that hard work.

Bevin's story, continued: "Spike is talking!"

It takes enormous effort to learn Zeus's entire speech to Hercules well enough to just say the part about the "heart of a hero." But our kids do this. What was once just a blur of intonation punctuated by a word or two we could understand, later sounds like a real sentence, once the extraneous noise has been eliminated.

This is the essence of mitigation—breaking down the entire speech so you can just say the part that matters, the part that resonates to you: "Diamond in the rough!"

Bevin had mitigated such gems when he was eleven and spent many months at NLA 2. When we left his story back in Chapter 2, Bevin had been working at NLA 3 for a couple of months: isolating and re-combining single words. And now, as we pick up his story six months later, he continued to work at NLA 3 but had begun experimenting with beginning grammar. As a twelve-year-old, it was hard work. But he'd discovered a method that worked for him: he'd go back to "the source," usually well-known and well-loved videos, and extract particular vocabulary and concepts. Other times, he'd practice two- to three-word combinations, often in matching sets.

Bevin found some success with simple grammar. Scoring his language became a dilemma, then, because when the grammar was correct, it was difficult to determine if the utterance was a Stage 4 grammatical construction or a Stage 1 gestalt. But what a nice dilemma! When the grammar was wrong, however, these valiant attempts were clearly Stage 4. During this time, it was impressive that Bevin was quite open to the grammatical models of the clinician, but only if they matched his intention and were useful to his purpose.

The following is a complete transcript, with each utterance marked as NLA 1, 2, 3, or 4, as best determined from the context. The extreme detail of this transcript, and others like it in the rest of this book, is included because the coding was part of a teaching project designed to share the NLA assessment protocol with other SLPs. Readers simply interested in the flow of Bevin's progress from transcript to transcript are urged to ignore the numbering of utterances and to read these snippets of language formulation for the joys they are. Those who wish to know what each level signifies as they read along could pay special attention to the beginning grammatical utterances and notice how well they fit within the running dialogue. Bevin's utterances are not labeled 'B' unless there are two speakers.

The sample began as we were watching a video narrated by Jiminy Cricket, who says, "Let your conscience be your guide."

"Let your conscience be your guide."

1	**B**	**What are you doing?** [1 gestalt]
	M	[commenting to Megan, another clinician, about how B was sad because Tori was not here]
2	**B**	**She's going to Racine.** [4 grammar]
3		**What is Megan doing?** [2 mitigation]
4		**And always let your conscience be your guide.** [1 gestalt]
5		**Let your conscience be your guide.** [2]
6		**What are you looking?** [2]
7		**What are you doing?** [1]
8		**Hey!** [3]
9		**That's it—** [2]
10		**Come on now—** [2]
11		**Let's sing it!** [2]
12		**Whoa!** [3]
13		**I say—** [2]
14		**Laam pu.** [unknown]
15		**What happened?** [1]
16		**I'm gonna look.** [2]
17		**Here the rules are.** [2]

We then began commenting on several referents in front of us as well as the movie:

18		**Pinocchio.** [3, watching Guseppi call the cat]
19		**Those are flowers.** [2, pulling them out of the Pooh box]
20		**Pluto—so this has been a lot.** [2]
21		**Bad kitty.** [3]
22		**Bad day.** [2]
23		**Pluto's back.** [4]
	M	Let your conscience be your guide. (watching Pluto struggle between the angel dog and the devil dog)
24	**B**	**What?** [3]
	M	Let your conscience be your guide, not the devil.
25	**B**	**Not the devil.** [2]
	V	Now save him! (the words on the video)
	M	Listen to Jiminy Cricket.
26	**B**	**Now, save Jiminy Cricket.** [4]

	M	Good boy, Pinocchio.
27	**B**	**Someday, you'll be a real boy.** [2]
	M	You're a real boy, Pluto.
28		**Plihmbu.** (unknown)

"Someday, you'll be a real boy."

In the following, Bevin continued to comment on the videos, returned to the theme, then finished with further commentary on the videos:

29		**The Indians are coming**. [4, The children in the old Mickey cartoon were dressed like Indians]
30		**Pinocchio! Pinocchio!** [1] (B whistled a song once and then hummed it again in Donald's high-pitched voice)
31		**x x x guys x x x.** [2]
32-34		[1, long series of unintelligible self-talk]
35		**Huh? Huh?** [1]
36		**Here I am.** [1]
37		**That's it—** [2]
38		**Let's sing.** [4]
39		**And always let your conscience be your guide.** [1]
	M	[recounting the above]
40		**Ready.** [3]
41		**Let the fun begin.** [2]
42-45		[1, series of gestalts]
46		**Hey, that tickles.** [1, commenting on the video]
47		**But he should not be here when your mother's out.** [1]
48		**Stop, I say.** [1]
49		**x x x** [1]
50		**x x x** [1]

While this language sample is still somewhat difficult to understand, it represents a real landmark compared to the blur of vocalization a year and a half earlier. First of all, Bevin was intelligible, which reflected the fact that he was intentionally attempting to communicate and expecting to be heard and understood. The transcript above represents a total of 50 distinct utterances, only 11 of which were unintelligible with no evidence of intentionality.

Further analysis of the 39 intentional utterances included these totals: eleven were gestalts (22% of the total of 50); seventeen were mitigations (34%); six were single words or combinations (12%); and five were grammatical constructions (10%). Together, they represented a conversation about a topic of extreme interest to Bevin. That Bevin could achieve a conversation at all, given his late start in language development, was a real tribute to his tenacity. And within the context of an ongoing relationship where both partners shared a set of referents, the conversation had a measure of coherence such that Bevin maintained a nice mix of communicative utterances for the duration of the half hour.

Clearly, Bevin was a communicator and was making a concerted move towards developing generative grammar. Bevin's last year of elementary school year continued, and he continued to progress.

Eight months later

Bevin's therapy was described in the following excerpts from his progress notes at the time:

"Given his age, Bevin's progress has been excellent! He was so surprised to be taken seriously at first that this stunned him. After a few sessions … Bevin realized that the clinician would help him start to mitigate, since even he did not really want to say all those words he had to say to get to the part he wanted! Sessions … were always child-centered so the clinician could hear Bevin's gestalts and find out what he wanted to talk about. We worked together, back and forth, Bevin starting with a whole line, paragraph, or scene, and me helping him mitigate it or pare it down to what he wanted … When Bevin does not have another way to say something, he goes back to a selection in his internal video library and says it out loud. If someone is there to help him mitigate out the part he wants, he no longer says the original gestalt … if I say nothing, Bevin has no way to find the part he wants, and he will continue to say the entire gestalt."

Scribing what a child says lets him know you're listening but trying not to interrupt.

It also bears mentioning the value of scribing, or silently writing down what a child says, when taking vocal turns seems inappropriate. There were many times I felt that my vocal turn would interrupt the flow of what Bevin was composing, but I still wanted him to know I was listening. Scribing was the answer. I kept track of his train of thought; he knew I got it; and it was there to be played back when the time was right.

The school year came to an end, and Bevin had made striking gains in the eight months that had gone by. Bevin was 12 years, 8 months old at the time, and while he was older than his classmates, he had just left elementary school behind him. The following sample took place as Bevin arrived for a family sleep-over. The clinician had asked his family to drive around the block before coming up so we could have a first conversation together. After asking about this request, Bevin began talking about having worked all year long and being ready for summer, but he was wondering what the "map" says to do next! As the sample continued, Bevin moved into a celebratory mood and looked forward to the summer. While Bevin's language was not completely "transparent," its meaning could be deciphered if one knew the context and could read between the lines.

1		**What's the matter?** [1, asking why C made his family drive around the block before joining us, 1]
	M	(responds)
2	**B**	**Work year long.** [2]
	M	You worked all year long.
3		**What does the map say to do and?** [2]
4		**x x last time.** [2]
5		**x x come on, you know.** [2]
	M	We have things to discuss all summer long.
6	**B**	**In summer.** [3]
	M	Uh-huh.
7	**B**	**In summer, it be nice.** [4]
	Video:	X marks the spot. (referring to a Treasure Chest)
	M	X marks the spot.
8	**B**	**X marks the spot.** [1]
		(video: secret treasures)
9		**Pull.** [3]
		(video: singing a rainbow song)
10		**We've made a rainbow, we've made a rainbow, and it's a really beautiful one.** [1, a Barney song]
11		**Wow, it's a beautiful rainbow.** [2 + 4]
12		**Oh, come on, kids.** [1]
13		**I will miss xxx.** [2]
14		**Come on, everybody.** [1]
15		**Yee haw!** [galloping to the side, 1]

The action then moved to Bevin's plans for the summer and the bag of dinosaurs he needed to fulfill his ideas. As Bevin's communication moved in and out of the pragmatic, likewise his language became more or less "colorful" and more or less "transparent":

16		**Next Tuesday.** [3]
17		**The lifetime Barney video.** [2]
18		**You just gotta believe.** [2]
19	**B**	**Big board—** [3]
20	**B**	**Bag dinosaurs.** [3]
	M	I'm trying to find the dinosaurs.
21	**B**	**I'll show you.** [2, going and getting a bag]
22	**B**	**Come on.** [2]
23	**B**	**Follow me.** [2]

"And she said, 'Enjoy years.'"

24	**B**	**I need bag.** [4]
25	**B**	**Let me see.** [2] (into the office to ask for videos)
26		**Bring it home.** [2]
27		**I'll show you.** [2]
28		**Tuesday—pack it up, ready to go.** [2, finds Aug. 28 on a calendar]
29		**And she said, 'Enjoy years.'** [4]
30		**Thank you.** [1]
31		**It taste of paradise—a little big taste—taste of paradise.** [4, re: Sierra Mist]
32		**Next Tuesday: CD, DVD Dino Valley** [3]
33	**B**	**Marge's—noft you and get buy Jurassic.** [4]
34	**B**	**I believe—** [2]
35	**B**	**Where are you presents?** [2]
	M	[laughing]
36	**B**	**Be nice.** [2]
37		**And four seasons.** [3]
38		**And numbers.** [3]
39		**And ten, six, and ten.** [3]
40		**And season two in five, six, four, five.** [3]

A shift then occurred because of a topic the clinician introduced, but Bevin reasserted his original theme of the coming of summer.

"Hakuna Ma-Christmas."

	M	I lost my can.
41	**B**	**What happened?** [2]
	M	I don't know!
42	**B**	**What happened to it?** [2]
43		**Hakuna Matata; that means no worries; I just can't wait to be king.** [1 + 1]
44		**Hakuna Ma-Christmas.** [2]
45		**Can you feel the love.** [1, singing]
46		**It's in the world of other world.** [2]

In the following, "Bevin's space" referred to the clinic playroom, where Bevin had decided to have regular sleepovers. The conversation then moved to logistical questions about toys and the toy room.

47		**Only on Sunday, on Friday, in Bevin's space.** [3]
48		**I'll go to Bevin's space.** [4, to the tune of Hakuna Matata]
49		**And I'll sleep.** [4]
50	**B**	**On the weekend—I will go to Bevin's space.** [4]
	M	Wanna keep—
51	**B**	**Keep 'em here, wait till Mom comes.** [4]
	M	OK.
52	**B**	**Where's Mom?** [2]
	M	Work.
53	**B**	**No.** [3]
	M	Where's—?
54	**B**	**In the toy room.** [2]
	M	Ok—
55	**B**	**In a basket.** [2]
		(playing with dinosaurs)
56		**Here key.** [3]
57		**Oh, come again soon.** [2]
58		**Happy xxx.** [3]
59		**No!** [3]
60		**Yeah!** [3]
61		**No!** [3]
62		**Yeah!** [3]
		(seeming to mitigate the dialogue)
63		**You stay—again soon.** [2]

This final language sample of elementary school was fitting. The topics were celebrating, planning, and friendship. Besides this half-hour sample being 100% intelligible and communicative, many of the utterances were part of dialogues. Of the 63 total utterances, ten were gestalts (16%); 22 were mitigations (35%); 18 were isolated or combined single words (28%); and 13 were grammatical (21%).

Comparing these totals to those 8 months earlier, the biggest difference was in the complete absence of unintelligible utterances. The percentage of gestalts had dropped from 22% to 16%, and the percentage of mitigations remained essentially the same. The percentage of single word combinations went from 12% to 28%, however, and the percentage of grammatical utterances went from 10% to 21%. Even when gestalts were used, they were clear and communicative. Mitigations, too, were creative and expressive: **"Hakuna Ma-Christmas,"** for example, is the subject of an illustratration on page 220.

As a child moves out of Stage 1, the number of words he says decreases. This means intelligibility can increase.

Looking more closely at original word combinations, Bevin was able to assemble concepts with elements of time and place, some with grammar, some without: **"Only on Sunday"; "on Friday"; "in Bevin's space"; "In summer, it be nice"; "It's a beautiful rainbow"; "I need bag"; "And she said, 'Enjoy years'"; "It taste of paradise—a little big taste—taste of paradise"; "Marge's, noft you and get buy Jurassic"; "I'll go to Bevin's space, and I'll sleep"; "On the weekend, I will go to Bevin's space"; "Keep 'em here, wait til Mom comes."**

The following is a nice sequences of phrases, just emerging in their clarity but suggesting where Bevin might go next with his language combinations. The reference was to the particular Barney videos he wanted in order to complete his collection, and he was referring to them by seasons and series, not an easy concept to express with grammar: **"And four seasons; And numbers**; **And ten, six, and ten**; **And season two in five, six, four, five."** No, I didn't really "get it," but the idea was there, and the attempt was a good gauge of Bevin's ability to put concepts together in the sequential manner required for grammar.

Thus, while the accuracy of his self-generated utterances was limited , the variety and the confident nature of the attempts was gratifying. And it was this variety that suggested that Bevin had not yet matched his potential for developing grammar; thus, we will return to his story in Chapter 15, as he continued to develop his language competence in middle school.

Before we leave this charming young man, however, this magic point in his life is best told by his mother, Linda, to one of our workshop audiences—and Bevin himself.

B	**Spike is talking!**
L	I can tell that.
B	**When he wants to—**
L	I can tell that too.

Among the messages Linda offered her audience were these:

"I didn't realize Bevin was talking **to me** with his movie talk; I thought only the direct comments were for me, like **"No school,"** or **"Cheeseburger."** Now that I understand that Bevin is talking to me, I can listen and hear things I never knew were there. Knowing there's more inside him gives me hope: hope for his future and hope for our family."

Chapter 14
Considerations for Elementary School Students

Take the first step

As the last chapter illustrated, the process of acquiring language naturally can only start once it starts! The kids who were able to undertake the process on their own have done so by elementary age. And if they have not done so, it does no good to delay. Here's the unequivocal message: just get started. Whether or not you feel you are ready to plan for anything beyond the first step, just take that step.

Knowing there is a progression to language development is the key. That's really all you need to know to get started. You don't need to know where your child is within that progression; that will come later. And before you figure out how to do anything more sophisticated, you will help your child so much by simply paying attention and listening. Don't worry about trying to do something with what you hear. Your child won't expect you to. He is quite used to not being understood, and he won't expect you to understand him any better now. But he will be so happy just to have you present with him. Be present, just "be," and listen in a very new way: peacefully, broadly, deeply, without judgment. When we suspend judgment, we can hear beneath the surface, and we find that the gist of something often lies camouflaged beneath the broad brush strokes of chatter we used to dread.

Be present, just "be," and listen in a very new way: peacefully, broadly, deeply, without judgment.

It is a leap of faith, to be sure. We are so used to bemoaning those repeated gestalts: "Oh no," we think; "Not that line again. How many times is he going to say it? I am so tired of hearing it over and over again." The alternative scenario requires a quantum leap of philosophy. Your strategy is to suspend judgment and listen between the lines. Believe it or not, there is a good reason your child is saying that line again and again and again and again. Don't block it out, as much as you would like to. Suspend judgment and just open your ears and let your brain stay fuzzy. We tend to take our kids' language so literally that we miss the message.

There is a good reason your child is saying that line again and again and again and again.

When Bevin first began the NLA process, his mother wrote in her journal: "Bevin began to see Marge Blanc and his treasure box began to creak open! Someone actually understands him fully and speaks Bevineze!" Well, not really, but I did know how to be present, to simply immerse myself in Bevin. I knew that Bevineze was in my future.

Speaking Bevineze

Let's be honest: I didn't speak Bevineze at first, but I knew it was a legitimate language and worthy of study. I had given up judgment a long time ago, 18 years before, and I knew that between the lines was where the heart of the message was. It was there that the treasure lay. Quite honestly, that kind of faith no longer required a leap for me. I know it does for you, so please be bolstered by my years of experience and know that it is the right first step, every time. In fact, I can even add this: without that first step, the others make no sense at all. We need our child's raw material in order to get started.

You need language that comes from your child in order to help your child mitigate language

There is no other place to start! So, begin now: suspend judgment and listen with an open mind and an open heart.

Our kids are just as intellectually, socially, and emotionally complex as any children, and when their means of self-expression and sharing are limited, beautiful gestalts may contain the richest and most emotionally-charged language they have available.

Let's try out an example. This one comes from Joey and was referenced in an earlier report as an example of his "perseverative delayed echolalia": **"Welcome to my world; welcome to my world; welcome to my world; welcome to my world; welcome to my world …"** Why did he repeat that so many times? Was it simply an example of perseveration? Or was there a message? When we listen without judgment, we can consider many alternatives. Was it because (a) he needed to hear a heartfelt "thank you" for the kind invitation? Again and again because he didn't believe it? (b) He needed to have it said back to him as a reciprocal invitation? Again and again because people came and left in his world all too often? (c) He needed to express this welcoming nature of his because he was afraid some of his behaviors might seem to suggest otherwise? And he needed to be told directly, again and again, that he was not too much trouble as a friend, in spite of his health and social challenges? (d) He needed to hear someone say what a welcoming person he was? And until someone said it and meant it, he held out hope that someone would? (e) He needed to remind himself of the scenario the line came from and reassure himself of the world's goodness through that image? Again and again as his health challenges seemed to get the best of him? (f) Some or all of the above, mixed with other factors that are too myriad to list economically?

Our kids are just as intellectually, socially, and emotionally complex as any children, and when their means of self-expression and sharing are limited, these beautiful gestalts are often the richest, most emotionally-charged language available. Joey also knew how to say, "I want computer, please," but this hardly captured the beauty, inclusion, and openness of "Welcome to my world." We have often considered our kids the literal ones, but we are the culprits when it comes to this type of scenario. We tend to jump straight into "Oh, no, not that again" or "I wish he would say something else." Well, if our kids are just starting the NLA process, they don't have something else available to them to say. To say something more specific that would answer the questions above, they would have to generate something like "I hope you don't think I'm too much trouble to be with; I know my body doesn't function the way we all wish it would, but please know that I am a loving, caring guy and have an amazing inner life. I welcome your friendship."

Step 1: get started by knowing how to listen

Yes, there are many steps that follow step one, but step one is imperative to the rest of the process, so we need to take some time to understand it. There are many parts to listening well, and the following will help you know what it means.

1. Listen without judgment

Your work in suspending judgment will be much easier when you do two things: (1) Remember that your child is complex and deep. He is far more thinking, feeling, and aware than his body will allow him to demonstrate or that his language can communicate. (2) Remember that reading between the lines is much more important than reading the lines themselves. Don't allow yourself to get trapped in the literal!

Your child is complex and deep.

This is the time to listen to the heart of your child. Listen through the words but not to them. Suspend judgment and develop some hypotheses about the thoughts and feelings that might be suggested by them.

Reading between the lines is much more important than reading the lines themselves.

Remember that this is not about your child alone; he is not being "tested." You are doing this together, and, together, you will find the hidden meanings.

2. Listen deeply

Bevin's favorite word is "imagination." He learned it from Barney when he was young, and it has served him well ever since. Adults forget to imagine—imagine the child inside; imagine the depths. You will be helping a child like Bevin, who has never been able to plumb the sound tracks in his head to isolate the communicative language. Keep your eye on that prize: the gems within the sound tracks your child has in his mind; the ones he keeps saying. They house the prize.

Listen between the lines, among the lines, and below the lines. Let your mind imagine, so it can hear. When you have a thought, or just a glimmer of a thought, note it to yourself; better yet, write it down. What do you feel when you listen? Do you hear confusion? fear? anger? frustration? hope? joy? Listen with your heart and keep a diary of all you hear. Your child's thoughts, his diamonds in the rough, don't need to become any more polished to be diamonds. Listen, and you will discover that you have found some. Treasure them; they are the stuff of narrative—your child's narrative of himself. Know that he will eventually be able to polish them, at least somewhat, but until you mine them together, he can't. Nor can he have the enormous benefit of sharing the rough diamonds with you!

Listen with your heart and keep a diary of all you hear.

3. Listen broadly

Listen over time. Remember repeated lines later on. Write them down and try to keep the general strands of language—or thought—in mind as you continue to listen. Pay attention when you hear something later on, later in the day, the next day. When themes emerge, take them seriously. You may be onto something important.

4. Listen to the story

Weave together the strands of thought from your child. It will become a story, your child's story. Build the narrative your child is living. Jot it down; let your child know you are doing this. It assures him you are taking him, his language, and his story seriously. Say something if you have something to say: just a word, an acknowledgement, a smiling repetition of a meaningful line. But don't feel like you have to say anything—until you have something to say.

5. Listen peacefully

Be peaceful and give it time.

All this listening, plumbing, and mining takes time. Be peaceful and give it time. You actually have no choice: if your child senses you don't have time or are impatiently trying to move on, he will quickly sense he doesn't have the audience he has needed all his life.

6. Listen with an open mind to the future

Grammatical constructions are not the only form of legitimate language.

Consider the "prize" you are aiming towards: flexible, self-generated grammar. At the same time, however, don't be fooled that grammatical constructions are the only prize, or even the best prize. Consider that grammatical constructions are not the only form of legitimate language. Yes, we hope our kids get there, but even if they don't, mitigation can be a semi-flexible and beautiful form of self-expression.

Consider the following mitigation Bevin composed that summer between elementary school and middle school. Yes, it is the Barney song. Yes, we were all somewhat tired of the Barney song. Yes, we thought Bevin should "outgrow" it. Listening with an open mind, though, I received this prize and many others like it. This is the one I received that summer:

> **You are my friend.**
> **We're best friends.**
> **Fun with my sister.**
> **A beautiful world.**
> **To eat and sleep and be with the people you love and care about.**
> **You love me too.**

It bears mentioning that this poetic treasure would not have come to be without some peaceful listening—it took several turns—and some scribing. Scribing always seems to work well as a way of making visible and permanent what kids say. Many kids do not relish hearing themselves played back with speech; but they do value being heard. Scribing what kids say is, then, the perfect alternative. It does not interrupt; it allows kids space to search their mental encyclopedias; it lets them know, in no uncertain terms, that they were heard.

Scribing lets kids know they were heard, but it does not interrupt—so kids have the freedom to continue to think.

Before Bevin left elementary school, his mother wrote in her journal, "Bevin is talking much more since seeing Marge and has so much happening in his head!!! His scope of awareness around him is now about 30 feet and he is even nosy." Bevin's mother's comments suggest the benefits derived from Step 1: (1) the student knows he is being heard and taken seriously and that his talking matters; (2) he learns that his language has communicative value, even in its unabridged form, and so he pays more attention to it; (3) as he pays attention to his own language, he begins to move naturally from Stage 1 to Stage 2; (4) as he pays attention to his own language, we can see some Stage 2 processing that has already taken place.

As we have said many times before, it takes two to communicate, and when we join our children as active communication partners, they become communicators. Our kids begin talking more, and they begin talking more to us. It may take days, weeks, or months, but gradually, as they become more conscious communicators, you become ready for step two.

Step two: listen to the loud parts of Stage 1 gestalts

Once our children are talking openly, without hiding or feeling like they are just talking to themselves, they often become more intelligible. Then, we can start to hear the difference between language they intend to say and language they are trying to skip over. The loud parts may become louder, and the slurred parts quieter. We can more easily figure out which parts kids are trying to extract or mitigate and which parts they are trying to slough off. We then find out how aware they are of the fast-forwarding process that leads to successful mitigation. As we have said, it's tremendously difficult to fast-forward through a full-length movie, and it is so much harder than just the few words little kids have to rush through to mitigate. So we need to be patient with our older students and help them by putting a "book mark" in periodically to "hold their place" for them.

We need to be patient with our older students and help them by putting a "book mark" in periodically to "hold their place" for them.

When Bevin first realized I would help him mitigate, he was dumbfounded but eternally grateful. I would simply jot down the loud words and phrases, and when he was ready to hear me, I would read them back. He thought I was pure genius, but I was just listening for the loud parts and bookmarking them for him.

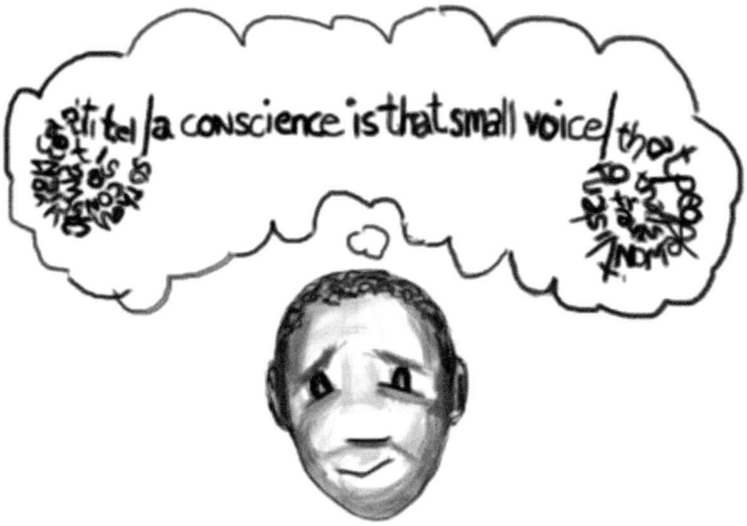

Step three: keep track of the mitigations

Once kids have successfully isolated some phrases and sentences they want to say, it makes sense to put together a list of them. They will not all occur with any regularity, but once you start keeping track, you will find out which ones do. If your child loves to write, he may enjoy keeping track of his own mitigations, maybe even cataloguing them. Even if it's you putting together the list, a visual display of them is usually empowering.

Step four: share the mitigations with others

Our kids so appreciate being heard, and when others begin to understand what they mean by their quirky phrases, they can become effective communication partners too. It makes your job so much easier when the phrases your child loves are part of the family's shared dictionary. Once kids' intentions are understood, communication takes place.

Step five: build some easily-mitigable gestalts into your daily language

Just like we do with younger children, we can build some useful gestalts into our language so our older kids have the benefit of some easy-to-mitigate phrases such as "Let's …," "It's …," and "I'm …." Making sure our older kids have access to a nice variety of each of these phrases makes their mix-and-match process so much easier.

Step six: watch for signs of Stage 2 mixing and matching of phrases

Spontaneous mixing and matching is a sure sign that Stage 2 is working well. Some phrases that are quite handy may show up all over the place, and kids get considerable mileage out of them. For Bevin, we got used to hearing phrases like "You'll ..." as a request form, for instance, and "What kind of ... ?" as a question form. Other phrases only get to be used occasionally, such as "Hakuna ma-Christmas," and a student inexperienced in mixing and matching might be misunderstood as simply trying to recall the line from the song. I'll have to admit I was surprised when Bevin came up with that one.

Step seven: watch for signs that it's time for Stage 3 single-word isolation

Once mix-and-match sentences predominate, gestalts begin to fade away and kids often use new ones only to explore new intellectual and linguistic territory. It is usually about that time that they are ready to try out Stage 3 single-word isolation. Recall what that stage was like for the little kids and think about how awkward it was for them. Imagine, then, how strange it sounds to older kids to use two and three-word phrases. It will be helpful to have an experienced SLP partner with you with this stage, as our profession is well-versed in this type of single word mixing and matching. SLPs can make it fun, and older students don't need to feel odd using these short forms of language.

Step eight: watch for signs that it's time for Stage 4 beginning grammar

Again, your SLP will be invaluable here, as our profession is quite used to making this determination and knowing when it is time to begin basic grammar. From here on, your job will be easier, and you will have the fun job of helping your child generalize his new constructions at home. One of the basic strategies for supporting grammar development is modeling many examples of a few constructions in the same time period so none is overlearned as a gestalt or mitigation. The idea here is another kind of "mixing and matching," but this time with a few grammatical forms at the same developmental level.

Model many examples of a few constructions so none is overlearned as gestalt or mitigation.

Step nine: keep developing grammar at Stages 4–6 as long as possible

You and your child's SLP will want to continue to promote the development of grammar for as long as it is possible for your child. There will be individual differences in that time line, of course, but even when no further development of grammar is possible, your child will still have a lifetime of continued language growth: pragmatic, semantic, narrative, and conversational.

Step ten: know that language growth can flourish after grammar development has ceased

You and your SLP partner will want to explore all the types of language use that maturing students can develop as your child continues his journey as a life-long learner. Section 5 will cover these areas of language growth and use in detail, since these areas are part of the experience of individuals of high school age and beyond.

Summary

We are now ready to move on to Section 5, where we will continue with the stories of our kids' progress in natural language development once they have taken their first steps in elementary school. The ten developmental steps outlined in this chapter are still relevant in middle school and high school, of course, but there will be so much more to those students' adventures. Even after grammar has ceased to develop sometime in the teen years, continued language learning and expanded language use will be a part of all students' development throughout secondary school. Like the rest of us, our kids are life-long learners, and language and communication continue to be defined and refined as our students mature into adults.

Afterward: starting the NLA process in middle school

As we complete Section 4, we should add a few words about starting the NLA process in middle school and even high school. Is it possible? In a word, yes. And while the method of assessment will be reminiscent of the way one would start in preschool or elementary school, an older student will be much more entrenched in a well-established way of talking. If his echolalia has not been acknowledged by middle school, it may have gone underground by then, and well-practiced scripts may be all anyone gets to hear. It is still well worth the effort of an assessment of natural language in middle school and high school, however, for two reasons. One, there may be remaining potential to develop mitigation and word-combining, even if true grammar is out of reach. Two, even with limited remaining potential for grammar development, assessing the student's natural language is important in establishing goals for pragmatic language growth.

Chapter 15, on middle school students, will not contain a separate protocol for starting the NLA process, because it would be the same general protocol described at the end of Chapter 1. There are additional notes about assessing older students in Chapter 17, however, so if you are contemplating assessing a middle schooler's natural language for the first time, you will want to read both of these descriptions. Your methodology will be a creative, individualized combination of these two.

With that caveat in mind, then, we are ready to continue the journey of those students who began the NLA process in elementary school.

section 5

Older Students: Middle and High School, Life-Long Learners

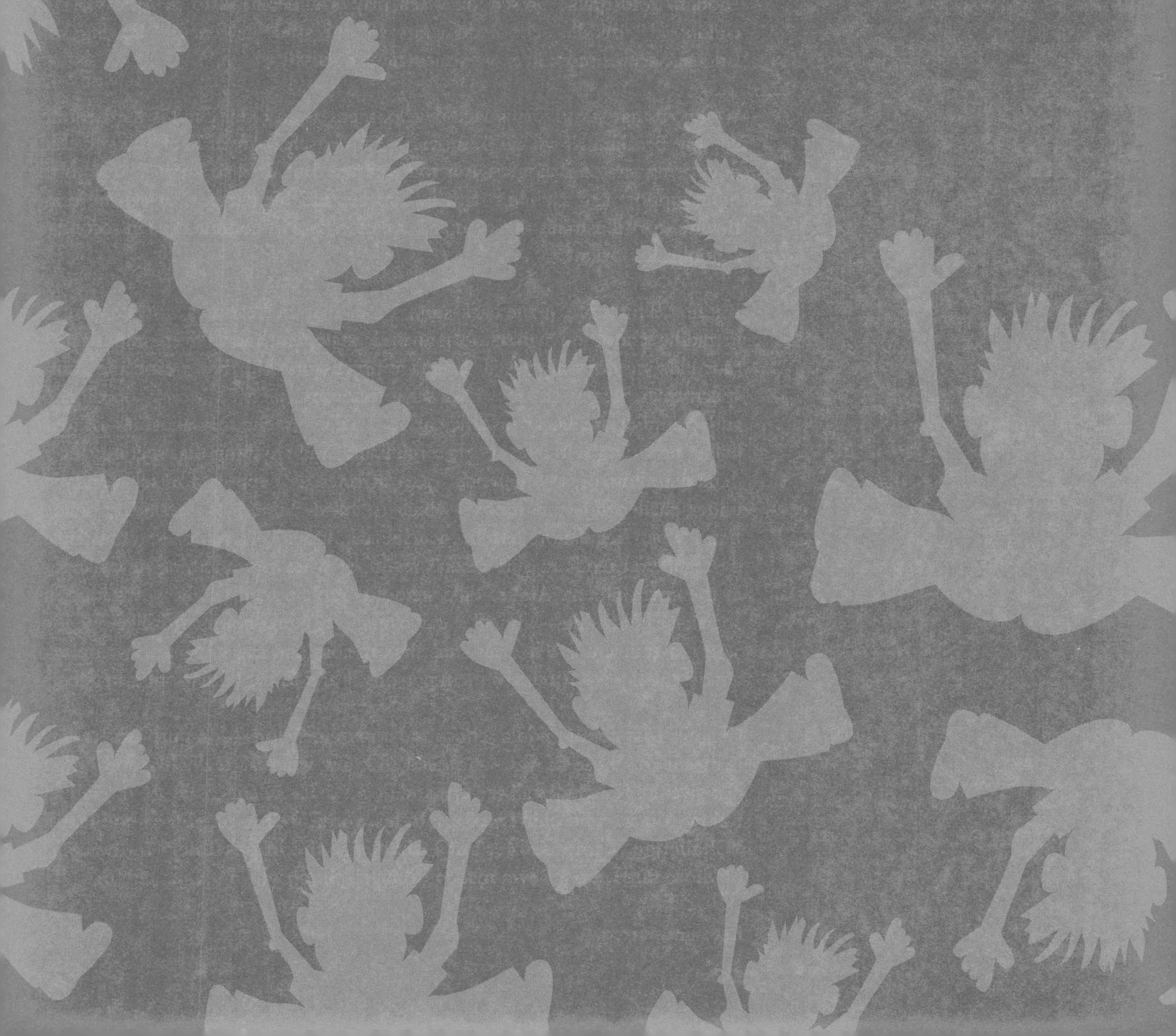

Introduction

There's no clear cut-off age for grammar development .

Clinical experience shows that kids who are behind in language development have years, often many years, to continue developing rule-based grammar. We used to think that if a child's grammar wasn't fully developed by age six or seven, it was too late. But we are finding that when it's delayed, there isn't a clear cut-off age for grammar development. This is good news for our ASD kids!

Returning now to Bevin's story, as he approached his teenage years, it was quite apparent that his grammar development wasn't about to stop any time soon. I could see the signs of new grammar emerging even as middle school ushered in new challenges to self-regulation. It was good that Bevin had time on his side, because his sensory defensiveness and lagging motor skills were challenge enough. And unlike preschool, when play is understood to be "the work of childhood," middle school demands all our students' energy. Playing with language seems more like an extracurricular activity.

Breaking down whole movies is immensely more difficult than breaking down snippets of dialogues at a younger age, but with the right support and a child's faith in himself and his partners, it can be done.

We know that starting language development as an older child is hard enough anyway. Breaking down whole movies is immensely more difficult than breaking down snippets of dialogues at a younger age. But we also know that with the right support and a child's faith in himself and his partners, it can be done. Bevin's story illustrates this complex equation, and its continuation in secondary school is important.

But first, a bit more of the back-story: to say that life becomes more challenging in middle school and high school is an understatement and an over-simplification. Our kids are not only gestalt language processors, but they are on the autism spectrum, which means they have sensorimotor challenges. Motor coordination and planning are likely insufficient to adequately support activities of daily living, including self-care, sports, organizing, and anything that requires motor demonstration of competence. Also affected is support for self-regulation under challenging conditions—which is the definition of secondary school. Even when regulation has been achieved under one set of circumstances, dysregulation tends to surface and resurface whenever anything new happens in the environment. And middle school is replete with newness. It's loud; it's social; it's confusing—with all the dynamics changing hourly. It is like one long series of transitions. That our students can continue any language development amidst the din is a tribute to them personally and to the human spirit in general.

Chapter 15 is about middle school and is extremely long—on purpose. Its detail is meant for those of you who need to know what it's really like and how to not give up. It includes all the ups and down that students really go though and follows Bevin, who didn't give up. In his words, well-selected for good reason: **"Challenge is impossible, but I challenge the impossible."** In the course of those three years, Bevin made it to high school, which is Chapter 16.

Let's get started.

Chapter 15
Developing Language in Middle School

When we left Bevin's story in Chapter 13, he was twelve and a half years old and about to enter middle school. It makes sense to review his progress here, because after a few months in middle school, Bevin's life turned upside down, and the undulations became the main event he had to contend with. Language took a distant last when faced with pure survival. But it started out innocently enough.

First, let's review Bevin's progress since he began the NLA process at age ten, with his wealth of Stage 1 language spoken at lightning speed and only fleeting evidence of communicative intent. That he responded quickly to intervention demonstrated that his communicative intentions were not far below the surface. Over the two and a half years before middle school, Bevin developed greater language flexibility, grammar, and conversational timing, all of which served him well. His last language sample taken the summer before middle school revealed 100% intelligible, communicative utterances. Of these, 16% were gestalts, 35% were mitigations, 28% word isolations and combinations, and 21% grammatical. Bevin got a running start on grammar before middle school, and that was a good thing.

Between the ages of ten and twelve, Bevin benefitted from community-based PT and OT services that focused on self-regulation from a sensory-integrative perspective. When those therapists moved away, Bevin was still able to maintain fair self-regulation for almost another year. As he became a teenager, however, his needs increased, and the services provided at school just weren't enough to make up the difference. School itself had become a challenge in every conceivable way, particularly to Bevin's tenuous self-regulation. Bevin's hyper-acute hearing was taxed more and more with each passing day of hallway cacophony, and he began wearing noise-busting earphones more and more often.

But on one particular November afternoon in sixth grade, Bevin was happily looking forward to the winter holidays and preparing to borrow some of his beloved toy animals from the clinic. We had a long, playful discussion that particular afternoon, and Bevin presented arguments from four different perspectives: his own, mine, his mom's, and the toys' themselves to try to convince me the animals would be better off at his house.

The conversation began in the toy room of our clinic, with Bevin negotiating on behalf of himself and the toys. The preciousness of this conversation became quickly apparent, and I decided to offer him a deal: if he would allow me to videotape him, something he intensely disliked, he could take home the entire herd. He agreed, and, after utterance 16, I had the benefit of a recorded version. Without that record, I might have missed one of the most clever parts of this conversation: the inclusion of so many perspectives.

1 **We must pack it up.** [2, presenting his opening argument]

2 **I will tell a story.** [4]

3 **That was not possible.** [2, speaking for Marge]

4 **My mom said, "It was too cold."** [4, presenting the "Mom" perspective of his wishful thinking]

5 **They must not stay.** [4, continuing that perspective]

6 **We must pack it up after playing.** [2, his own perspective]

7 **A bags—we will pack it up.** [4, continuing from his perspective]

8 **We must pack it up.** [2]

9 **There 'st much time.** [1, one of his frequent gestalts]

(A few moments later, Bevin continued the argument)

10 **I was not safe.** [4, from the animals' perspective]

11 **I must never, ever stay here.** [4, same]

12 **It was not wrong—cannot stay.** [4, not completely accurate, but understandable; from Bevin's perspective]

13 **For two 'm we won't pack.** [4, speaking as himself, being selective about the characters he wanted]

14 **Get these smellies or grouches.** [4, using mitigated vocabulary to explain why some characters were not included]

15 **They're staying until September.** [4, apparently staying home until September]

16 **They're staying until September.** [4]

(After agreeing to tell the story again while I filmed him)

17 **You are not taking the toys home.** [4, Marge's line]

18 **It will stay until Thanksgiving, please**. [4, meaning stay at home]

	M	(glosses B) And then what happens?
19		**We will get our toys now!** [4]
	M	(gloss) And—
20	**B**	**And then make of life.** [2, his oft-repeated long-term plan]
	M	And where is that life going to be?
21	**B**	**In the bag.** [2]
	M	(glossing him)
22	**B**	**In the bag.** [2]
	M	Is it going to be outside?
23	**B**	**In the bedroom.** [2]
24	**B**	**In Bevin's room.** [2]
		(Another scene, in the toy room where the animals are)
	M	(gave an introduction)
25	**B**	**OK, it was too cold for toys.** [4, returning to his mom's supposed argument]
26		**We just cannot stay.** [4, speaking for the animals]
27		**It was not—it's not possible.** [2, Marge's position]
28		**Marge's: we're not taking more toys home.** [4, Marge's is my name, mitigated from "Let's go to Marge's"; my perspective]
29		**It was not possible.** [2, continuing from Marge's perspective]
30		**It is not possible.** [2, correcting Marge's grammar!]
	M	(questioned his mother's position)
31	**B**	**It was too cold for toys.** [4, offers his mom's argument]
32		**We just cannot stay.** [2, from the toys' perspective]
33		**And then, just pack it up. Twenty—25 toys, go home in two weeks.** [4, an originally-formulated idea]
34		**Summer, we will pack up to ready to go.** [4, meaning to return them]
35		**Make a—make of life.** [2, a common desire of Bevin's is to "make a life" for animals]
36		**Make a life of land.** [2, Bevin, the environmentalist]
37		**Live in the nature.** [4]
38		**Of the life.** [2]
39		**The end.** [1]

It was a privilege to be a part of this dialogue, one that stretched every fiber of Bevin's fledgling grammar. It was stilted, to be sure, a sign that the building blocks of these original utterances had just recently become mitigated from elsewhere. The use of wording like "I will," "It was not ...," "I must ...," and "We just cannot ..." etc. suggested an older student, certainly, but one who had not yet acquired the contractions and colloquial forms common to teenagers. The language sample lacked the natural sound of well-oiled generative grammar and made it abundantly clear that Bevin would have to use his new skills in many situations before they would have the ring of "natural." But all beginning generative language users face the same challenge. We are reminded of younger speakers who have just acquired the ability to formulate and come out with pearls such as "Daddy doed her beards" and "I not gets more." Bevin's language was just as endearing to me, and I was thrilled we'd captured it on tape.

As it turned out, the school year never produced another such gem, one that continued for so many turns. Bevin's strong communicative intent had ruled that day, and he pulled out all his linguistic stops. The result demonstrated the power of language, of intention, and of thought. It proved to be a window into Bevin's emerging competence that showed us how much pure grammar he had developed and how much more we needed to do to make his progress accessible and useful in daily life.

Progress during sixth grade

Bevin made good progress throughout middle school, even though he had precious little time to practice his language in the crunch of daily life. Once a week throughout his sixth grade year, Bevin came to our clinic with a full agenda, and he and I talked for several hours straight. He no longer had outside PT or OT services, but he used the sensorimotor equipment in our clinic well and always orchestrated a complete experience for each of our sessions. In addition, Bevin teased his sister every day and engaged in several meaningful conversations daily with each of his family members. When blessed summer came, Bevin went to day camp and talked to his counselors all day long. Bevin was motivated and continued to blossom.

Following are excerpts from Bevin's progress report six months into sixth grade. That report noted measurable progress in Bevin's development of mitigated language, generative grammar, and the pragmatic use of both in conversation, including narrative, explanation, and drama. Those details are included here to give the reader an intimate feel for what progress actually looks like when an older student is engaged in the process of language development. Specific examples are included to give the reader a realistic idea of what might be expected as students explore with their new-found tools.

> Bevin now produces Stage 2 and higher language 90% of the time during his therapy sessions, an increase from 80% nine months ago. This means that he uses a combination of mitigated forms (isolated from the gestalts they originally

came from in Bevin's mind), mix and match utterances made up of mitigated parts, and self-generated sentences almost exclusively.

At Stage 2, Bevin practices certain long mitigations many times during most sessions, often to understand the words embedded in them, to commit them to memory (for future reference, making them more accessible than the original gestalt), or to communicate something particular.

Gestalt language (in the form of Stage 2 mitigation) is still highly relevant to Bevin, and it is apparent, once he draws from several in the short span of a few moments, how important Stage 2 still is to him.

Bevin produces Stage 3 and higher language 70% of the time during his sessions, an increase from 50% nine months ago. This includes isolation of single words, and constructions of two or more words, whether or not these constructions are grammatical. It remains important that Bevin continue to explore and work with his mitigations when he needs to and to combine words creatively.

Following are a few examples of how Bevin has used a combination of Stage 2 and 3 constructions in the last two months to explore ideas. Utterances are grouped by common phrases:

> **This flood for you.**
> **It very funny for you.**
>
> **It's called 'out of control.'**
> **It's called 'Daddy's in control.'**
>
> **This is gonna be trickier than I thought—this is gonna be conscience than I thought.**
>
> **Mean animals—** (watching elephants on a video)
> **Man, are they ugly—African plains ugly.**
>
> **Very happy means.**
> **Excusy means.**
>
> **Very spitting means.**
> **Very brutal means.**
> **Very clown means.**
> **Mountain very means.**

The progress report continued by commenting on Bevin's progress at Stage 4, and it tempered these comments by noting the continued place that Stage 3 practice had in his continued language development. Older students have missed this kind of thought-combining at a younger age and need ample opportunity for this practice.

It is clear that language at Stage 3 and higher is now merging into Stage 4 language and that grammar is now playing a greater role in Bevin's language development. It is still important that Bevin try out combinations of thoughts (and words) at Stage 3, much like the examples noted above.

Bevin produces Stage 4 language (DSS Levels 1–3 or higher) 35% of the time during his sessions, an increase from 15% nine months ago. While his use of grammar is expanding nicely, his accuracy is just beginning to become a target of therapy. His grammaticality depends on whether or not a particular piece of the grammar has been isolated (Stage 3), how well-practiced a construction is, how salient it is to the communiqué at hand, and how well-regulated Bevin is for the task.

Following are some examples of grammatical constructions from DSS levels 1–3 used in the last two months. It is notable that Bevin often is able to produce a particular grammatical construction but not to finish the sentence:

Put all the movies in the bag. (Bevin can deliver directions with ease)
Draw dinosaurs and conscience—Draw him and him—
Draw them.
And you get big things: candy and gingerbread and lollipops—gingerbread house.

It's Shaggy. (use of "'s" contraction)
It's come true.
It's not a good guy.
No, it's not.
It's the worst case—
It's called a 'ha ha ha.'

This messy room is not fair. (use of "is")
This worm is very means.
It is a terrible—
Who is he?
Isn't very, you'll—

Where are the jelly beans? (use of "are" and "'re" contraction)

Those sharks are dangerous.
They're monsters.
And they're too—
Bears is, are a little funny.

It was a big huge— (past tense, "and")
Videos got flooded.
Everything dried up.
Made a chair.
Had to be fun.

Dinosaur and Flintstones and other Bevin's movies.
It's like angry and boo.

It was gratifying to find Bevin using more "natural-sounding" language, in striking contrast to just four months earlier. The accuracy of his sentences was lower than in the language sample where the toys asked to come home with Bevin for Thanksgiving, but Bevin sounded much more like the teenager he was. His report continued:

The following was part of a series of utterances, each different from the other and all exploring ideas and grammar:

It's called a bad guy really different.
It looks a bad guy—It's called quiet.
It looks to be a bad guy
It's gonna be a fat guy.
It called really different.
Bad dreams, are they ugly!

Bevin regularly uses two sentences in a row, in narrative and discourse, twice during a session, an increase from once per session nine months ago. Following are a few examples of narrative or explanation during the last two months:

It's called Valentine's Day. Get all the friends around the table, all in one place. (planning a party, which took place at CDC with 4 other boys)

In March, it will be flooded. Those Bevin things are flooded. (making a case for taking some toys home, to save them from the impending flood once the snow on the roof of the building melts—we did have a leak!)

A recent dialogue illustrates Bevin's conversations:

B	**It's like belly ache—a hospital.**
	(humorously talking about a dried up marker)
M	Should I throw it away?
M	What did you call it?
B	**It's called old.**
B	**Throw it in the garbage.**

The report concluded with a table of the grammatical structures Bevin had mastered, those he was still working on, and those he needed next, developmentally. It was a nice list, but clearly lean in the "mastered" column.

Stage 4 grammaticality is assuming more of the focus of his therapy. Following are the grammatical constructions Bevin has mastered (1), those that are emerging (2), and those he needs to round out his grammatical base (3). Attentive listeners should listen for categories (2) and (3) and use those constructions themselves:

	Verbs	Pronouns	Other
(1) Mastered	is contraction: 's are contraction: 're	it this those they he	not and Where?
(2) Emerging	am verb (+s) was past tense *(did, went,* etc.*)* let's gonna will can	I me we you us	like after Who … ? Why … ?
(3) Needed	wanna gotta hafta regular past tense ('ed)	that us she our their	Is it … ? Are they … ? Was it … ? Were they … ? Am I … ?

Table 19: Bevin's Stage Four Grammar

The progress in sixth grade was notable, but Bevin had a long way yet to go.

I'm a real boy

In spite of any lapses in grammar or other linguistic skills, Bevin was feeling proud of himself in sixth grade. For as long as I had known him, he had questioned what it would take to become a "real boy." At about the time of this progress report, Bevin announced his coming-of-age, saying, **"I'm a real boy!"** I was so proud of him! The following was another version of the story:

B	**Someday, Bevin the only one to meet is a T-Rex boy.**
M	(glossing)
B	**I T-Rex—the only one. I wanna be is T-Rex boy.**

Bevin's emergence as a real boy that spring came complete with many treasures: he drew amazing dinosaurs after not being willing to draw since he was expected to when he was little; he invited participation in joint activities, which was new; and he engaged in group activities if he was allowed the freedom to come and go at will. Two other students about his age joined us from time to time, and Bevin seemed able to reenact the school scenes from his old favorite Barney movies, stating, **"Barney—it's love."**

As summer approached, Bevin began making plans:

> **Summer and Mother, and—will be—videos and dvds—and big and beautiful—and fall—and then fill it up and fill the up and—and fall will be dreams—And then we filled up—Fill up and—you'll, we'll be a man and get along. All of us—we'll be full. And try again, we'll be full. Never fear. And we'll be, we'll be—magic carpet ride. We'll be magic, beautiful. We'll be 14—big—14 years old. And then we'll be filled. And the way top, bottom. I'll be a big full. I've been a big story. I've been a big magic. I've been a big supplies. I've been a big artist. I've been a big play doughs. I've been a big magic wand. I've been a bit magic wand, Legos. We'll be full by September. We'll be free—hooray. It will be full. We'll be summer: June, July, August.**

It was fortuitous that Bevin had made so many wonderful plans by then, because things started to fall apart after that. As his sensory defensiveness escalated, Bevin talked about **"the means"** and resorted to pinching and biting at school: **"I've been biting forever; babies forever."** But summer came, biting stopped, and Bevin regained his good nature. **"Tah dah,"** he declared, **"It's wonderful! Nice long summer. We'll clean up in August."** Over the summer, Bevin experimented with story-telling, including this alternative version of *Horton Hatches the Egg*: **"Hello, Horton. Now, now what have we here? Bye** (to the bird). **A hay truck—a build a straw. He's in trouble. Oh no, he broke it!**

Don't not—it more kinda a— (M: Don't get off the nest!) **She stole it. Call the police! Hey, I know. Hello—hello, beast. I just follow my father."**

But don't listen too closely

Fall came, and seventh grade hit Bevin hard. His intensifying need for more concerted OT/PT services became evident. After a summer of regulation bliss, the dawn of the next school year hit like a wet wash rag. Bevin's comment on his own regulation needs was this: **"Bumps are bites,"** and clearly the bumps of September resulted in pinches and bites to all those within reach. I found him a community-based PT by October and an OT in the spring. PT worked on core strength and motor planning, and OT addressed Bevin's severe auditory sensitivity. It was a hard year.

A progress report three months into his seventh grade year noted the following:

> Bevin continues to make steady progress in his generative language development and his social language use as long as his self-regulation needs are met. During the summer, Bevin was consistently well-regulated as he attended YMCA camp daily and was relaxed and focused when he came for his weekly sessions. Once school began, however, Bevin was faced with the challenges of middle school, and came to his sessions in an over-aroused state, one where conversation was simply sensory overload. Bevin's school team found his behavior problematic enough to institute a Behavior Intervention Plan at the time of his IEP.
>
> To meet this regulation need, the clinician and Bevin's family arranged for weekly Physical Therapy sessions to occur at CDC, and after four sessions, Bevin's parents reported that his wellness had increased measurably and that he was accessing his core muscles for all activities, notably sitting and reaching, and his teachers were reporting increased use of his arms as well. Bevin's biting and pinching behaviors decreased markedly almost immediately, and his smile has been broadening as time has gone by! Conversation can again occur without the fear of sensory overload, and Bevin is again addressing his speech and language goals.

The report continued:

> Bevin now produces Stage 4 (DSS levels 1–3) language in spontaneous sentences 50% of the time (increased from 35%). He now takes two turns using original sentences in conversation at least five times per session. He uses three sentences in a

row at least once per session to narrate or explain. In general, Bevin's language has the sound of "self-generated but delayed" if you don't listen too closely. His production of self-generated sentences converges fluently with his useful gestalts and mitigations in such a way that the casual listener could think they were all self-generated. The more discriminating listener might just say that Bevin sounds "odd" or imprecise. Bevin also uses an inordinate number of sound effects and single-word exclamations, so the overall effect of his verbal expression is dramatic but "unusual."

Following is a series of utterances Bevin produced recently to set up a session. They are labeled: O (original), M (mitigated), or G (gestalt):

Stegosaurus next. O
Think about it. M
I don't have any stripes. O
Uh, I don't finding xxx. O
Too much corn—'cause of the heat. O
Relax! M
I'll get something else. O
You'll get the rest of it. O
Here you go. M

The following were Bevin's turns in conversation with his mom about school:

'Cause I'm not—because I not hurt the people. O
I hope not hurt people. O
Thanks for listening. M
Thank you, Jesus, for this truth. M

Following are some dialogues:

M	Would you like to listen to the Spanish subtitles?
B	**No, I learn the Spanish alone. O**
M	Thank you for sharing that with me.
B	**Maybe I'll talk to the mom. O**
M	Are you going to have a party?
B	**It's a birthday party. It's mean. O**
B	**I been so mean lately. O**
B	**I hope you're satisfied. G/M**
M	It's not mean unless you feel mean.
B	**All right; OK; I'm up—happy. M, O**

B	**I was just trying to help. G/M**
M	I know that.

Some turns in dialogue:

M	I would never insult you knowingly. (I was laughing at his happiness.)
B	**I'm not insulted; I'm happy. O**

B	**Got some honey bees. O**
M	(commenting)
B	**I feel some my head. O**
M	(commenting)
B	**How many honey? O**
M	How many honey bees?
B	**I feel my head in a quandary. O, M**

B	**Which is worse to live with, a tiger or a gorilla? O, M**
M	I think a tiger.
B	**A gorilla-tiger! O**

Some nice compound and complex sentences with 'and':

You get chips and soda and videos, and hurry back. O
You go get chips and soda; I'll go pee and I'll be right back. O

M	You got tired today.
B	**Yup—I'm sorry. O/M**

M	I almost said 'Jiminy Christmas.'
B	**I think he's a cousin. O**

Me hurt everywhere

Winter break came and went, and going back to school was tough. By the end of January, Bevin was well-practiced in the art of asking for others to be quiet. He'd learned to reject a bellowing **"Shut up!"** as it didn't promote much good will, but tried more sugary versions of it such as **"Now shut up, ok?"** as he tapped me on the shoulder. And he found more socially-acceptable alternatives that worked: **"Sh! Listen!"** and **"Hush!!"** On the flip side of asking for others to be quiet, however, Bevin began engaging in louder-than-usual sound effects and non-stop self-talk that seemed designed to drown out the din from outside his head. While I have never used the term "movie talk" to describe gestalt language, even the language taken directly from movies, this was clearly "movie talk." It appeared that Bevin had turned on his favorite movies inside his head, and was hearing and saying the sound track to comfort himself.

Then came the self-diagnosis: **"Me hurt everywhere!"** This line was delivered as part of the dialogue from *The Land Before Time*: **"I'm ok; I'm ok; Are you ok, Petrie? Me hurt everywhere!"** which made it safe to say. In this cute way, Bevin dared to talk about the immense headache he had from all the noise surrounding him all day long. I had seen it coming for a month; the pain was getting worse. It had to be nearly unbearable for Bevin to make it an issue, but, finally, he was asking for my help.

What I could offer him was acknowledgement and hope. And I knew who to call. I did not consider myself an expert in sensory defensiveness, and certainly not an expert in auditory sensory defensiveness, but I knew who was: Sheila Frick, co-author of *Therapeutic Listening* (2009). Sheila is renowned as an expert in listening therapy for sensory modulation, and we were fortunate that she maintained a practice in the Madison area. I called her the next day. It took two months for Sheila to find a place for Bevin in her program, but she then coordinated with me and Bevin's PT for the rest of that spring. Bevin continued to work on his core muscles, added considerable vestibular input to his growing body, and added daily listening therapy to his home program. Following are some excerpts from his Progress Report four months later, as his seventh grade year was about to end:

> The last reporting period has been one of personal growth but one of enormous challenges for Bevin and his family. Bevin's auditory defensiveness became almost unbearable at the beginning of the calendar year. His availability, both socially and physically, declined, and, by mid-February, he was wearing his headphones most of the time. Only in the last month has the world periodically quieted enough for Bevin to continue his social progress.
>
> During January, Bevin continued to develop linguistically, and his growing repertoire of gestures increased his communicative success. His language became more and more reflective of the severity of his sensory defensiveness, however:
>
> **I didn't know he's going to Papa.**
> **I'll pinch you.**
>
> **Silence!!—What was that?**
>
> **Hush!!—Much too hard on him.**
>
> **B** **I'm being ok.**
> M You are; you're being funny.
> **B** **No way—now listen!**
>
> **I'm afraid xxx—nothing can stop it.**

Super sonic ear boy

His family's notes from this period of time are telling. His mother wrote in his Functional Listening Questionnaire: "Bevin has always had auditory sensitivity ... He is super sonic ear boy ... It has gotten worse and worse. Now it is critical. Bevin can not tolerate anything where there is an auditory component without his headphones, especially his loud school environment. Bevin is a very good boy. He attempts to go through all the parts of his life and can mostly hold it together, if he has his headphones on. Recent private PT has helped immensely, but listening therapy is clearly our next need. The hardest time of day is throughout his school day. It takes him two hours to recover every day after school. The impact on Bevin is that he doubts his own abilities to be a 'real boy' when he bites someone." One of his mother's comments about Bevin's biting was especially poignant. She noted that the deafening sound Bevin hears is scary. She wrote that when Bevin was "too scared to find his words, he bites to stop the scary scenario quickly."

"The impact on his family is that we are remaining sane ... just barely. Bevin has trouble settling to sleep and staying asleep. He wakes up 5–6 times during the night. He screams, plays with toys, goes to his parents' bedroom, talks to himself, wanders around, eats, and takes the house apart. Nothing helps him get back to sleep."

In the clinic, too, Bevin relied on his headphones until he had gotten enough physical input. The spring report contained these notes from early in the semester:

> On another occasion, Bevin had his earphones on for the first 30 minutes and didn't converse at all. After a half hour of intense bouncing, he seemed to be able to muster at least a few disjointed gestalts. After an hour, Bevin could engage in a truncated dialogue about his need for summer vacation:
>
> | | |
> |---|---|
> | **B** | **Summer vacation.** |
> | M | It will be better then, I know. |
> | **B** | **Got it?** |
> | M | I do understand how you need that time outside. |
> | **B** | **Jungle (xxx)—** |

That's what friends are for

The power of being acknowledged, respected, and offered hope cannot be overestimated. Once Bevin knew that his family and I were going to help him, he relaxed, and was able to be happy again. The following notes relay a sense of that hopefulness.

You know something—you're all right!

M	We've got our Todd.
B	(big smile)
M	Then we'll get our Sheila.
B	(big smile)
B	**That's what friends are for.**

Even though it took two months to get started with listening therapy, Bevin had hope and worked hard on regulation and the parts of language he could tolerate. His sound effects increased, as did his "talking over" his growingly noxious environment. Bevin dared to continue talking about his pain, but his language was always punctuated with hope, love, and good will. Bevin participated socially in spite of, and sometimes because of, his discomfort. Sometimes his thoughts were embedded in layers of opaqueness:

Action—it's gonna be scary.
I got a—mood—running here.
Will be—rescue.
I think my plan worked.
I can't breathe.
I can't my wings.

Other times, Bevin's language was completely lucid and transparent:

M	(trying to spell Dipolosaurus)
B	**I'll try to show you.**
M	I wonder why Crusty hangs out with them.
B	**He's Crusty Turtle.**
M	Yeah.
B	**The Crusty Turtle was old and mustachy.**

Bevin accepted new physical challenges he was ready for and rejected those he was not:

Never! (responding to the idea of play wrestling)
I gotta move away from here—how to handle this thing?
(responding to the side-to-side movement of a bolster swing)

He also found hope when he felt better:

I'm OK—better. I up—happy—bouncing here.

And he resisted things that seemed threatening:

Here—over there—don't come up with that thing.

Also, during this time, his mother reported that Bevin talked about me and

CDC daily and commented to a friend on the phone that because of me, he could **"take care of"** his school challenges and they could look forward to summer camp together.

Then one day, almost two months later, Bevin entered with: **"Hi Marge! I'm back!"** and, for the first time ever, proceeded to gather up all his things in the office to bring to the play room. The session was notable for Bevin's upper body dancing while he bounced on the big ball and the fact that he accompanied his performance with dramatic facial expressions. Later, he played invisible drums along with a movie. This performance confidence was new and part of his progress even when other qualities were not progressing. Even though gestalts and sound effects had become more prevalent as a way of "drowning out" the sounds of the world, movie narrating seemed to be the one arena that Bevin could maintain with his generative grammar. And, to his considerable credit, Bevin was able to maintain his sense of humor throughout this difficult period. After lots of gross motor activity, Bevin chose a fine motor one and proceeded to string plastic monkeys together on the trampoline. He laughed:

> **It's a funny: xxx I got a plan: stay home!**

Bevin was even able to maintain a fairly long conversation about finding another activity:

M	(bringing back some blocks)
B	**Take 'em away!**
M	(brings another activity)
B	**You're stinky.**
M	Sorry, bud.
B	**I'll get it.** (leaving to find an activity he likes)
B	**I suppose they was a try them.** (agreeing to try my 2nd selection)
M	(laughing)
B	**It was a long time ago.** (referring to having tried it when he was young)
M	I know; but you're ready now.
B	**What's the name again?**
M	It's just a fine motor activity.

But then after pinching a teacher at school, Bevin's gestalt comment was understandable:

> **I'm looking for a safe place to spend the night.**

And he actually talked directly about hope:

> **On Thursday, it will be hope.**
> **Now listen: Just a couple days, just a couple days will be spring break!**
> **Look everybody! Check it out! I'm bouncing! I'm OK—so remember, I'm OK!**

One caveat should be mentioned here. While Bevin did engage in longer conversations at times, and that language does appear fluent once it's on paper, it was spoken much too rapidly for most listeners to understand. Putting it on paper gives it an air of legitimacy, which it deserves, but also belies how difficult it was to hear in the midst of his sound effects and movies blaring loudly at the same time.

B	**It's called sticky, sticky goo.**
M	(taking a turn)
B	**I think—I think three more.** (requesting I find more jars of goo)
M	(commenting)
B	**What am I do—sticky goo.** (making a rhyme)
M	(laughing)
B	**I'm sticky and gooey.**
M	(commenting)
B	**It's not my fault.**
M	It's the goo's fault. (taking a stab at the meaning)
B	**No goo's fault.**
M	(maintaining the idea)
B	**Enough of this.**

That was beautiful!

Finally, after two months, Bevin began his listening therapy, and his first comment at Sheila's clinic said it all: **"I love, I love, I got a lot of love in here!"** After trying out a couple of CDs, Bevin tolerated listening to a third and commented: **"It's wonderful; that was beautiful!"** After listening as long as he could tolerate, Bevin applauded: **"Bravo, bravo, that was wonderful—and now—"**

Bevin then composed an **"I'm sorry"** song for his family and spent the remainder of the session exploring all the fine motor materials in Sheila's clinic, saying, **"Sorry, it's Bevin's day,"** as surely it was.

Bevin began his home listening program, and the next week, he came in without his headphones on and hugged me. He left them off for 20 minutes, until he started climbing. After 10 more minutes, he took them off again and listened to a movie at a level so quiet, I couldn't follow it. Then Bevin proceeded to compose a beautiful song about the movie I had failed to find for him. His maneuvering on the yellow swing around the trampoline was fluid, and his intonation was gorgeous. He said:

B	**I'm OK.**
M	You're awesome!
B	**And still I'm sorry—even more adventures.**

After three weeks on his listening program, Bevin's speech was clearer, and he came in with no headphones on at all while exploring the toy room for books and fine motor toys. He commented, **"I am a man. It's called 'I am a man.'"** He had no video on while playing with dinosaurs on the trampoline, and his voice sounded casual: **"Oh, very pretty!"** A half hour later, he put in a video but announced: **"Playing with the bigger boys now!"**

Additionally, Bevin seemed to have no real use for large motor regulation activities that day, calmly playing with fine motor things on the trampoline. He was, however, quite ok with assuming some postures that would challenge his core while he played. When the PT suggested that Bevin might be ready for some different kinds of things, Bevin responded: **"I'm fine—don't worry; I know exactly what I'm doing,"** and left the room. Before leaving CDC that day, Bevin added: **"I'm not ready yet."**

After a month, Bevin's positive changes waned, and he was clearly ready for a change in his listening program. His headphones were on more, and he was again "talking over life." But, interestingly, his syntax was growing more sophisticated, with question forms we had not heard before: **"What are you doing?" "What's that?" "What do you do with that?" "Why did you not . . . ?"** In the midst of the din, language was still developing. His family saw this too, and his mother commented, "Within the tumult inside of him, Bevin is growing inside with his language." And even as Bevin was needing some things to change in his life (like summer to come!), his faith never waned. His mother reported, "Bevin woke up this morning with, **'Hellooooo, Mama. I go to Marge's. Oh, happy day today! It's OK, Mom, I can do it. I will take care of you, of Bevin, happy, big, tall boy!'**"

Summer was good; Bevin took part in a daily YMCA camp again and also continued his listening program, his PT program, and his speech and language program. In the middle of the summer, I commented to Sheila that Bevin was more "available" than he had been for six months and that the goals I had set for him a half year ago were finally appropriate again. But it was hard to keep up with his listening program during the summer, and by fall, Sheila saw regression and recommended he begin it all over again.

Eighth grade: fright, fight, or flight

The year started out rough and was marked by an inconsistent school special education program. His OT listening program just wasn't enough, and Bevin checked out. His headphones were on more often than not, and Bevin got used to talking more to himself than to others. People got used to not listening to him. But again, in spite of it all, Bevin continued to make progress in language development. It's just that it was hard to see amidst the "movie talk," and few people really got to hear the best of Bevin. In a report to his school in November, I wrote the following:

Under more usual conditions, when Bevin is trying to protect himself from auditory and other sensory bombardment, he typically 'watches' a favorite movie in his head and produces the sound track. It takes a quiet, predictable, safe environment for Bevin to take off his (literal or figurative) headphones and allow his left brain to engage with (real time) language.

This is a classic 'fright, fight or flight' scenario ... Bevin's regulation fluctuates widely, and can change quickly. Because his auditory sensitivity is so acute, Bevin simply cannot comfortably exist in an environment that is too loud! If he wears his headphones and can engage in non-stop self-talk (say the movie tracks as he watches movies in his head), he can manage to remain in the environment.

If one of those two survival elements is not 'allowed,' Bevin is at severe risk of being dysregulated to the point that he will be in immediate 'fright, fight, or flight.' What this means is Bevin will 'flee' if allowed; he will panic if not allowed to flee; and he will 'fight back' if he cannot flee. At that point Bevin will pinch or bite out of desperation. While he is incredibly sorry to have done so, and will say, **"I'm sorry, I'm sorry, I'm sorry,"** he is then dysregulated to the point that he is desperate. As we know from the sensory integration literature, a bite is grounding like almost no other physical input ... last Friday he wanted me to find the movie, *Amazing Miracles*. As Bevin told me, **"I was wishing for a miracle."**

It went on like this for months, with his outside programs unable to offset the challenges inherent in middle school and growing up, especially growing up in a noisy environment that had too little program support to offset it. Bevin's private OT, Sheila, felt Bevin desperately needed deep vestibular input, and she was challenged to find ways to provide it with the intensity he seemed to need. As Bevin said, **"It's like my head's in a vice—I've been too hurt—I need a movie."**

But as the fall went on, things got better. At school, his program evened out, and in PT and OT, vestibular input was starting to register. Plus, the holidays were getting close.

Winter holidays

Like they had years before, Thanksgiving and Christmas breaks offered Bevin hope again, and we had good sessions all through November and December. One treat was that Bevin was developing enough body awareness and motor planning that his gestures were coming alive. As delayed as his language was, it was always ahead of his nonverbal communication. With gesture, though, Bevin was becoming a "ham," acting out stories he watched in front of the mirror.

Watching the walls of Jericho tumble down on his TV screen, Bevin paddled himself away, saying, **"Let's get out of Jordan!"**

And as his body began catching up with his brain, Bevin also seemed to be developing a fledgling sense of himself as a player in his own life. When he was young, he used to become upset at the movie protrayal of people flying. He would demand that I understand that he felt he could not fly. But, after receiving PT and OT during these intense growing years, Bevin not only seemed to come to grips with his developing body, but, more basically, that he had a body at all. This was our conversation as Bevin bounced high on the therapy ball:

B	**That's fly.** (watching himself in the mirror)
B	**I can't fly.**
M	Yes you can—you can fly in your mind.
B	**I can fly!**

But the conundrum continued:

B	**It's time for me to get back to business.**
B	**When I can sit still—**
B	**You can fly: that's a lie.**
M	It's not a lie; it's an idea.

During the session before Thanksgiving, as Bevin paddled away from Jordan, he watched himself in the mirror, bouncing on a giant ball and declared,

> **"Look, I'm flying!"**

And later in December, Bevin one-upped himself with a deliberate pose with outstretched arms, declaring, **"I can fly!"**

Bevin also explored feelings and their expression both sincerely and playfully. He play-acted along with movies, watching himself as he made faces, hugged himself, looked incredulous, and glared at an unseen impostor. He gestured with dramatic emphasis and added nonverbals to support his verbal communication. His mother's description of him was priceless: "He is naughty every day, takes one look at my mush face and then kisses me and says, **"Do this, Mom. Look, the lips go up and that is happy. The happy face is a good choice, Mom. I am sorry sorry, your highness: I will never, ever do it again. Mama, show me lips up now."**

Use your words

That winter, a scary incident occurred in Bevin's neighborhood. Unbeknownst to his family, Bevin had heard about it and it must have spawned a nightmare. Bevin surprised his PT and me by talking and drawing about it for one hour straight one day. We knew little of the incident itself, so were really only able to offer sympathetic partnership, yet Bevin worked it himself. A few of his sentences are included here, to give a sense of the conversation: **"I had no idea … these kind of stinks ran in the street … Stinks, bad dream … And a trouble here, princess bride … I had no idea these kind of trucks run in the streets … Eyes of mean, young man … A fly … boo a run … run, hide … boo run … whatever … Really stinks … run hide! That girl … and by the king of command, that girl's gonna be a princess bride! … and by next Friday, you should see princess bride … Be back later … big trouble: sad, sad … And by sad figure … We better fly; don't run; sad princess bride … By the king of command: sad face, bad dreams … Shoo shoo! Get out … I know you: you're the famous diamond back. I'm warning you."** "Use your words," we say; Bevin did! Think of it as "talk therapy."

Suddenly, a new-born king

As Christmas approached, Bevin's interest in the Bible expanded beyond Jericho and the miracles. Bevin often revisited old Sunday School lessons and re-watched the videos he'd not fully understood the first time around. He wanted me to witness these stories so I could help him unravel parts that never quite made sense. The Old Testament proved difficult, but with the help of his family, who'd gotten him these videos in the first place, we got through it together. "Use your words," we say; Bevin continued to.

A long way to go

As the second semester of eighth grade began, Bevin was still in pain more often than he could cope with. He tried to escape into the movies in his head and spoke the movie lines non-stop. Even though communication faltered, the occasional dialogue revealed how much Bevin realized his challenge. **"I've got a long way to go,"** he'd say. **"And you're going to take me there, and not give me any trouble—right?"** Bevin's January goals were telling, as it wasn't until Goal 6 that language was even mentioned. Most of the goals were about re-finding that place that supports language; that's how basic our language program had become. The goals are included here as testimony to the struggles our students face and we need to face, for the sake of our students:

1. Abate, monitor and decrease sensory defensiveness
2. Develop primary muscle awareness and use
3. Increase development and use of fine motor skills
4. Continued development and use of motor planning skills
5. Develop awareness of challenges to positive social interactions
6. Regain tolerance and productive use of language models
7. Increase percentage of self-generated language
8. Continue development of self-generated language
9. Continue development of functional use of social language

I wanna get back to the laughs

As motivated as he was to do well, Bevin was clearly counting the months until summer:

M	Bevin's counting the months till summer.
B	**Five!**

And he had some pretty strong feelings about winter:

B	**ABC winter—XYZ winter.**
M	It's just gone on too long.
B	**No.**
M	No?
B	**It's ugly.**
M	You're right about that.
B	**Winter's OK once in a while.**

Bevin spent his productive language time engaged in stories. He explored Nemo, swimming in groups, escaping, and growing up. As he said:

B	**They're in a school.**
M	Yup, they're in a school.
B	**Of course, I go to college. Yes, sir!**
M	Of course you will, smart Bevin!

His sense of the future re-emerged, and even though our PT was leaving, Bevin took advantage of the last month of his company. Bevin would get well set-up and announce, **"I wanna get back to the laughs."** To his credit, he was able to say things like, **"I'm free; I'm free; I'm alive!"** And he was quick to acknowledge my part in his life:

M	You did it!
B	**We did it.**

He was proud of himself, seemed to have lost his self-consciousness, and no longer had to hide. Through OT and PT, Bevin had become aware of his body, and a conversation with Sheila showed just how aware.:

S	(reading an explanation of how a music CD was intended to integrate the right and left sides)
M	Two arms, two sides of your brain, two legs.
B	**And my body too.**

Another conversation with Sheila was revealing:

S	(telling Bevin about how the ear is the integrator of the body)
B	**This mean—trying to get his rest.**
B	**Can you hear me, Doc?**
B	**Like I got my head in a bottle.**
S	It'll get better.
B	**That's the patient!**

Another OT session was successful in introducing Bevin to some intense vestibular input. As Sheila predicted, it did affect his ears, as his lowered head was at the center of the movement. His language was telling:

My ears ringing. Boy, my ears ringing

As the session continued, Sheila attempted to introduce Bevin to a follow-up activity on a scooter board. Bevin's response was clear:

S	That's cool.
B	**It's not.**
M	Not yet?
B	**I did say 'not'!**

Along with Bevin's increased use of his body in his self-expression came timing and intonation. Up until that time, Bevin's intonation was all about the source of his language, as he would take on the tone and timing of the original gestalt. But as he started to become the actor in his own drama, Bevin gave more and more of his own voice to his words. He experimented and practiced nuance and tried on all kinds of voices. He was becoming himself, but he was working on figuring out who he actually was!

Taking stock

Bevin still used his sound-track language to mask the world's noise more often than not. So while evidence of grammar development was still there, it only showed up in bits and pieces. Meaning really mattered to his need for grammar, so one day in January, when Bevin really wanted to understand what was happening, he produced these questions:

Where we gonna go?
What do with them?
Where am I go? Go back to school?
Where did we go?
Where'd everybody go?

Realizing that these tenuous, beautiful question forms represented yet-emerging grammar, I was excited. But I was also aware that there was not a reliable way to take a language sample that would demonstrate Bevin's growth and capture his current competence.

So, by the middle of the spring semester of Bevin's eighth grade year, I had assembled all the grammatical structures Bevin had produced since Christmas, and I wanted to share them with everyone in his life. Each session had a theme or two, and, when he wasn't hiding in "movie talk," Bevin only had time to work on the particular grammar that lent itself to the topic of the day. For this reason, it was impossible to inventory all of the grammar Bevin had within his competence short of looking at a two-month period of time. But once it was all assembled, we held a family-and-friends workshop to look at the various categories of grammar and formulation and brainstormed ways we could help Bevin use each more, practice it with a variety of vocabulary, and master it.

Recognizing that only the SLP reader might be truly interested in this list, it is still included to give a more complete picture of what Bevin was actually doing with his grammar at age fifteen. This still sounds almost like an oxymoron, but, it's not: this mid-teenager was still developing grammar.

Of the total inventory, a few categories were well-practiced, and Bevin could produce this grammar frequently and with ease. It helped to start a sentence with one of these structures so he could give himself time to produce a unique ending. And it helped immensely that he could put "It's ..." and "It's called ..." with virtually any of his vocabulary words and take part in conversation. Then there were some sentence starters that took just a bit more self-regulation to access, but Bevin usually could say all the pronoun and verb forms listed below. Following is a sample of utterances in the most important categories.

Table 20: Bevin's Grammar - Pronouns
It's: *It's fixed; It's a sorry; It's full of Pumba; It's too heavy; It's late;* etc. (numerous examples, including occasional advanced vocabulary: *"It's nauseating."*)
This is and That's: *This is fun; This is powerful; This is trash—this is the color of trashy; That's bad; That's really stinks; That's bad news; That's right; That's not right; That's really funny; That's what I call 'that was fun'; That's mine?* (numerous other examples)
I: *I lost; I said 'trouble'; I don't like it; OK, I'll try; Excuse me, I'm shy.*
You: *You're up; You are stay here; You sure? It's you, Barney; And you best friend; I trusted you.*
He: *He's grouchy; He did it; I know he's somewhere; He said it's own way; He said it's all right.*
We: *We did it! We don't need it.*

Table 21: Bevin's Grammar - Verb forms

Verb commands: *Take it down; Sit there; Stop it; Stop singing; Leave my friends alone; Leave weed whackers alone.*

Am (to be verb): *I'm shy, I'm going back home; I'm happy about this; I'm thinking … think this funny; I'm free; I'm free; I'm alive; I'm feeling like a valentine.*

To be: *I want to be a Walter.* (his dad)

Present tense verbs: *That sounds like Walter; That sounds like a boy; That tickles; You are stay here; So you are scary fight.*

Future tense verbs: *It gonna work; This is gonna work; We're gonna stop that; Gonna get stripes out; Gonna be a 'be careful'; It will be soon; I will never again; Paradise—will be running very fast; I'll go around—then trash; I'll do it; I'll check it out; I'll take the water home; That'll work.*

Past tense verbs: *That was a whole year long; That was fun and good; That was scary, the holy ghost in heaven; Bevin was shy; I lost, I said 'trouble'; Gorilla said, 'Diamond in the rough'; Eagle said, 'Aaaah, wonderful, wonderful, beautiful'; I saw them; Then Tarzan moved and fight back; It sounded like he in trouble; She's not feel a little bad about that—I dreamed about.*

Secondary verbs: *I think I didn't; I think I do; I think I'm gonna be here all day; He said you can do it; We gotta try to stop him.*

Passive verbs: *He's got hands; It's called …* (numerous examples)*; I got caught.*

Table 22: Bevin's Grammar - Question forms

What: *What's funny? What's goin' on here? What's that? What is that? What is the matter with her? What is it, Mom? What a stranger here? What are you looking at? What are you doing? What are you thinking about? What kind of drum? What kind of song?* (many examples)*; What do with them? What? I did listen the teacher—I did!*

Where: *Where's Mom? Where's Papa? Where's my couch? Where's Tarzan? Where we gonna go? Where am I go?*

When: *When does he get a chance?*

Who: *Who are you?*

Why: *Why are you stopping? Why? Why is the body go? Why the flying go?*

Others: *Do you see that? Is the 'shut up' out of the bag?*

Table 23: Bevin's Grammar - Negatives

Not: *That's not so hard; I not see him anywhere; It's not an ogre—it's a stegasuarus; Not yet, please.*

Don't: *Don't bounce me on the tops; I don't like this; I don't like that; Please don't!*

Can't: *I can't see; I can't fly; I can't a bee; I can't, over there; I can't even be—the boy.*

Others: *No, I didn't; Doesn't look stranger; You shouldn't have to go.*

Table 24: Bevin's Grammar - Conjunctions

And: *That's another Bevin's hats left over—brown and red and white; I'm a boy and I'm sorry; That's really funny—can't talk—there he is and there he is; Hairy and dinosaurs and Barney and like that.*

Combinations: *I know it here somewhere; I'll do this, you move the trampoline; What I am—person; That sounds like 'crazy'; That sounds like he's in trouble; That sounded like he's in trouble; That's what I call 'that was fun'; Just a little bit, then take 'em away; That was country—that was heaven—that was world around; One good American boy—an American—green blue and the earth—out there, the earth; OK, I'll go round, then trash—satisfied; Ball, then swing, then go—you go.*

Table 25: Bevin's Grammar - Other formulations

Phrase starters (verb forms, Just, And, Maybe): *Tastes like mango and …; Tastes like horrible; Tastes like vermin funny; Sorry about a wise and scary; Just a wise and scary—get a beat up; Such a wise and large and danger; Sort of wise and scary—danger; Just want the purple, different; Just when the Bevin is careful—just Bevin is careful; Maybe sharptooth eat them; Maybe birdbrain stink 'em; Maybe crazy jaguar; Maybe a stranger.*

Grammatical competence in real life

Reading over this composite list, a few comments are in order:

First, Bevin's competence with grammar was evident more or less of the time, depending on the circumstances. If he had good self-regulation and could take his time, he used his well-practiced grammar flexibly and allowed himself the freedom to experiment and reformulate. The next example is illustrative. Bevin's OT, Sheila, had wanted to try a different swing for vestibular input. Bevin loved the purple swing but wanted to use it in a different way, one that he could control. He maintained his head in an upright position almost all the time and was not comfortable relinquishing control when he couldn't see out of the lycra and didn't know how his body would feel. So he said:

> **"Just want the purple—different."**
> **"Just when the Bevin is careful—just Bevin is careful."**

Secondly, if you read closely, you will notice that the vocabulary content of the grammatical sentences was typically limited. When Bevin used grammar accurately, he used easy-to-retrieve vocabulary, although occasional higher-level vocabulary occurred with "It's …" and "That's … ." On the other hand, the phrase starters and other favorite formulations like "That sounds like …" provided a vehicle for some "mix and match" of automatic form and more difficult-to-retrieve vocabulary. Interestingly, looking ahead to the next year, Bevin ultimately spent hours and hours on this aspect of his language development: using the grammar and sentence starters he had and combining them with a constantly-growing vocabulary. He used a pattern similar to the following sequence as he looked out the window:

> **Someone stranger here; Here's a someone; Maybe a stranger; Doesn't look stranger.**

But at the time of the spring workshop, I was just excited to share Bevin's grammatical competence and emerging forms with his family and other team members so they could help model and monitor them. At the same time, however, one caveat was given to Bevin's family and friends: don't be surprised to find colorful gestalts still alive and well, and embedded in otherwise grammatical sentences. Sometimes Bevin had no useful or retrievable alternative; sometimes they just said it best:

> **Almost spring be our guest.**
> **I've got sweet savoir faire.**

Conversation re-emerges

It was mentioned at the beginning of this chapter that Bevin's long conversation on behalf of the toy animals was unique in sixth grade. Actually it was unique during all of his middle school years, given how much of his energy he used just to get by. Bevin resorted to self-talk when he needed to escape and communicated as best he could the rest of the time. He often engaged in two- to three-turn conversations, but rarely seven or eight. Seeing the end of middle school in sight, however, was occasion enough to stimulate a ten-turn conversation, although the level of both grammar and vocabulary was minimal:

B	**Four months about—March, April, May, and June.**
M	Really three months till summer now.
B	**And then—**
M	And then three months of summer!
B	**And this almost over.**
M	Yup, your last spring of middle school!

B	**And this mean—**
M	It means—
B	**Escape!**
M	(laughing)
B	**It's over!**
M	It's good to have spring break too—just to relax and think.
B	**Think very well.**
M	You do think very well!
B	**Five days from school.**
M	Right!
B	**It will be soon.**
M	It will be, buddy.
B	**Soon!**

Looking at the limited language within this conversation makes the toy dialogue from two and a half years before even more significant. Had Bevin not completed that dialogue in sixth grade and had I not been able to record it, I might not have been able to demonstrate to myself, to Bevin, and to his family how far his grammar development had come. I was grateful all through Bevin's middle school years for that conversation (a "window" into his competence), and how I'd resisted the temptation to just say "no" to his initial request. His middle school life might have been so different if I had been more worried about the clinic's collection of toys than his communication.

Conversational dialogue morphs into ...

Bevin had long used favorite movies as beginning points in many ways: sometimes narrating over them to offer his own take on the subject, sometimes providing his own "voice-over" with the sound turned off, and often to ask a question or to share a referent with the clinician. Following is a portion of a 17-turn dialogue during which he was playing a Timmy the Tooth movie. The theme was familiar: the trouble with school. The Cavity Goon was never mentioned by name, but his influence was indeed felt:

B	**I don't need the stinkin' all day.**
M	I know you don't.
B	**Come on, check it off.**
M	I know, it's so structured.
B	**It's time for us to go.**
M	And we will this summer.
B	**As we gather—**
M	Yup, we'll gather up all the toys and take them outside.
B	**I am sorry 'bout this.**
M	Nope, it's a worthy plan.
B	**Four years, all work, sorry.**

M	You're right, Buddy; summer will be great.
B	**Have—have to stop.**

The following is an example of a conversation in which Bevin asked a question about the main character in the movie, Kiki:

B	**The queen—but she's queen.**
M	I think she calls herself a witch, because she has powers—not bad powers, good powers.
B	**It's not fair.**
M	Not the right term to call her a 'witch'?
B	**Get rid of it.**
M	And call her a queen? OK?

Another kind of exploration occurred with topics that had special meaning to Bevin: gorillas, animals in captivity, adults, and dogs. Following is a portion of a conversation about dogs—one dog in particular, I learned. After each of Bevin's comments, I'd either take a turn or not, depending on if I'd figured out the theme or question and had anything relevant to say. The background here is that Bevin's family had owned a dog, partly to give Bevin experience with dogs, which he'd been afraid of. But when they learned it needed more room and exercise, they had to give it away. In the following conversation, I learned that Bevin didn't understand this and thought it had run away. Apparently, Bevin felt real guilt about not "following this dog," but after this conversation, his family was able to give Bevin the reassurance he needed to assuage his guilt:

I was thinking about the dog.
Scared—those dogs.
Running with dogs.
Running after the dogs.
And I followed this dogs.
Doggie.
Dog was you.
That was—June is—ruff ruff.
Leave the dog here.

Story evolution begins

While he watched the old cartoon of Bongo, the captive bear who goes to live in the woods, Bevin also combined his theme of summer freedom with dogs and home:

You can't get away.
I gotta get away.
Ah—that's what I call a freedom boy.

Bevin then mimicked wearing a straight jacket as he looked in the mirror, and opened up his arms:

> **I'm free boy.**
> **I'm free—** (howling)
> **I'm coming back home.**
> **Come, boy.**

And as he 'rode' away, with a dramatic look of bliss on his face, he added:

> **I'm a Bevin, a boy.**

In another version of the story, Bevin shifted characters, being himself for one utterance, then an unnamed adult (A) for the other. As himself, he was 'handcuffed,' and as the adult, he assumed an authoritative manner and voice:

A	**And then listen, listen conscience, Bevin boy.**
B	**Catch you later.**
A	**Hey, Bevin boy.**

Bevin then practiced this narrative/monologue for the naive Bongo on the TV screen (V=video scene and video narrative). In this exercise, Bevin first provided an alternative monologue for Bongo but then began narrating in the third person, returning to monologue momentarily:

V	This is the life.
B	**This stinks.**
V	Ah!
B	**And I don't know—**
V	(Bongo lying down)
B	**You're free.**
V	(Bongo falling asleep)
B	**I'm free.**
V	(scenes of Bongo in the forest)
B	**The dawn of life.** (etc: bits of mitigations)
V	(birds chirping)
B	**Oh, geeze.**
V	(Bongo meeting Lulu Belle, the girl bear)
B	**Wonderful.**
B	**Trees and clouds.**
V	(the same scene)
V	(Bongo meeting the natural bear)
B	**Hello!**
V	When bears are really in love, they say it with a slap.
B	**Be rough and tough and mean and growls.**
V	(rewound to repeat that scene)
B	**Time to growl again and scare—**

This narrative/monologue continued, and then Bevin selected other movies such as *Mickey and the Beanstalk* for creating narrative/monologues. Over time, these stories morphed more and more into true third-person narratives, which Bevin continued to practice during the summer.

The first of the following comments is Bevin narrating *Aladdin and the King of Thieves*. This was difficult. The next three are his stage directions to Aladdin. These were easy:

> **Flying forward in time. Put them in flying forward time.**
> **Run, that's him over there!**
> **Man, go back!**
> **Now look, gorilla!**

In this way, Bevin continued his grammar development while working on things he cared deeply about: story-telling, story-creation, and subjects that were important to him.

The central character in his own story

Bevin practiced a lot that spring. Since he was less and less self-conscious about being seen, heard, and even video-taped, he sometimes enjoyed seeing his creations afterwards. But as his long-time friend and confidante, I knew my role was a privileged one, and I didn't want to "wear out my welcome." I tried to be judicious in my feedback and just deliver it when I thought it would be truly useful to Bevin. Above all, I wanted him to continue to live his life in front of me and with me.

Categories, vocabulary, and more

Another area that developed during that last spring of middle school was Bevin's vocabulary, albeit a fairly idiosyncratic one. Some of his words had a long history: they were the particular words he associated with feelings, good and bad. "Bester" was the actual family name of his favorite relatives, and "besters" were those things he liked best. Camels were his favorite animals because they were in the Bible, so "camels" came to stand for an entire group of animals he loved. "Desert," too, was the place of the Holy Land, so all things "desert" were in a class of their own. "Pumpkins" were a bit more difficult to figure out, but seemed to mean special things to look forward to, like Halloween pumpkins that Papa would keep in the garage until the special day when they emerged. Other categories developed over the summer: wolf-catchers, life, Fun and Fancy Free, God, What have you done?, China, and 'I told you.' When things didn't seem to fall into a category and were sort of a hodgepodge, Bevin labeled them "gangwar," which seemed to be a phonetic rendition of "gangway," with the same sense of chaos.

Bevin's mother once claimed that I "spoke Bevineze." Well, I didn't for a long time, but now "camels" was a category I found myself applying to my favorite animals: pelicans, blue herons, and wolves. For Bevin, though, a "wolf catcher" made up an entirely different category, so we didn't necessarily share all aspects of vocabulary.

Picking up the pace

As Bevin's self-regulation improved that spring, so did his availability for language models. It had been almost three years since his openness had been this great, so I tried to take advantage of the opportunity without stepping on his toes and ruining my potential to help continue his language development. The following is the kind of dialogue we had in which I provided judicious, but useful, language models:

B	**That was whole year long.**
M	It was a long school year.
B	**Coast is clear.**
M	Almost clear.
B	**It's almost clear.**

Another way I unobtrusively modeled language was by writing down what Bevin said and then inserting missing words or my turn in the conversation with a different colored marker. Bevin loved the written word and always read the completed conversations out loud. This is the type of completed conversation he read:

B	**I thought I was blue. I don't belong.**
M	I'm sorry I was gone last week.
B	**Sorry alright!**
B	**Go on, go on—Bevin go on now.**
M	We can both go on now.

Two more examples are:

B	**Bevin was scared.**
M	Words can hurt.
B	**Tell us a story from the good book.**
M	Words can heal.
B	**I've learned to live with it.**
B	**One week ago—**
M	I was gone. I was sad. I'm happy to be back.
B	**I was happy.**
B	**Missed our talk.**
M	Me too—I missed our playing.

Bevin's longest oral conversations occurred around figuring out the logistics of something, such as play equipment. One particular swing afforded occasional conversations, where Bevin used my input to modify his language. In one instance, he took fourteen turns to get some lycra to work the way he wanted. A part of our dialogue was:

B	**Take this swing away.**
M	It's floppy.
B	**It's too floppy.**

Bevin's directions and commentary lasted for eleven more sentences, with his last sentence: **"That's better; it's satisfying."**

As the middle school experience began to dim, Bevin began to believe in himself again. For the following, Bevin selected a video to establish the topic of conversation. My words are not included here, but this conversation gave me the opportunity to comment on Bevin's intelligence and his readiness for the future.

V	There are some things I can't do.
B	**I can't; I can't.**
V	I want things the way they were.
B	**I'm not stupid.**

He also commented: **"Gorilla—maybe—he can talk. Who cares? I know he will."**

Bevin still had occasional bad days at school during the spring. On one, I picked him up from school to go to OT and he observed, **"It's a grey day; let's get out of here."** But after a half hour of therapeutic music, Bevin said, **"Thanks for helping; thanks for your help."** After intense vestibular input at OT, Bevin commented: **"I'm breathed,"** and at the end he said, **"This is an awesome world. That was wonderful—thing."**

Finally, at the end of the school year, Bevin's own words described the push-pull of growing up and entering another phase of life. He had made the choice to go to a school dance on a Friday night instead of being at the clinic with me. He loved the dance, but missed the security of being at the clinic. His juxtaposing of comments was a perfect expression of the push forward and pull backwards that is growing up. The past is "jail," but it's "safe." Here are his words: **"I'm safe in here. I'm never going out of this jail again. I'm safer here. I will never not go out this jail."**

But "out of jail" Bevin did emerge.

Grammar and other developments

Looking ahead to the next year now, Bevin's grammar continued to develop through the summer and during his entire first year of high school. This meant that grammatical development continued until Bevin was seventeen years old. And while his continuing acquisition of syntax was exciting, it mattered more and more that Bevin was honored in his high school and supported to use his grammar and the other parts of his language to communicate, to create, and to demonstrate his intelligence and learning.

High school was a wonderful time for Bevin and truly paved the way for life-long learning—the topic of the next chapter. What made high school work for Bevin was that his OT, his listening therapy, his speech and language, and his summer camp all continued, but especially that his school team really appreciated him. They found him smart, spirited, and funny, and the opportunities to explore the world of social interaction and vocational possibilities appealed to Bevin.

It was evident that Bevin had come a long way since his early mitigitaion days three years before. One phrase from those days is illustrated here (language sample on page 175). It was clever, but Bevin was beyond clever. In his own words, Bevin was now beginning the journey from **"Bevin, the boy"** to **"Bevin, the man."**

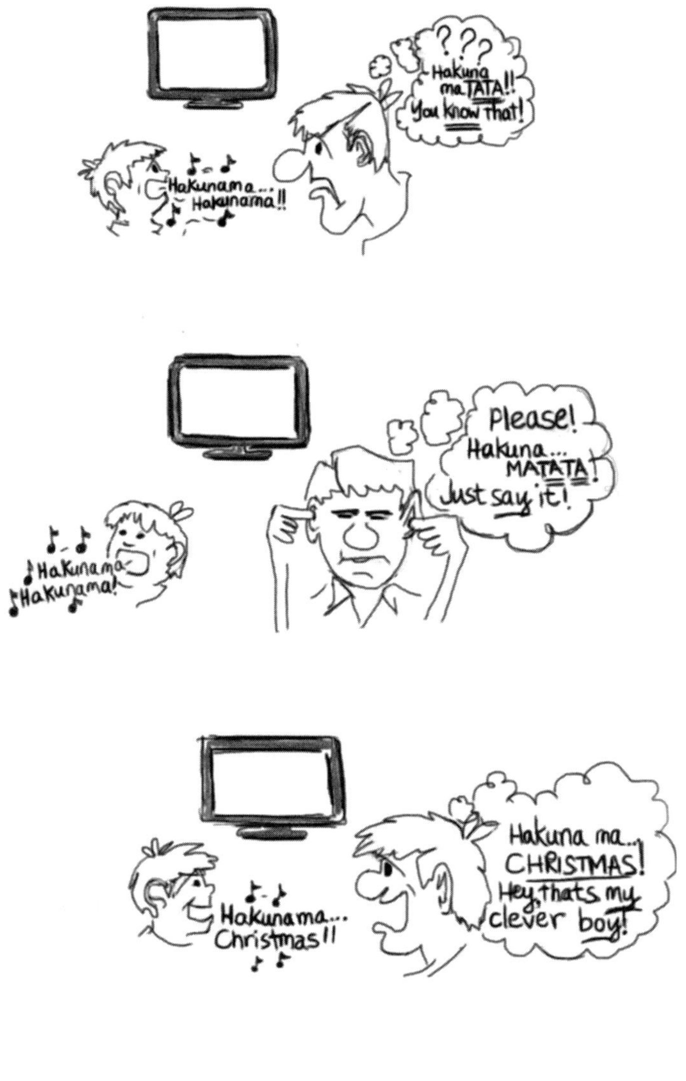

Chapter 16
High School and Lifelong Learners: Functional Communication

Grammar: it's all about how we use it

Our journey in this book is paved with grammar. But grammar only describes the paving bricks; it's the journey along that road that matters. So even before grammar began to develop, we were watching for what would motivate our kids to set out on that journey. We were paying attention to what was important to our kids and what would help them see it through. We were watching for signs of communicative intent, non-verbal or verbal. And along the way, as our students developed grammar, we were making sure they had a wealth of life opportunities to develop functional uses for that grammar: seeking information, sharing opinions, interacting with friends, and developing self-advocacy skills, but also more advanced uses like playing with ideas, postulating, and testing hypotheses. And all along the way, we tried to make sure our students were having fun.

Regardless of whether our students' language was Stage 1 echolalia, Stage 2 mitigation, Stage 3 words and phrases, or Stage 4–6 sentences, the salient quality was always how that language was used.

And later, after our students' development of grammar ceases, we know that their use of language will continue to grow for the rest of their lives. Throughout their teenage years, their young adult years, and all the years after that, their use of language can expand to meet the opportunties of the environments they find themselves in.

When our kids were in third grade, their language was used to tell and write personal stories. By middle school, language was used for demonstrating knowledge. This will only expand in high school and beyond, when language will be used to present one's self to others and to learn and share the tasks of life and work.

So, what can we do to support life-long learning with language? On the one hand, we need to make sure that language tasks are tailored to each student and that they can be achieved with the grammar a student has. On the other hand, we need to pay attention to whether grammatical competencies are being fully utilized. In other words, if a student has mastered Stage 4 grammar, he has all the basics of sentence formulation within his competency plus the ability to form basic compound sentences. Let's look at how his writing composition can sound: "The kids all went to the water park and stayed there all morning. They left at noon and brought souvenirs back with them." It's not fancy, but with

Stage 4 grammar, sentences such as these can be constructed for most basic tasks.

If a student has Stage 5 grammar competencies, he can use all the basic conjunctions and can form temporal constructions such as, "The kids all went to the water park, but couldn't stay very long. They had to get back to school, so they got souvenirs to take home." If a student has Stage 6 grammar, there are no grammatical limits to the constructions he can assemble, even with the temporal order mixed. He can use embedded clauses as in this example, "The kids all went to the water park, and before they left to go back to school, they each bought a souvenir to take home."

Grammar enables complex expression. If grammar is incompletely developed, it limits that complexity. But, even with basic grammar, composition is usually adequate for relating experiences, narrating stories, and explaining ideas sequentially. With advanced grammar, the sky is the limit.

The older a student is when he masters grammar, the less practice he has using it.

It should be remembered, however, that the older a student is when he masters grammar, the less practice he has using it. Think for a moment about the typically-developing child who has Stage 6 grammar by kindergarten. Complex constructions at that time of life are about the childish things of life, and few demands are placed on the child to construct stories and explanations. He uses his grammar quite naturally and easily all day long. When a child has had a chance to practice naturally, the demands of school are then developmentally appropriate and appropriately challenging.

Grammatical competence is one thing; ready access to that competence is another.

But our students who have mastered grammar by third grade, fifth grade, or tenth grade face challenges enough simply incorporating that grammar into daily life. Using newly-acquired grammar to write, to tell stories, or to explain are not appropriate expectations until that student has developed automaticity with the regular use of spoken, conversational grammar. Grammatical competence is one thing; ready access to that competence is another.

Similarly, functional communication needs practice time.

Functional communication over time

We need to be purposeful in building in communicative opportunities for our kids and sympathetic to how little practice they may have had along the way.

While our kids are growing up, we always want to make sure that the communicative functions they are expressing with language are expanding along with their skill in using higher-level language. But just as grammatical development is delayed for our kids, so, too, is their functional use of language. What is typical for the beginning kindergartener is not present for our kids until third grade, fifth grade, tenth grade, or even later. While we need to be watchful and purposeful in building in communicative opportunities for our growing kids, we need also to be sympathetic to how little practice they may have had along the way. "Finding" language when it hasn't been there for very long is a challenge and requires thoughtful attending to one's self. Regulation and a supportive environment help students come up with their best language. But when the chips are down, it is the old language that often resurfaces. Newer grammar takes time to find.

But time is on our students' side. Unlike grammar, which has a neurologically-defined capacity, functional skill-building can continue for the rest of our students' lives. As adults, we all continue to build skills as we to adapt our communication to the circumstances of our changing lives. So, too, will our children as they become adults. Form and function are partners, but function trumps form as the skill set we all can continue to build for the rest of our lives.

Bevin prepares for high school

We left Bevin in the last chapter as he was regaining his self-regulation and gaining motor skills—and his functional language was blossoming. And he was about to embark on high school, which was very supportive of his continued growth.

The summer before high school was one of exploration, when Bevin was able to work on bringing together the parts of himself that were developing: his sense of his body, his sense of space, his emergence into fine motor skill, his motor planning, his grammar, and, most importantly, his sense of himself as an actor in his own life.

Our sessions that summer were spent outside as much as possible, and tended to go longer and longer into the night as he had so much he wanted to accomplish. As we mentioned in Chapter 16, some of his progress started the previous spring as Bevin began practicing original dialogues between himself and others. His first were with the movie characters, Bongo and Mickey Mouse. Then he expanded by role-playing as if dialoguing with people. As the spring came to a close, Bevin was developing his stance vis-a-vis the adults around him. In these snippets, B is Bevin speaking for himself, and A is Bevin speaking for an adult:

A	**Beware of—anywhere.**
A	**Come over here, Bevin!**
B	**Born to be wild!**
A	**That's better.**
A	**Well run along—push!**
B	**That's right!**
B	**I don't need no stuck in all day.**
A	**Why you little means!**

Negotiation was also done in real life, as Bevin had the following kinds of conversations with his OT as they jointly figured out just the right input to his feet (S=Sheila):

B	**Yeah, we're flying—**
B	**Take your hands—**

B	**Ow; owchie, huh?**
S	Sorry.
B	**Perfect.**
B	**Where are my toes?**
S	Right here.
B	**Soft and breezy.**
S	How about the other foot?
B	**You find these feet. They're out there.**
S	(manipulating his left foot)
B	**You are so stop it!**
B	(pulling away)
B	**Stop this racket!**

The summer began with great relief, as his parents noted in an email in June: "Bevin came home beaming and happy and relaxed and slept well. He woke up relaxed and happy, packed his own bag and lunch, got ready by himself and waited outside, and then he went camp giggling and silly. He came home and said, **"Mom! I went to Marge's, Mom!"** Thank you, Marge, for helping to save him."

Bevin's progress peport in July noted the following:

> Bevin has had a wonderful summer so far. He triumphantly met the end of the school year, declaring that he was free! His language changed gradually from talk of 'means' and 'hyenas in the Pridland' and being 'sorry'—to rainbows, relationships, and, increasingly, storytelling. The transition to summer also included an increase in fine motor activity, first at the end of his OT sessions and then throughout all his CDC sessions. His progress during the summer has been remarkable!

Particular areas of progress were noted:

> 1. Bevin has increased his awareness of his own state of sensory comfort and uses several strategies to increase his self-regulation:
>
> - Given maximal support (environmental, physical, emotional support, and social permission), Bevin moves freely to vary his distance from others and keeps himself adequately self-regulated.

- Given moderate support (less environmental, emotional, and social support, but maximal physical activity), Bevin moves within the confines available and achieves adequate self-regulation. Settings include YMCA camp with trained, familiar counselors; home environment under low-demand conditions; after-school program with trained staff in the gym and the library.

- Given minimal support (few environmental or physical supports, fluctuating emotional support, and increased social challenges such as high noise levels at school), Bevin tunes out the world around him with headphones or watches internal 'movies' and moves within the confines available, but never achieves adequate self-regulation.

2. Engagement in social conversation with the adults close to him, using language (as opposed to sounds effects) 75% of the time and grammar at DSS levels 3–6 80% of the time with 40% accuracy. Bevin has drastically increased the time he spends engaged in social conversation with adults close to him and has achieved the use of language 75% of the time when maximally supported by one of these familiar adults! One barely recognizes 'the new Bevin' without his headphones and his sound effects!

- Bevin's use of grammar at DSS levels 3–6 fluctuates with the topic and the availability of specific linguistic information (written, provided by the partner, etc.), but has reached 75% of the time during limited conversations, given maximal support. The accuracy of Bevin's grammar fluctuates with his familiarity with the particular grammatical structures used, but reaches 40% during limited conversations, given maximal support.

- Examples of basic level grammar, often sentences with newer vocabulary words:

  That's weird.
  It was a long time ago; it was an inspiration.
  They fail, couldn't kill.
  They're life; it's love.
  Rizzo the Rat here: "That boy's in trouble!"
  A bat from a jungle out there.
  I'm thinking.
  Please stop fight.
  Put her down and put her down and put me down.
  I told you about 'em.

- Higher level grammar, without newer vocabulary words:

  The nose is gonna be hurt somebody.
  This could be in a circus.
  Run—It could run—It'll be run.
  I don't know how you do that.
  We act like that.
  I can't stop laughing!
  I been looking—that way.

Progress with conversation

The summer report before high school continued to describe Bevin's progress with conversational skills in the form of a treatment goal addressing "engagement in reciprocal conversation with important adults at least fifteen times per session."

Bevin has achieved a nice, free-flowing, conversational style this summer. Many examples were notable:

- The following described how the beef jerky was:

B	**It's pretty yucky.**
M	Is it?
B	**It's pretty great.**
M	It's OK, just—
B	**Kinda hard, hard—**
M	It's pretty old.
B	**What kind of old?**
M	It's so old, it's dried out and hard.
B	**It's old and hard.**
M	Right.

- The following was after we laughed at a Baby Bop and BJ scene till we cried, and Bevin was able to spit out: **"I—can't—stop—laughing!"**

B	**You know what? It's for pleasure.**
M	(laughs)
B	**—when you laugh.**
M	That's true.
B	**You know what?**
M	What?
B	**It's empty.** (referring to his pop can)
M	Oh yeah? (laughing)
B	**You know?**

M	Yes.
B	**I thought so.**

Progress with narration

The summer report continued to describe Bevin's progress in relating his own experiences, narrating stories, and explaining himself at least four times per session, using at least three consecutive sentences each time:

> Bevin's skill in this area is just emerging, allowing his humor, drama, and emotional sensitivity to be expressed in the process. Bevin often brings up old stories, as if to explore the meaning that was lost on him when he was younger. One week this summer, Bevin referred to a movie within a movie we were watching:
>
> | | |
> |---|---|
> | **B** | **A little rat—A long time ago. It's too much.** |
> | M | A long time ago— |
> | **B** | **Long, long way ago—many years.** |
> | M | Yes— |
> | **B** | **It's too young then. It's a reason to grow.** |
> | M | It's hard to understand when you're young. |
> | **B** | **Nobody explain anything.** |
>
> - The following dialogue occurred the week after Bevin missed his session because he was sick. His mom had called to see if we might make up the session, but I never got the message and never called them back.
>
> | | |
> |---|---|
> | **B** | **Come back—I dunno.** |
> | M | I never called you back; your mom called but I didn't get her message. |
> | **B** | **—call the rules and no one say anything.** |
> | M | I know; I never told you I couldn't see you on Friday. |
> | **B** | **I dunno.** |
>
> The conversation continued after a little pause:
>
> | | |
> |---|---|
> | **B** | **Next week.** |
> | M | (looked at Bevin, not understanding the referent) |
> | **B** | **I mean next year—fall.** |
> | M | Right, we'll go back to Wednesday and Friday in the fall. |

B	**Next year, I'm going the bigs.** (referring to high school)
M	I know, buddy.
B	**You will be sorry!** (meaning, I think, that this summer is when he is the most able to work on language.)

One other example, told in the third person, seems to relay Bevin's own thoughts about trying, failing, and reflecting:

> **They will listen—they will do their jobs—they did mistakes—they sorry.**

Bevin's progress in narration is emerging with great creativity! Bevin is truly telling stories, as illustrated by the following. Note that grammatical accuracy decreases when the vocabulary load is high.

- In the first story, Bevin assembled farm animals to resist the wolf, who was clearly angry (and, we learn at the end of the story, righteous!). The clinician took minimal turns to facilitate where useful, and the story stopped and restarted several times.

> **They're gallop as fast as they could.**
> **The wolf was very angry.**
> **Come on, men! Get ready to attack.**
> **The scavenger was scramble, scramble.**

B	**One page at a time.**
B	**Come on, guys** (putting cows and pigs together)
B	**Pigs are afraid. Come on guys—'fraid, attack!**
B	**The three little pigs and it was time to attack.**
M	Did you guys make it?
B	**Cows and pigs a ran—as fast as he could.**
B	**You're a little pigs and that's just what—**
B	**Attack!**
B	(fighting sounds)
B	**The wolf is very angry with a brown cow, moo.**
B	**America's at the door.**
B	**A stick too strong much, but a wolf can down side.**

- On another occasion, Bevin told a very different style of story with a preponderance of vocabulary words and minimal grammar. These lines emerged without a break:

  Moon and stars tonight.
  A light.
  Millions of stink.
  A rat—villains and—three vegetables and stink.
  And barbeque and mustard.
  Onions, garlic, tomato, cheese and pumpkin.
  (drawing a picture at this point)
  And then walrus: "Arr, arr, arr!"
  And seal: "Wrar, wrar, wrar"
  It's about—flowing, easy.

The report went on to set goal areas for the fall semester in high school:

Summer has been restorative, confidence-building, and has given Bevin hope for the future. The problems to be addressed during this next six months focus on the significant challenges of returning to school, particularly his first year of high school. The problems to be addressed in this Plan of Care have to do with helping Bevin achieve a sense of his potential under maximally supportive conditions so he can:

- Continue to access his skills and continue to develop them in the fall during after school times with maximal and moderate support.
- Achieve a comfortable state of self-regulation under the minimally supportive conditions of school.

The problems and goals to be addressed with this POC are:

1. Severe sensory defensiveness under minimally supportive conditions: Bevin will generalize his awareness of his own state of sensory comfort to school and seek support from school personnel when he is uncomfortable.
2. Functional use of developing muscle awareness and skills for self-regulation: Bevin will use his growing sense of his muscles and skills for self-regulation under a variety of moderately-supportive conditions to achieve comfortable body proximity and body orientation 50% of the time at home, after-school activities, and social groups where social distance is allowed.

3. Functional use of developing fine motor skills for activities of daily living and vocational training: Bevin will use his fine motor skills functionally for ADLs and vocational training by demonstrating ten new fine motor skills in areas such as hygiene, self-care, animal care, and cooking in the clinic and at home.

4. Functional use of developing motor planning skills for ADLs and vocational training: Bevin will develop the functional use of developing motor planning skills for ADLs and vocational training by demonstrating ten new motor routines in areas such as those above.

5. Continuing engagement in positive social interactions once school starts, with those people who will continue to support Bevin maximally and moderately (his respite workers, family, etc.). Bevin will engage in reciprocal conversation with these adults by taking three turns at least 20 times per day.

6. Continuing tolerance of language used and modeled by others once school starts, with those people who will continue to support Bevin maximally and moderately. After a break to decompress and regulate after school each day (using appropriate equipment and activities), Bevin will choose to take off his headphones and find the language used by others to be tolerable and useful. Success will look like 2/5 school days.

7. Continued use and development of self-generated language once school starts, with those people who will continue to support Bevin maximally and moderately. Bevin will engage in social conversation with the adults close to him, using language (as opposed to sound effects) 50% of the time (reduced criteria because of school starting) and grammar at DSS levels 3–6 80% of the time (same criteria). Bevin's accuracy will be at least 50% (increased criteria).

Later in the summer, Bevin's mother wrote in an email: "Bevin is so happy lately he is almost delirious." After three years in 'jail,' well-deserved delirium.

High school

As the fall began, Bevin was delighted to find that he was acknowledged for being smart, for being funny, and for being creative. He blossomed—and continued to bloom for the entire year, when the telling of his story necessarily closes with the advent of printing this book!

The first several months of high school brought with it new language models straight from the teens around him. Bevin was open to all the new language and came away with new phraseology and new social expressions that helped him sound like the happy high-schooler he was. Bevin's fine motor skill also blossomed, and he was able to pair language with the fine motor activity of creating with play dough. The following is a short snippet from several minutes of talking about what he was doing as he created:

> **Beautiful—oh well, the magical, go little butterfly.**
> **Butterfly and the magical.**
> **Oh well, I'm not, I'm not alone.**
> **Hello, little fellow. What happened to you?**
> **Sprinkle, sprinkle, sprinkle—you think it's enough?**
> **I gotta, I gotta, I gotta—**
> **It's magical; it's magic.**
> **Come on, little magic.**

Minutes later, he was still creating and narrating his creation:

> **I just made the world.**
> **Love all the world.**

Bevin wanted to do everything himself, more and more as the fall went on. He joyfully saved things to bring to the clinic, **"to help the Marges,"** packing them all and resisting help. As he said to his mom when she realized how independent he'd become: **"I, a diamond in the rough, in the rough. Thanks, Mom."**

Language development continues in high school

Bevin's next progress report was written after his fall semester in ninth grade, when Bevin was already seventeen years old. The following comes from that report, summarizing the six months before:

> The summer allowed Bevin the opportunity to maximize his self-confidence under highly-supportive conditions (Camp Adventure, CDC, OT, home), to prepare him for his first year of high school. This semester has been far better than anyone could have predicted, with a staff who finds Bevin delightful and funny and who thoroughly appreciates him! Staff has worked together to address Bevin's occasional less-than-socially-conducive behaviors in a consistent way, and his blossoming speech and language skills have been promoted in his English class, his Speech/OT group, and other school venues.
>
> This clinician saw Bevin twice a week, with our Friday sessions lasting many hours; the slow, unhurried pace was key to the progress Bevin made. His regulation was first and foremost,

of course, and Bevin spent an hour with movement activity, assembling everything he needed for the afternoon/evening (food, seating, etc), and organizing the materials he would use (movies, books, writing materials, manipulatives, art supplies, etc.). Once he had shed the stresses of the week, Bevin settled into a venue that included his self-assorted library of old movies, old and new books, old and new action figures, and old and new manipulative and art materials with which to create. Always, Bevin practiced language; sometimes, through his actions, he explored an idea or posed a question; sometimes he practiced narrating familiar movies; throughout the entire six-month period, Bevin expanded his work on his own self-created stories and explanations.

Following are excerpts describing Bevin's progress on his 6-month goals:

Goal 1: Coping with severe sensory defensiveness under minimally supportive conditions: Bevin has successfully communicated his need for his headphones or a quieter environment 75% of the time at school, in his own way. Bevin essentially "retreats" from social engagement by talking to himself, moving away slightly, or walking to other parts of the room, thus alerting staff of his need for quiet. Clearly this is two-way communication, with his understanding teachers and aides ready to help him achieve regulation.

Goal 2: Functional use of his growing sense of his muscles and skills for self regulation under a variety of moderately-supportive conditions to achieve comfortable body proximity and body orientation 50% of the time at home, after-school activities, and social groups where social distance is allowed: Bevin has achieved this goal at a higher level than anticipated, estimated at 75% of the time when social distance is allowed.

Goal 3: Functional use of his fine motor skills functionally for ADLs and vocational training by demonstrating ten new fine motor skills in areas such as: hygiene, self-care, animal care, and cooking in the clinic and at home: Bevin has achieved this goal, and the venues can now expand!

Goal 4: Functional use of developing motor planning skills for ADLs and vocational training by demonstrating ten new motor routines in areas such as those above: Again, Bevin has achieved this goal, and is now ready for greater efficiency, accuracy, and complexity in his motor routines.

Goal 5: Continued engagement in positive social interactions once school starts, with those people who will continue to support Bevin maximally and moderately (his respite workers, family, etc.). Bevin will engage in reciprocal conversation with these adults by taking three turns, least 20 times per day: Bevin has surpassed our hopes for social engagement and has not only achieved this conversational goal with the usual supportive people in his life, but regular, positive, single-comment verbalization with those at school as well.

Goal 6. Continued tolerance of language used and modeled by others once school starts, with those people who will continue to support Bevin maximally and moderately. After a break to decompress and regulate after school each day (using appropriate equipment and activities), Bevin will choose to take off his headphones and find the language used by others to be tolerable and useful. Success will look like 2/5 school days: Bevin's success has far exceeded our expectations. No only has he kept his headphones off for most of his school week and tolerated the language used by his usual conversation partners, he has used the casual and modeled language used by others in school and out of school!

Goal 7: Continued development and use of self-generated language once school starts, with those people who will continue to support Bevin maximally and moderately. Bevin will engage in social conversation with the adults close to him, using language (as opposed to sounds effects) 50% of the time and grammar at DSS levels 3–6 80% of the time, with accuracy at least at 50%: Bevin has met parts of this goal, using language 50% of the time under well-supported conditions, but the percentage of time spent using accurate, generative grammar at DSS levels 3–6 has fluctuated widely. Rather than develop consistency and accuracy with grammar, Bevin has been exploring the use of generative grammar to tell more lengthy and elaborate stories. It appears that Bevin's own path to language growth is taking a different course from the one this clinician anticipated, but the benefits to Bevin's self-expression, communication, social interaction, academic growth, and creativity are more like Bevin himself: holistic, meaningful, thoughtful, and fun!

The report included quotations from Bevin that reflected his growing awareness of his body and his body in space. He referred to himself more, even expressing positive feelings about sensation as he experienced his body in space and developed greater self-regulation and confidence:

Looks like me.
Got dizzy in purple.
It hit me.
I'm got arms like this.
My wish—round and round—push—my push wish.
It's me!
It's me—I smell!
It's not me now.
This brush is a good.
I don't feel funny.
I can't see a thing.
I 'member something.
I gotta practice here.
Now I really look like a Bevin boy.
I know about that.
Maybe just a little sleepy—

The following was a well-considered conversation about himself from December:

B	**I'm pretty good.**
M	Yeah, you are—at a lot of things.
B	**I know about faces.**

Self advocacy depends on self-concept. Socially-effective self-advocacy depends on adequate self-regulation to choose polite language.

Self advocacy depends on self-concept, and socially-effective self-advocacy depends on adequate self-regulation to choose polite language. Bevin advocated for himself with useful language on more and more occasions:

Come on! We gotta get back! Move!
Swing a little bit—school program later.
Marge's, take off! We're out of here! See you Monday!
Wait! Not willow! Just nature, right?
Where's things—things from yesterday?

Self-regulation = language access

Self-regulation improved as Bevin's sensory defensiveness moderated and his use of space became more fluid. As he felt better, Bevin was more available for auditory input and verbal output. This translated into more tolerance of the language used by others, more inclination to incorporate that language, more multi-sentence turns, and more multi-turn conversations. A new target emerged: conversational contingency, that is, the idea that conversations are built on each turn being 'contingent' on the one before it. The clinician's daily notes from December stated that it seemed that, for the first time, Bevin could talk and listen at the same time and still integrate what the clinician was saying!

The following demonstrated his growing repertoire of and access to socially-acceptable ways of achieving self-regulation and advocating for himself:

M	(laughing about the story Bevin had created)
B	**No laughing!**
M	Sorry, Buddy; I was laughing because I liked the story.
B	**Just the Barney's farm is laughing.**

Reciprocal conversations were commonplace throughout the semester. A few will be noted here, just to capture the different qualities expressed. All these conversations came during the last month of the semester. The first was when Bevin was soliciting help finding a category of movies and then commented on them.

B	**Where's nature?**
M	I think it's over here.
B	**Nature is good.**

The next was a simple conversation that illustrated the same 'contingency' quality:

B	**They play.** (referring to a movie of crabs on a beach)
M	Uh huh.
B	**—to learn.**

Following is another commentary:

B	**He's kinda cold at the South Pole**
M	It sure is.
B	**Pretty cold.**
M	Yeah, it is.
B	**Humans warm it up.**

The clinician was judicious about asking questions, but Bevin was usually able to offer a thoughtful answer as in the following conversation:

M	What's your favorite bird?
B	**Like birds like eagles.**
B	**Like flamingos.**

Other conversations explored humor and joking. The third example in the following series showed Bevin's growing flexibility in modifying language for the benefit of his partner, who was starting to take his joke seriously:

B	**What was that?**
M	I don't know.
B	**Stomach growls.**
M	(laughing)
B	**That was a monster.**
M	Listen to that penguin colony!
B	**Like a peanut gallery.**
B	**You hit me in the butt.**
M	That would hurt.
B	**Somebody hit me in the butt.**
M	Who did that?
B	**Nobody.**

A funny, multi-sentence 'skit' took place at Sheila's clinic, where Bevin was trying on a blue body sock but started eyeing a red one:

> **Oh, my gosh! Maybe was a ghost around here. Where'd she go?**
> **Whew! I'm not a ghost.**
> **That's pretty pretty good, but the big red is over there.**
> **This is good. We have central.**

The next comment was an interesting take on the range of human potential:

M	It's too cold for humans. (referring to Antarctica)
B	**Some humans have it. Some humans don't.**

And the following dialogue offered a moment of candor, something new in Bevin and highly valuable:

B	**Where are they going?** (referring to flamingos)
M	They're staying there, don't you think?
B	**Staying there.**
M	They don't have to migrate, do they?
B	**They can't!!**

As Bevin became less sensory-defensive, his tolerance of other people's language increased. He incorporated the following social phrases that had not been heard before:

Uh oh!
Ahhh!
Wow!
Whoops!
Oh, my!
Ai yi yi!
Let's see—
Whew!
Aw!
Oh my gosh!
Cool!
Of course—
Good!

Bevin also tried out various types of voices and varieties of intonation, as well as mitigation of some new expressions. A few of his new expressions were:

It's all about—
He's all about—

How different.
How about that one.

And there were numerous examples of Bevin incorporating the clinician's language:

B	**These are good.**
M	It's a good collection.
B	**Good collection.**

Use of self-generated language to narrate

While Bevin had not developed the accuracy of grammar we expected, he chose to use his self-generated language in much more creative ways. Using the grammar within his competence, the language of his environment, the written word, and the gestalts in his mind Bevin began crafting narratives, action sequences, explanations, and other multi-sentence compositions that expressed his thoughts and ideas.

Throughout this first year of high school, Bevin practiced story-telling with manipulable play characters. For years, Bevin had periodically tried to work on narrating familiar movie sequences first by talking along with movies, then narrating from the third person perspective. Bevin also "viewed" movies in his head, saying the words and sound effects of the sound track out loud. But it was only in high school that Bevin could coordinate words with his body's actions. Using gesture and manipulating characters, usually animals and dinosaurs, Bevin usually began with categories, places, or habitats, assembling props and plants within each. Always giving them verbal labels that were relevant to his conceptualization, Bevin might refer to such categories and places as "fight box" (with a set of weapons), "scary" (particular animals), "scaries over there" (another set), "spirits," "garden," "desert," "God," etc.

During each session, the clinician tried to make new characters available to Bevin, as his creativity was supported with this novelty. Bevin also had access to all the toys in the clinic and used wild animals and dinosaurs in some way at least every other session. While the action of characters was still limited, Bevin used our outdoor sessions to promote action, for instance, going over a "mountain" to simulate the journey of Horton the elephant with other animals. It was gratifying to see Bevin's language and his actions begin to coordinate.

In one story, Bevin narrated the adventure of some animals he had assembled in a scene. Using vocabulary that represents his categories of animals, Bevin referred to those that represent God and those that were 'wolf-catchers' as follows:

> **Long ago, the world was filled with giants.**
> **You fellas hit the road.**
> **God, and does the thing, the farm.**
> **Wolf catchers are way over there.**
> **But the wolf catcher.**
> **We take off, then get 'em.**
> **Move out—then let the work and play.**
> **Fellas!**
> **Farm—these God hit the road.**
> **Santa, that's when I was little.**
> **"Better watch out—"**
> **Barney's farm is coming to town.** (sung to the tune of 'Santa Claus is coming to town')

Witnessing his story generation and beginning to understand what these stories meant to Bevin was a true joy. As the semester continued, Bevin's stories became more and more creative as he juxtaposed his categories such as dinosaurs and Christmas. The following is a segment of a much longer sequence of sentences Bevin produced.

> **Years ago, Hanukah.**
> **Look at that Christmas.**
> **Looks like me, years ago.**
> **He's got giant, lizard-like dinosaur.**
> **Looks like a million years ago, like a dinosaur.**
> **It like a plant-eater dinosaur.**
> **He look like a little—he sleeps.**
> **Sleeps like a dinosaur—spirit.**
> **Like trips—spirits is you.**
> **This is for Geo Kids like Zoboo, like a Zoboo, like a special one—like a spirit.**
> **These are like dinosaurs.**
> **These are sleepy.**

These are sleepy, way over there.
These got Christmas-like dinosaur.
These got carol-like dinosaur.
Looks like a giant Tyrannosaurus Rex, like a boy.
For the garden carol.
Carols and gardens—wow!
Boy, garden, Christmas.
These are all giants.
Wow, he's got giant lizards.
These are all giants.
He's got giant teeth like dinosaur.
Wow! Wow! Wow! Wow! Wow!

Bevin's stories were spoken rapidly and were over all too quickly. To really understand them, one had to focus intently, and it helped to jot them down for later reading. During his last session of the semester, Bevin talked for about 30 minutes straight, using virtually all self-generated sentences to narrate an original story. All about dinosaurs, Barney, Christmas, and himself, the following segment, extending to the next page, illustrates Bevin's creative story-generation, as difficult as it was to follow in real time:

There is trees and trees—fun, fun—fire in there is heat. That's trees, fun—This is trees. What kind of Barney? What is it? Cool! Red. Don't you know anything? Hello! Roar! Bye, bye, Barney. He's a biggest Hanukah-like Christmas. This is plain fun. Look at this guy. He's a celebration. That was a big celebrate and sky. Celebrate and celebrate. Blue sky and sky, the hall sky. Celebration the sky—the hall. Wow! Wow! He's the biggest of dinosaurs. Wow. He's a big as a giant. That's a big giant. Beautiful, cool. That's will be come back.

That's will be come back as boys. Oh, hello! Oh, hello! Oh, hello! Ai yi yi. Hear from that one. That was hear from that one. Deck the hall. What the hall. These a giant roars. He's a big dinosaur. That was scare me. Wow, he's a biggest dinosaur. He lives in a special, in a school. That was name of a lizard. Express camel as a special dinosaur. He's a Tyrannosaurus Rex, like a dinosaur. China—that was China—her and special. Celebration. These are live in the special in the school. One dinosaur named was Tyrannosaurus Rex. That was camel, and camel. That was special in a school. What in the world? Here and now. He was a plant eater. Of course, there were great plant eaters. What in the world? His name? Ah, got it! (read from book) Chinese star. You're changing like me. (Bevin moved to look out the window) I'm here and remember: I love you!

Some elements of interpretation are speculative, but the clinician was familiar with Bevin's category, "camel," which referred to gentle animals and perhaps gentler versions of scary animals, including dinosaurs like Barney. The reference to "China" and "Chinese star" seems to be the "star in the east," and Hanukah seems to be a reference both to prehistory and pre-Christmas. It is interesting that the roar of the meat-eater seems to be overshadowed by the Barney version of a T-Rex, and that peaceful plant-eaters may be metaphorically related to the Christmas story.

Development and use of semantics

Bevin regularly added vocabulary to his useful language repertoire during the fall. Place names were new, as in the following example, referring to places where dinosaur bones are found:

The rocks is underneath—like Texas and Utah.

S	You want the purple swing?
B	**This name raspberry.**
B	**Raspberry name.**
S	Oh it's the raspberry swing.
B	**That's right: cold and dark.** (commenting on animals hiding in the shade)
M	Uh, it looks dark and cool.
B	**Cold is never trouble.**
M	Hmm—
B	**Easy and safe.**
B	(narrated the meerkat stoy on the TV)
B	**I'm pretty good with it.**
M	You are, Buddy.
B	**Shade—oh, that's shade.**
B	**I hope this works.** (referring to the meerkats hiding)

Development of speech clarity

As Bevin's confidence increased, he was more often willing to be filmed, and by the end of the semester, he even asked to re-do his expository about dinosaurs so he could make it more clear on the tape. As his confidence in himself increased, so did his willingness to be seen and heard. His speech became more deliberate and clear at the same time.

Life-long learning

Bevin's pride in his high school success was palpable. His own words summarized his post-elementary school years best:

B	**I was so angry!**
M	But you're better now; you made it!
B	**I was brave!**
M	You sure were—and you succeeded.

Bevin began high school with NLA 4 competencies—but not accuracy—and had other grammar at NLA 5 and 6 which he could access when regulation was optimal and constraints were minimal. Elements of new grammar emerged throughout the school year, and some were practiced enough to be part of his competence. In his own narrative version of *Horton Hatches the Egg*, he used conjunctions more regularly than I had heard up until then. His words follow, with the conjoining words in orange. This story also included the prepositions 'for' and 'to,' a variety of verb forms, and a quotation:

> **I don't understand: out of the jungle that's all good. It stinks where we're going. I'll handle this for you. This very mean but I'm a stranger here. 'It's mine,' scream the bird. All biz as you are. I am a least as you. You stupid xxx feathers. Is it time to—Magical—years—that stinks. This stinks around here. We're not gonna eat.**

Bevin's style was not to work on consistency and accuracy of grammar out of context, but he constantly practiced using his grammar to talk about his ideas. In the story above, Bevin expressed that to leave the jungle was sad, and to voluntarily leave was incomprehensible. Horton had a duty, however (**"I'll handle this for you"**). Capturing him was very mean. **"But I'm a stranger here"** made it even more defiling. The bird's line was delivered, and Horton retorted that he was all business and at least as good as she was. To miss his magical years truly does stink, but no one is going to eat that egg if Horton has anything to say about it.

Older students feel immediate pressure to use their newly-acquired grammar.

Developing a grammar is one thing, but using it flexibly to express oneself is another. It takes time to use one's grammar in a great variety of meaningful contexts before it becomes automatic. The more it is used, the easier accessing it fluently becomes. Young children who have already developed grammatical competence have lots of time to practice before they are called upon to talk or write under pressure. But older students in whom grammatical competence is just emerging are under pressure to use that grammar almost immediately. No wonder Bevin liked to just play with his new structures, creating jokes and songs and playful games and stories. No wonder he liked paraphrasing favorite movies with language he constructed himself. Bevin was developing ease of access.

This last year of Bevin's language acquisition story illustrates how fluent his commenting and his narrating was becoming, at least when support was maximal and self-regulation was optimal. Looking back over his eight-year journey, it is apparent how much support and self-regulation mattered to this process and how rarely they coincided in real life. Educators talk about students' "teachable moments," and with ASD students, these can be rare indeed. But brave kids like Bevin are motivated to use them well.

Practice makes better

In the course of this last year of Bevin's story, practice paid off. Meaningful self-exploration, idea generation, and storytelling were important to Bevin and afforded him the opportunity to practice flexible use of grammar, vocabulary, and all the intonation, timing, gestures, and drama he'd been amassing in his sizable expressive repertoire.

Because this book is still mostly about grammar and its development, this segment of the chapter will be devoted to the bits of grammar or their use that emerged during the last semester of Bevin's story. It is included here because of the significance of Bevin's still-developing and solidifying grammar and because of the hope it can give readers who care about an older student like Bevin. Here are some of the notable utterances, grouped by type of notable quality: (1) grammar, vocabulary, or form, (2) coordination with his body, (3) comments about himself, (4) self-advocacy, (5) narrative construction, and (6) creativity.

(1) Grammar, vocabulary, and form (grouped by common features and important because of verb forms, embedded clauses, prepositional phrases, indirect objects, conjunctions, question forms, and colloquial expressions):

I said it doesn't work!
I'm all brave and courage.
I was just checking—I checked.
I don't see anyone anywhere.
To everyone: I am sorry!
I gotta teach you something—remember!
I understand he's mad.
I'm righter than you.
I'll eat 'em in a little bit.
I got a question for you.
I've got something—muppet dinosaurs.
I put 'em back so tight.
I'll be right back, before you know.
Mattress says, I gotta stay here.
I hadda go back.
I told you she was all right.
I'm sorry I was lost.
I just know he will.
I don't think he will.
I thought you farted.

My brain is getting lessons.
My hairs are, oh dear, as short as mine.
We'll call you 'Utah.'

Don't worry about it now.
It was too hard on him.
It's ripped apart.

It's a big gooey, got gums like monster.

It's growing—like a stalk.
It's no funny either.
Of course there's fossil in Utah.
Oh, this is delightful.
That was courage angel—
That guy—well—ugly.
These dino Rexes will come back as boys.
They're not bullies; they're friends.
That sounds like a brother and sister.
King of dinosaurs are everywhere.
These bees are still buzzing around every day.
Something's not quite right here.
Something bad is happening up there.
Take a picture of that.
Watch me get it.

Like a T-Rex or a camel.
Sounds like a man's talking.
That's a Barney-like dinosaur.
A bird, a pelican, like a toucan, like a flying pilot eagle.
He's got a letter Z like a Zabu.
You're acting like crazy.

Maybe except migraines: he's always mad.
My mama told me, my papa if I can't even be a loudrock.
I check out what this is.
That's what it's for.
Just checking about what's underneath the ground.
Let's see what we got for now.

But, you're right.
But, that is dino.
But, she wasn't feeling well.
But, I'm sorry.
I'm happy, but who are you?
No, because it stinks.
'Cuz it's impossible.
So, we did the Bob one.
So, I'll call you orange and black.
So, when the blue faces are dark.
Then one day when blue scar was fall down cliff.
When I grow up, I'll go to the desert.
When I grow up—I'm gonna be a Sampson dinosaur.
When I grow up, I'll get a job.

What's a stink? Must be somebody else.
What's name? Cats.
What's her name?
What happened, spilling?
What are you laughing like that?
What you wanna do?

Who cleaned up?
Who took my cup?
Where'd that come from?
Where she's gone?
Where's the fossils? It's here somewhere.
What'll we do?
Is name of costume, right?
Would you like a picture?
You'll do it later?
How are you, Sampson dinosaurs, and your bugs?
How's your race, Bob?

Let's see—
That's for sure.
What in the world?
Gee, thanks.
What about this?
But, wow!
Good idea!
Oh boy, so ridiculous.
I get it!
Have a look—
That's silly.
You know what?
Oh my gosh—

(2) Language coordinated with his body as he was creating with playdough, essentially saying a phrase or sentence with each part of the creation:

> **Bat's his name—jam and jelly. Like a big giant: there's a head, a one big head, a ears, two ears—they're wings. There's wings I call them. Fruit bats, like a big vampire bats, like a dinosaur. There's a head, body: vampire bat!**

(3) Language about himself and his opinions:

I spin myself.
I'm a good swimmer.
I love that.
Two things: swing and music from months ago.
That's it: my toes.
Ah, that's better.
Next week, I promise you I'm talking to you.
I made up stories.
I's your best friend.
I'm pretty good at spooky.
Where you goin': Utah!
Last time I couldn't understand. It was a long time ago.
Think bullies are not very nice.
I'm gonna bring you a little peace.
My butt is so purple.

My belly is so aching.
Our teams are spirit of soar.
But my belly still feels bad and my throat feels fire.
Someday, I'll teach them a lesson. I'll teach my story.
Now take a picture of me.
I wish, I wish—my teeth is fixed and back to normal—like before.
In June, back to normal.

B	**I was gentle.**
M	You were gentle very recently; but you got touchy.
B	**I thinking I was touchy.**

Someday, Bevin writes his name: Iguanodon Camel.
What's it called? Hey fever, huh?
This is the last time you swollen, understand? (to his dental abscess)
I hate this swollen. It stinks.
I'll be a dream, cross the road, this summer.
You hurt my heart; you hurt my ears—you hurt my feelings.
My feet is all wobbly.
You know, fossils are scary to me.

(4) Language used for self-advocacy:

No, I don't think so.
OK, I'll do in a minute.
I'm busy by now.
I talking myself.
I got my own way to go: Bevin brain.
Don't say anything; now just wait for the end.
Please don't do that.
Don't touch it, all right?
Cut it out.
Please don't yell.
Easy, take it easy.
Wasn't stinky before; always nice before; that's better; my back, it's fixed.
I hate noise.

(5) Language used for narration:

That's big problem; I think we're home some big problems—and troubles, still have 'em.
Just a voices, a big scary—but is bushes—first is hunters all around.

Bevin could sound the attack: 'Ruff, ruff—ruff ruff.' That's me with a sound the attack. Sound be's the dogs!! Sound the attack!

They're three fish up on the rocks. They're three spots: one with stripes, three spots by the Rex right now. Find out it's a leopard about now! A alley cat—looks like a large and stinky —Wait a minute: I'm a boy! But I'm a sorry boy. I mean, that's all right. Wait a minute: I'm a mouse! Cats?! I'm a boy! But, eagle! Poor Bevin.

A biggest ferocious roar; use teeth and long sharp claws. One day, coming closer. Comes at me, eyes are red and glowing; Suddenly, they're coming closer and closer. Suddenly they're coming closer! Whoa! Gangwar! How many time I told you. I think it's coming in a minute. I got to be afraid of 'em. Not here! I'm scared.

You will come back as boy. That Rex boy will come back as boy. Men come back as dinosaurs. Gallimimus you a long time ago. Gallimimus, mother lizard, thunder lizard.

We don't like being blown up; We're smashed!

Dinosaurs outer space; It's coming closer; It's my conscience; Mama, it's coming.

(6) Language used for creativity and poetry:

Blow the horn; Growl, growl, roar; Trouble, trouble to the Lord, take the sword; Please blow your horn; Troubles and troubles: throw them away!

Sweet dreams, is that you? Sweet dreams of mother. Sweet dreams is you.

Someone will be; someone who stinks; Stinks like ugly; Ugly funny.

Utah, wonderful! Yoke bomb. Utah was a fossil. Take care of them very funny things.

Red is a warning. Red is as cook. Red is warm. And gangwar. And flashing—I'll call you. Red is calling. Red is separate as a sandbomb. Explosion, that's right. Dinosaur planet, beginning of the world. This was a big explosion. Beware, it's a red. Flashing as a big bomb. It's glowing. This is the story of the whole world.

One story deserves elaboration, because it was a revisiting of an earlier conversation, when Bevin had expressed his sadness that he had not "followed this dog," his dog that he mistakenly thought had run away. The further significance was that this story was one of several that occurred in a single session, obviously a "window" day!

B	**What do you think? I think—**
B	**I think I'll never run; Oh, I think he likes me; Come back, come back, dog; Please come back.**
B	**All dogs are God, bad guys.**
M	Are they bad because they run away?
B	**Runned away.**
M	(explaining how his dog had not run away but had to be given away to a family with a farm)
B	**I don't think so.**
M	(explaining the reasons for this and how the dog, Rosie, is happy there)
B	**Thank you, Marge.**
B	**I was never run as a dog; from my imagination.**
M	I know you didn't run after him, but you thought about it afterwards.
B	**Right; have to follow the dog.**
M	You can have a dog again someday when you have enough space.
B	**I understand; she understand.**
M	Right. It's still sad.
B	**Too sad.**
B	**I'm sorry.**
M	I'm sorry too.
B	**I'm sorry, sad.**
B	**He's understand.**
B	**It's OK.**
B	**Someday, a dog.**
M	Someday, you'll get a dog again.
B	**After a man, college.**
B	**Charlie barking dog April.**
B	**I'll call you Charlie Barking Dog someday.**
B	**It's all right the dog.**
B	**Bingo, I'll bring him back someday.**
B	**What's his name?**
B	**I'll call you Charlie Barking Dog.**
B	**I'll find you later.**

Finally, a few series of utterances were important as parts of a self-portrait. In the first situation, I inquired if Bevin had a way to play a CD I had gotten him:

M	Do you have music in your room?
B	**I got my computer.**
B	**I got my own.** (pointing to his head which housed a huge collection of music)

Bevin could talk about his brain; he knew what he was capable of; he was proud.

The second series came when Bevin returned to a common theme: being safe vs. stepping out in the world. He began by saying, "Someday," then went on:

B	**Someday—**
M	Right, you'll have adventures.
B	**But I'm safe.**
M	Right, you don't need to do it now; when you're ready.
B	**I'll be a construction worker.**
B	**I'll be a Walter.** (his dad)
M	You will, buddy.
B	**I'll be a good jobs.**
B	**I'll be a freedom.**
M	You will earn money for yourself.
B	**And remember—I always right.**

The third series referenced his future dinosaur dig in Utah. Bevin was holding two small human characters who were having a conversation (B = Bevin; A = Bevin rold-playing an adult):

A	**Bevin, that is a big dinosaur.**
B	**Come on, boss; let's go.**
A	**Come on, boy; let's go.**
B	**The biggest of dinosaurs: T-Rex.**

The fourth was about my idea to have an art show exhibiting Bevin's clay creations and his photography:

M	So you think we should have an art show?
B	**I think so.**
B	**I think pretty good.**
B	**I think so, pretty good.**

The fifth involved a dialogue Bevin attributed to his father: **"My father once told me—my father said—I was always right."**

The final series returned to Bevin's thoughts about his future job, this time expressing that it could be in either of his favorite habitat areas, the desert or the jungle. 'Bob' refers to construction work, as in *Bob the Builder.*

B	**Bob and desert and jungle.**
M	Are you going to have a construction job in the desert or in the jungle?
B	**I don't care.**
M	Oh, sure.
B	**Bob is name is Africa and India, India desert.**
M	Right.
B	**South American jungle and Central.**
M	Sounds excellent.
B	**What can I tell you?**

Clearly, Bevin was feeling proud of himself, and believed in his future. So did I!

But daily life continued relentlessly, of course, and Bevin's regulation ebbed and flowed accordingly. The spark that always remained was bright, however, and Bevin had proven he could maintain his sense of self under all kinds of conditions. I had no doubt he would thrive.

It is time now, to take leave of Bevin and his continuing story. Standing back, we can consider the lessons that speak more universally. There are many here for you to take away and consider in light of your own student's situation. The beauty of Bevin sharing so generously of himself is that there are many parts of his story that resemble those of other amazing people. Please consider the parts that resonate with you about that special student you know and love. All the nuances of Bevin's story are here to learn from. They are unique to Bevin, of course, but the challenges and strengths he learned to work with are more universal. His humanity is broad, and as you immerse yourself in his story, in his life, you can draw strength from his tenacity and know that a special kind of tenacity exists in your student too. All the best to both of you!

In summary

As the telling of Bevin's story comes to an end, one thing is apparent: his story is far from over. Over the course of eight years, Bevin had developed enough competence with grammar, access to vocabulary, self-regulation, and conversational skill to be a modestly-flexible communicator—under supportive conditions. More than two thirds of the time, Bevin was able to use transparent language people close to him understood, to use polite language to self-advocate, and to use colloquial expressions that allowed him to blend in among a select group of peers. The rest of the time was up and down in all these areas, but Bevin and the people in his life knew how to alter the environment to help

Bevin communicated when people gave him the benefit of the doubt and applied the patience to read between the lines.

things swing back up again. Bevin had been trying to communicate all his life, and now his timing, tolerance, and self-selection were such that almost everyone around him recognized he was communicating. He was successful when people gave him the benefit of the doubt and applied the patience to read between the lines. Bevin's natural sense of humor was intoxicating, and he could command an audience everywhere he went. Bevin was a communicator—one who had the skills, drive, and creativity to continue to be a successful life-long language learner.

As we now close Bevin's story, we are ready to present some general principles that have been gleaned from the experiences of a variety of older students. With these in mind, along with Bevin's words and drawing below, you can approach your own student and support him in his own journey.

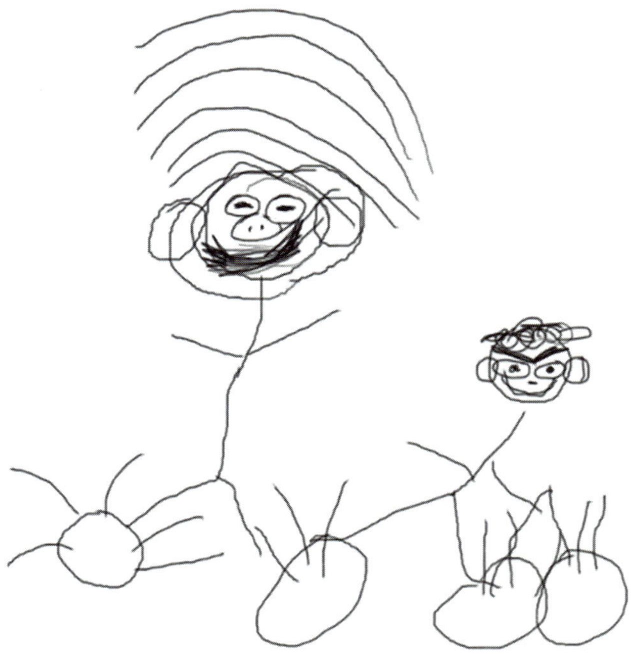

"That's me and you. Magical rainbow. Love each other."

Chapter 17
Considerations for Older Students and Life-long Learners

Language development started a long time ago for each of our older students. NLA was part of that process, and may still be. But, at some point, we know development of grammar stops. That doesn't mean that language development ceases, however. In fact, functional communication growth and language learning will continue for the rest of our student's life. Like all of us, our student will learn to converse in new areas, learn new vocabulary words, develop new linguistic concepts, figure out how to tell more captivating stories. All this is the continuation of life-long learning that will help our student function—and become—his or her very best.

Development of grammar will stop for our older students, but growth in other areas of language will continue for the rest of our students' lives.

Functional communication is about expressing what matters to the individual student. For those of us who support students, it means being aware of the person's language profile, including his combination of grammar, mitigations, and gestalts, and supporting him to communicate within the myriad venues of life. Some students have a complete grammar system; some have a partial one; others have only mitigations; still others only gestalts to work with. Finally, some students have never had their natural language assessed. This last scenario is perhaps more common than we would like to think. Some students have only been acknowledged for their use of the scripts, survival phrases, and vocabulary they have learned to say and generalize. If a student has only had learned-language to communicate with and his natural language has never been fully acknowledged or understood, you may be the first person to consider assessing it.

Functional communication is about expressing what matters to the individual student.

So before we consider the functional communication goals for students whose natural language has been acknowledged along the way, let's take some time to outline an assessment for the student whose natural language has never been assessed. The first consideration is like that for a much younger child: notice natural communicative intentions, ways of communicating that are outside the cued scripts, and words and phrases the student has been taught to say. Look for ways of communicating that harken back to the natural: intonation, gesture, body proximity, and mumbled "movie talk." You want to figure out what a student might be communicating spontaneously, so, more than anything, we want the student to be himself: to be natural and to express himself spontaneously. We want to honor that person by accepting and embracing him, just as he is, and truly being there with him.

If an older student's natural language has never been assessed, here's an outline of what to do.

With that in mind, please try these things to set the stage for your assessment:

1. Sit back, smile, and just be in comfortable proximity with this young person

in a setting that is supportive and pleasant for him or her. Maybe it's the OT room when it's half-occupied; maybe it's the library when no one seems to be paying attention. Whatever it is, find a space that supports your student to be herself.

Follow your student's lead.

Notice and support choices and happy sounds.

Respond to communicative attempts by smiling and listening.

2. Expect nothing, but be ready to follow your student's lead on the trampoline, in the ball pit, on the floor, in the pool, into the box of Legos. You are establishing the terrain for spontaneous communication to take place. You want to see your student at his communicative best, so you are setting things up for that to happen.

3. Notice choices, happy sounds. Join the student and help with regulation so the choices and sounds continue. This lets the student know that she gets to be herself—to spontaneously make noise and decisions for herself—and that she doesn't have to try to figure out what you want from her.

4. Notice communicative attempts; respond warmly with your actions but not your words just yet. Words might seem like inadvertent "judgment" to him, so wait until you know what to say that will not be misinterpreted. Listen and keep smiling: you are letting the student know you understand he is attempting to communicate and that you are trying to hear the message. Simply trying goes a long way towards helping the student continue his attempts. You are on the road to assessment.

5. Honor communication in any form. Try to follow the student's lead, non-verbal and verbal. Have fun—together. Be sure to let the student know whenever she has successfully communicated an intention, even if the message itself is still fuzzy. This creates a social bond and an atmosphere in which communication can continue.

6. When you can, without changing the atmosphere, jot down some notes. You might want to wait until the next time you are together, but whenever it happens, you are assessing spontaneous communication. Your notes will remind you which situations supported communiqués; they will tell you what your student found important enough to try to communicate about. They might even tell you the form and the function of certain nonverbal, and even verbal, messages.

Assessing language

If you are an SLP, the last section in this book is designed to give you the tools to complete a full NLA assessment. Even if you are not an SLP, the above outline is intended for you, because anyone with an open mind and an open style can witness our older students communicating spontaneously. Once you have achieved all six steps, however, you will want to partner with an SLP who is experienced in listening to students talk, as it can be daunting to decipher rapid, under-articulated speech, especially if a student is speaking in sentences, echolalic or not.

Also, if the student is new to you, you will want to compare your observations with someone who knows the student well. For that reason, one of the guidelines for NLA assessment is watching a home movie that shows the student in a variety of natural activities at home. A home visit might be part of the assessment protocol as well, depending on the extent of the information gathered elsewhere.

Establishing communication objectives

Know that your assessment will be invaluable in determining the language level you can target and/or the level you should use in establishing communication objectives. You will probably want to read the first chapters of this book to remind yourself what a pure NLA progression looks like. But even though the progression is the same for older students, Chapter 15 made it abundantly clear how murky the water can look for them. Even with Bevin, language levels could have been missed completely had it not been for certain supports that were added to his life at crucial times.

Know also that important communication objectives can be written for any student at any NLA level, with or without remaining potential for grammar development. Regardless of how much grammar a student has the competence to use, using language for communication is always the most important goal. If a student has some generative grammar, it will be useful in setting goals. Even if a student does not have generative grammar but has a nice variety of mix-and-match mitigations, using them flexibly enhances communication. Temple Grandin has maintained that her own language is made up of mitigations, mixed and matched for the occasion. And many of us have witnessed myriad occasions in which Grandin's communication was enormously successful. Matching one's best language to each life situation is key to social communication.

Regardless of how much grammar a student has, using language to communicate is always the most important goal.

Establishing communication objectives requires making a survey of the ways a student currently uses natural language to communicate, other communicative intentions she displays non-verbally, natural language she might use to express those other intentions, and the communication opportunities that could be provided for her. We often target intentions such as requesting things we want and need, calling others, requesting help, and asking factual questions. But the more social communicative functions often prove most salient to our students: sharing experiences, ideas, thoughts, and feelings; asking opinions; and asking for input. We sometimes make the mistake of thinking our ASD students aren't socially-inclined, when their social intentions simply remain hidden until they have accessible language with which to intelligibly express them.

The social functions of communication often prove most salient to our students: sharing experiences, ideas, thoughts, feelings; asking for opinions and input.

With an attentive communication partner who is committed to reading between the lines, students can achieve important communication objectives even with basic grammar, mix-and-match mitigations, and short gestalts. You will want to partner with an SLP to map it all out, but it can be done. Your student will benefit from your faith in the process and your modeling of how such conversations might sound. Even more important than modeling, though, is partnering with your student to create conversations when they matter the most to him. Your feedback establishes a way for back-and-forth conversation to take place and provides a vehicle for addressing all of the student's communication objectives into the future. In your partnership, you will practice and perfect a method for your student to engage with you and others as conversations on life's important topics come up, whenever they come up, during her lifetime.

Using conversational feedback

The part of a student's language that is at Stage 1 or Stage 2 can't always be taken literally. You both may take several turns in conversation before you understand a particular intended message.

The part of a student's language that is at Stage 1 or Stage 2 can't always be taken literally. You both may take several turns in conversation before you understand a particular intended message. Your feedback lets the student know that you are willing to work with him until you "get it," and in the process of taking conversational turns, he learns how you are interpreting his message so he can modify it. If the language a student is using is echolalic, he might be saying words he's only heard other people say before. In the following conversation with Bevin, I first misunderstood his intention because I took it literally. Once he modified his language, I understood that some of his words reflected what he thought I might feel, and some were his own reaction:

B	**I'm so disappointed.**
M	You are, with me?
B	**I'm so disappointed and sorry.**
M	Oh, am I disappointed in you? No, I'm not. You didn't do anything wrong. You don't have to be sorry.

One mark of the 'bingo' moment when a student feels understood is that he can then move on.

The message trumps the language—every time.

Bevin was worried about what I was thinking, but did not have access to the question form he needed. He had access to this emotion-packed comment, however, and might have continued saying it, more to himself than to me, had I not understood. But I gave him relevant feedback, and the conversation continued. Its most telling feature, however, was that it then ended. One mark of the 'bingo' moment when a student feels understood is that he is freed up to move on. In the case cited here, Bevin felt understood, and he did move on. It might take longer than two turns each for a conversation of this importance to communicate. If the student begins with an echolalic comment whose source is unknown, his partner might need to posit a few mitigations before the conversation can continue. This means is that such conversations can take time. But the detective work is well worth it when our kids finally feel understood and freed up to move on to other areas of interest.

One important take-away lesson here is that the message trumps the language every time. Acknowledging our students when we understand them is imperative. It always is. If we understand, truly understand, we are serving our students and promoting their social conversation and well-being. Correct language or not, sharing and understanding are what matter!

Remember how long it has taken our students to get to reciprocity—so resolve to 'stay in the conversation' with them as long as possible.

Our students demonstrate tenacity in their willingness to continue trying in the face of difficult odds. It helps to remember this, even when their language begins to sound more flexible and "normal." What they are dealing with mentally and emotionally is taxing, which makes access fluctuant and often difficult. We need to remember how long it has taken many of our students to get to a place where reciprocity is possible and resolve to stay in the conversation with them whenever we—and they—can.

Considering sensory and learning history

In both assessment and goal-setting with older students, it is also important to remember where they came from and what they were like when they were younger. Their sensory and learning history is important, even if some of it no longer seems as relevant. When a student was sound-sensitive as a youngster, it affected her ability to integrate language experiences. When a student spent years gravitationally insecure, exploration and play were restricted. When tactile sensitivity limited sensory experiences, skill development lagged. When a student limited her input to the visual, bridging to the auditory world took time.

Whatever backgrounds students have, it behooves us to remember that they weren't always able to tolerate their environments as they well as they can now. A common scenario is the inability to tolerate more than one input channel until later in childhood. Even as an adult, Temple Grandin describes the translation process from one channel to the other that is part of her thinking. Words conjure up pictures, she does her real thinking in pictures, then she translates the pictures into words for expressing thoughts verbally.

Older students weren't always able to tolerate their environments as well as they can now.

Grandin's teachings are now legend in our autism community and deserve reflection as we assess our older students. "I think in pictures," she famously wrote. "Words are like a second language to me. I translate both spoken and written words into full-color movies, complete with sound, which run like a VCR tape in my head. When somebody speaks to me, his words are instantly translated into pictures," (Grandin, 1995, p. 3). The phenomenon is hardly singular to autism. One of my SLP colleagues described his own processing as similar, especially when he was younger. Zadock Cropper noted that he processed language very slowly because he painstakingly translated whatever people said into pictures. He then did his "real" thinking in pictures and had to re-translate back into words so he could take his turn in conversation. "When I was in elementary school," he said at a workshop, "and the teacher called on me to answer a question, I had to translate her words into pictures in order to figure out the answer. Then I had to translate the visual answer into words so I could tell her. All this took some time, and by the time I was ready to answer, she had moved on to someone else. No one thought I was very smart in elementary school." Later, as an adult, his processing time became quite rapid with casual conversation, but at the time he shared this, he said he was still uncomfortable with more detail-laden exchanges (Cropper, 2000).

In our clinic's experiences with kids with ASD, we have found that most of our classically ASD kids tend to be excellent visual thinkers, many of them extremely talented. Kathy, the parent of one of our children, told us that her son "always had the ability to re-visualize … always to play back everything in his head and to store and to memorize everything … I feel that when he is pulling videos out of his head that he's actually placing himself in the video, that these people are actually around him, that it's colored, like he could reach out and touch and move through the movies as he's seeing them" (Kathy Schroud, personal conversation, 1998). As our students, particularly the older students, become more and more accustomed to using words, we can support them best when we realize how difficult, and even foreign, words have been. Again citing Temple Grandin, from her book, *Animals in Translation*, we would be wise to

Some of us in education are guilty of thinking that words are the ultimate goal for our students, but words can compete with the rich thinking that is possible without them.

realize how much mental work is possible and better without words. Some of us in education are guilty of thinking that words are the ultimate goal for our students, but Grandin reminds us that words actually compete with the rich thinking that is possible without them (Grandin, 2005).

We should also realize that by the time our students are older, they have spent quite a long time forming concepts. In *Thinking in Pictures* (1995), Grandin described this process for herself: "… my thoughts move from video-like, specific images to generalization and concepts. For example, my concept of dogs is inextricably linked to every dog I've ever known …" Grandin also talked about imagining new images: "I'm always forming new visual images when I invent new equipment … I can take images that I have seen, rearrange them, and create new pictures. For example, I can imagine what a dip vat would look like modeled on computer graphics … I take computer graphics I have seen on TV … and superimpose them in my memory. In my visual imagination the dip vat will appear in the kind of high-quality computer graphics shown on Star Trek" (p. 12).

Bevin provided me with a tangible example. In his last year of middle school, he began working on concepts in earnest. He assembled items that met his definition of "desert" or "bests" or "wolf-catchers" and then take pictures of them. Undoubtedly, he was creating new pictures in his encyclopedic brain, and although I could never fully follow the logic of his assemblages, I never doubted their usefulness to his thinking.

Take into account where that person has been and what the mental life of that person currently is.

So, in order to establish language goals for our older student, we need to take into account where each person has been and, as best we can, what the mental life of that person currently is.

Supporting language and communication

Language models should be at each student's language level, should be from his perspective, and should match his intention as best we can determine.

As older students, our ASD kids have learned to use input in different modalities, input that is processed in both cerebral hemispheres and input that comes not just holistically, but sequentially. But even so, our language programs need to take into account where our students have come from. Just as our older students still appreciate intriguing, relevant visual input, they still tend to echo gestalt language that is intriguing and relevant—especially language that matches their intention. For this reason, supporting language development depends, at least partially, on modeling the right language for the right occasion. To make sure it's not just a drill which promotes learning more gestalts, however, the language has to be at each student's language development level and truly from his perspective. That means language has to match a student's intentions, which can be tricky. How do we know the student's communicative intent? If the nonverbal clues aren't there, the verbal ones may be confusing: for example, a gestalt whose original context has been lost to time. Unless we know a student well, how do we know what his particular words might mean to him?

We can effectively deal with this conundrum by being honest and letting our older students know that we will try: that we will not be perfect, but that we care enough to keep trying. Students always seem deeply appreciative of our good intentions, even when first attempts are off-target. They learn to trust our understanding of them, not that we will always have the right language, but that sometimes we will. When students have learned they can take us seriously, they listen more closely and, when they recognize a language match, embrace it for themselves.

Here is a simple, but profound, example of how having the right words at the right time can pay off. Typically, Bevin did not echo much that I said; he echoed only when I said the exact right words for what he was thinking. Occasionally, I was able to seize a moment when Bevin was not only "teachable" but open to the acknowledgement of something very personal. The following exchange occurred one day when Bevin had done something particularly brave:

M	You're perfect.
B	**I'm perfect.**
M	You were brave.

I didn't get the opportunity to pay him this kind of compliment very often. So, it was particularly special to me that Bevin not only accepted my idea, but used the language I modeled to make it his own.

Unfortunately, "teachable moments" like this come less frequently than we would wish, and only when regulation is good. And as we well know, when regulation is less than optimal, nothing works.

Being regulated = available

Regulation issues may get easier for our students to understand and deal with as they work through them over time, but they don't seem to go away completely. Rather, they seem to resurface again and again as life's demands change. As our kids' bodies grow taller, they're harder to coordinate, and sensory modulation and motor coordination often have to be learned all over again. Plus, hormones race, emotions erupt, life gets more demanding, and sensitivities can explode without warning. As much as we would like them to be behind us, sensory diets are literally 24/7 throughout the teen years.

So it makes sense, then, to put a broader frame around regulation and to remember that even as neurotypical adults, our own regulation needs vary from day to day and even from hour to hour. We have only to remind ourselves about when we tend to stretch and yawn, when we sip our coffee, and when we find outselves fiddling with our hair to remember that all of us with our individual needs are part of one long continuum of humanity. It's just that our kids are farther to the end of that continuum and need our help to make sure that the materials for stretching and fiddling are as accessible to them as ours are to us.

Remember what regulation is and what competence is, and don't confuse the two.

Something else we can do for our student, and for ourselves, is to remember what regulation is and what mental competence is, and not confuse the two. At a minimum, we are chagrined by poor regulation, and sometimes we are scared by it. Our student is too. So, our attitude and strategies should remain steadfast when the chips are down: reach for the items in the sensory diet that have worked, and remember that your student has not lost competence. Remind him of that—again and again—and remind him that when his regulation is restored, so will his access to that competence be restored. Stay the course and don't succumb to panic.

Being regulated = language-accessible

We all forget what losing "access" to language is until we experience it ourselves. We know how to be nice; we know how to "use our words" to be polite in social situations. In the car, we carry on conversations with our kids in the back seat, occasionally reminding them, "Could you be a little quieter, guys?" We are so socially perfect—until an emergency. The storm cloud breaks, visibility plummets, and so does our demeanor. Once we feel the car start to hydroplane, we want absolute silence so we can think. Rather than say, "Oh, Darlings, could you refrain from talking for a few moments while I adjust my driving," we say, "Stop that talking now!" We might even pull out all stops and yell, "Quiet!" in a loud voice that belies our need for silence. What we are experiencing is lack of access to language—language we have been using many times a day, almost all our lives.

And even though we'd like to forget such experiences, remembering one is valuable when we think about our students who have had particular language within their competence for only a few years, or a few months. Maybe you've heard a student say something once or twice and even overheard him practicing it by himself many times. But then comes the inevitable: he tries to say it later, when he actually needs it, and he can't. He has been heard to say, "Not now!" But under duress, he yells, "No!" or just screams. You think, "He said it politely once (or twice or twenty times). Why can't he say it now?"

You have just witnessed lack of language access. Access is also called "language retrieval" or "word finding," even though the latter is misleading because it's really about language-finding. For our kids, retrieving recently-developed grammar or recently-learned vocabulary is always hard, unless it's during play or practice. But when a student is really trying to say it on purpose, it's almost impossible unless everything else is just right. When we talk about a maximally-supportive environment for our kids, that's what we mean. And that's what your student needs until the target language is so well-practiced under a great variety of supported conditions (both linguistic and life situations) that it becomes automatic when moderately supported.

Thinking and talking deliberately when the chips are down is close to impossible.

Unfortunately, life also comes with lots of minimally-supportive conditions and lots of challenging ones, and that's when language retrieval is the hardest. Talking automatically is one thing; thinking and talking deliberately is another. And thinking and talking deliberately when the chips are down is close to impossible—which segues to the next topic: augmenting language output when access is limited.

Augmenting language output

One has only to look at the media to realize how critical augmentative communication is within the autism community. The reader is referred to this author's column series, "Finding the Words … with Augmented Communication," *Autism Asperger's Digest*, for an overview of the topic. The reasons for using communication augmentation are myriad, but the common challenge is usually reliable access to intelligible language output. Challenges can be at the speech level: muscle weakness, incoordination, or motor planning (dyspraxia). Challenges can be at the auditory processing level: discrimination and sequencing of auditory input and matching it to vocal output. And as we know, they can also be at the language level: that is, access to language structures and vocabulary whose use is not yet automatic. Not only have our students with delayed language development had limited time with their new language structures, but "finding" them amidst the long-held gestalts takes time—and self-regulation. The teenage years are notoriously dysregulating for all students, especially those with sensorimotor challenges. This makes access to newer, generative language particularly difficult for our kids.

Many creative communicators have amply demonstrated the richness that can be conveyed through typing, keyboarding, and pointing to spell when oral language production is challenging. Visual-motor modalities are often ideal for language expression when oral output stalls. Char Brandl is one educator who has helped many young people move from Facilitated Communication to independent typing by gradually reducing the degree of resistance students need to achieve graded keyboarding (Brandl, 1999).

In *The Way I See It* (2008), Temple Grandin commented on Amanda Baggs, who famously demostrated her use of typing to communicate in a YouTube clip, "In My Language." Juxtaposed against a visual of herself rocking, humming, and slapping, Baggs then beautifully explains with typed language how her senses provide her a "constant conversation" with her environment (p. 86).

Another method of using spelling to communicate, the Rapid Prompting Method (RPM), was devised by Soma Mukhopadhyay. By pointing with their right hand to spell and placing their materials on the right side of their bodies, students access left brain concentration. The adult also stands on student's right side, so that her speech is being received by the student's right ear and left hemisphere.

"… and in the face of connectivity problems that prevent the right message from reaching the mouth, some persons with autism substitute alternative words and phrases that were practiced out of motor memory."

In her book, Mukhopadhyay (2008) explained her reasoning for using the pointing modality to bypass automatic speech: "Due to the social demand to reply verbally, and in the face of connectivity problems that prevent the right message from reaching the mouth, some persons with autism substitute alternative words and phrases that were practiced out of motor memory. Sam might say, "I want French fries," instead of, 'Please do not discuss me in front of everyone.' He reached for and got out a phrase he has uttered so many times that it is readily accessible to him through rote memory, even if it is not what he means" (*Understanding Autism through Rapid Prompting Method*, p. 58).

Mukhopadhyay included the story of 'Jack,' who had been doing well in school until the higher grade levels, but who then began experiencing increasing anxiety in the classroom as he wanted to take part in some subjects but not others. Mukhopadhyay (2008) wrote: "The teacher reported that Jack was becoming increasingly disruptive in the general classroom; his anxiety was resulting in overwrought verbalizations. In order to avoid embarrassment due to his difficulty in encoding variable situations and the challenges of more sophisticated textbooks, Jack had to take refuge in his old, restricted selection of phrases and subjects ... RPM provides a way to keep Jack integrated by pairing up his use of anxiety words with a lesson plan ... " (p. 102).

Mukhopadhyay went on to explain how Jack's phrase "I am scared" became "diluted" as he was involved with a RPM lesson about soldiers who were not scared. Mukhopadhyay attributed to Jack "an active, intentional form of vocalization with a deliberate function, to drown out the other auditory aspects of the environment." From the perspective of NLA, it would seem that Jack had retreated to saying his old (right-brained) gestalts as part of mentally watching internal movies with these phrases as the sound track. Through the left-brained technique of RPM, he was effectively pulled out of them and back into analytic processing..

Will was a CDC client during his teenage years, often balancing his gifted right brain's ability to hold and process several input modalities at the same time with his desire to communicate with sequentially-ordered language. Will effectively switched from beautifully-delivered echolalia to under-used, under-articulated, and stilted generative language. His family recalled that Will had used generative language as a young boy, but that it was often so soft and indistinct that few people heard it, recognized it, or engaged Will in conversation. Over the years, Will was taught to say a handful of scripted phrases and sentences, which he produced very clearly. This became the language those around him expected, and both his echolalia and his generative language were essentially ignored. Both were revived when Will began at our clinic at the age of fourteen. There, he created expressive songs, jokes, and stories and engaged in regular conversation, using his mix-and-match style. At the age of eighteen, Will was introduced to RPM, and a year later, he was composing his own stories by pointing to letters. Effectively bypassing his oral language conundrum, RPM offered Will direct access to his left-brain generative language in a way that was not reliable with oral speech.

Life-long learning and whole-brain thinking

Just as we all do, Will, Bevin, and other older students move back and forth between their cerebral hemispheres, depending on the task, the modality, and the goal. Temple Grandin explained that sometimes the shift is to engage in particular kinds of visual thinking. Will seemed to do it as he moved from processing linearly (with RPM) to processing holistically (when he created multiple media montages). Bevin seemed to shift from his left hemisphere to his right as he explored new language sources, performed his visual thinking, and added to conceptual categories. He seemed to shift back to his left hemisphere as he formulated grammatically, created stories, or wrote in his journal.

As students get older, they develop the ability to consciously do this shifting. As we all mature, we learn to shift at will. Cerebral transitions are sometimes difficult for any of us, though, and we might have to be dragged kicking and screaming from watching a movie, painting, or gardening in order to pay our bills, write a shopping list, or plan a trip.

For kids, especially ASD kids, these transitions are particularly difficult, and when children are young, they really have no awareness with which to steer back and forth. This developmental ability is known as "metacognition," meaning, "above cognition," or awareness of thinking. As we get older, it is what allows us the conscious choice to select what we think about and how.

Let's take an example. As a youngster, JP was decidedly right-brained and gestalt, but by second grade, he had developed whole-brained skills and good self-generated language. He had retained some flowery language in his right brain, which made him an excellent story-teller and emerging writer. JP had also learned how to make people happy at school by embracing his left-brained skills and curtailing his right-brained ones. Essentially rejecting one side of himself, JP felt he was more successful at getting along in a left-brained school system.

His parents were saddened by JP's decision, however, and by fourth grade, JP was mature enough to be metacognitive and happy with his parents' urging to revisit his other hemisphere. By integrating the two, JP finally discovered his "whole brain" and learned that he could rely on himself to do much more than just get along at school. His right-brained imagination enhanced his joy of learning, and as a gifted thinker, JP then had a multitude of right-brained ways to keep himself engaged when the redundancy of sequential tasks threatened to sap his creativity.

By the time we are in high school or college, most of us have learned that we can tap into disparate parts of our mind to meet all kinds of intellectual challenges. And when we look into the field of whole brain integration, we find that myriad programs are designed to help us pull together our left and right abilities. Fascinating in the ways that they focus on bilateral physical activity and crossing the body's midline and coming back again, we see how we are asking our brain to do the same thing. The figure 8 of Brain Gym, for instance, is a well-known way to wake up one's brain for a day at school (Dennison, 2010). As we get older, it gets easier, and by the time we are teenagers, we sometimes just need to quiet the part of our brain that is commanding all our attention and remember that the other hemisphere is still there.

Using—and not using—both hemispheres

Thinking without the left hemisphere sounds like an anathema after we have tried so hard to help our kids move to their left brains and ultimately achieve whole-brained thinking. But there are lessons to be learned from one interesting account. Because this happened to a woman who was able to describe it in retrospect, we can learn something about what might cause our kids to just want to 'hang out' in their right brains.

When she suffered a left-brain stroke, neuroanatomist Jill Bolte Taylor lost all language and sequential function. But after eight years, she recovered sufficiently to tell about her experience. In *My Stroke of Insight* (2008), Taylor wrote about the morning of the stroke: "The harder I tried to concentrate, the more fleeting my ideas seemed to be. Instead of finding answers and information, I met a growing sense of peace. In place of that constant chatter that had attached me to the details of my life, I felt enfolded by a blanket of tranquil euphoria … As the language centers in my left hemisphere grew increasingly silent and I became detached from the memories of my life, I was comforted by an expanding sense of grace. In this void of higher cognition and details pertaining to my normal life, my consciousness soared into an all-knowingness, a 'being at one' with the universe … In a compelling sort of way, it felt like a good road home and I liked it …" (p. 41).

Taylor continued to describe her sense of her body: "I was aware that I could no longer clearly discern the physical boundaries of where I began and where I ended. I sensed the composition of my being as that of a fluid rather than a solid. I no longer perceived myself as a whole object separate from everything. Instead, I now blended in with the space and flow around me" (Taylor, 2008, p. 42).

Language can mask and overshadow right-brained talents and perceptions.

While Taylor's perceptions the morning of her stroke are clearly more dramatic and extreme than what ASD individuals experience, it behooves us to learn something important from this astute observer. Those of us who tend towards balanced thinking or left-brain thinking can be quick to presume that ours is the best way to be and that it presents a worthy goal for our students. As Grandin has cautioned, though, language can mask and overshadow right-brained talents and perceptions. Without words in her head, Taylor felt at one with her surroundings and at peace. Thinking about kids who do not have a sense of where their bodies end and their surroundings begin, Bolte felt this fluidity was a gift. Taylor described a living-in-the moment feeling we seek in meditation but shun as planners and organizers in daily life. Taylor put a spin on right-brained thinking that we should keep in mind as we plan our strategies to change our students' brains with language.

Taylor did something else that was quite interesting. She wrote that in spite of her injury she retained some ability to observe her own thinking. It was this metacognition that prompted her to seek help and eventually recover full left-brain function. That same metacognition, she said, can allow any of us to choose where in our brains we "live" from one moment to the next: that is, the part of our cerebral cortex from which we experience life. By extension, if we learn to apply her lessons to ourselves, we might imagine helping our kids achieve greater metacognition and how they can choose to use their brains—from moment to moment, from task to task.

Life-long learning and metacognition

Many higher-level cognitive skills are learned best once students are old enough to be metacognitive. Language development is certainly not supposed to be one of them, but, for our older students, it often happens. There are trade-offs involved, some we have talked about in several places in this book. But the one advantage is that our older students can consciously choose when and how to practice their new language skills and what they want to achieve with them.

One of the interesting phenomena about Natural Language Acquisition is the mix of hemispheric activity that must be involved. We feel that we can see our kids beginning with right-brained visualizing and imagining as they mentally replay movies and life scenes along with their sound tracks. Mitigation brings in analysis, and we can imagine the hemispheric coordination involved in mitigating long gestalts and stopping and starting them like a human rewind. As phrases and words are isolated, shifts to the left brain must happen more and more until the left brain uses grammatical analysis to build original sentences. As the brain searches its store of visual images, movie clips, and poetic gestalts, there must be a rich blend of hemispheric activity. Even in daily conversation, the shifting from auditory processing to visual conceptualizing and back again is a complex and beautifully-orchestrated whole brain activity. Throughout life, of course, even after left-brained grammar development is complete, vocabulary growth and concept development continues, because it involves whole-brain activity.

Let's look again at Bevin, to see another way age factors into language development. We know that unlike toddlers or early elementary-aged kids, older students like Bevin experienced language development as more work than play. Recalling how readily a child like Dylan took to mitigating and to phrase formation, we see Bevin's experiences as more grueling and painstaking. He had to work at it. But what Bevin was not able to accomplish with light, childhood play talk, he was able to accomplish through planning and thinking and deciding what was worth **trying** to plan and think about and decide. Even so, the excitement of a potential overnight or an exciting idea for a story dialed the activity over towards the automatic side, and so a new set of play dough colors was a safe bet to prompt a flurry of semi-automatic practice with grammar. Keeping the activity at the level of the motoric "just right challenge" helped immensely, but it was also important to simply practice. When practicing new language, the written form helped make it less difficult. Drawing made it more whole-brained. But, ultimately, Bevin had to just buckle down, stick with his left brain, and practice talking. Yes, he could also assemble the visuals to match, take pictures of it all, write it all down, and applaud his success. But then he'd have to clean up and start the practice routine all over again.

Not so bad, really, but much much more work than what a young child of four or six or eight goes through.

As with so much of life, however, where the proof is in the pudding, the hard work paid off for Bevin, and that mattered tremendously to him. That he could sound somewhat like his high school peers often enough, that he could give a short speech in class about dinosaurs and have his peers ask him thoughtful questions, that he could plan his future digs in Utah and share his thoughts with his family and friends meant the world to Bevin—and helped him to move from the 'real boy' he knew he was to the real man he was becoming.

Examining the pudding

Question: if the proof is in the pudding, then what does the pudding look like? Answer: anything and everything each person wants—for the rest of his life. It's like that for all of us. We use our grammar in anything and everything we create verbally, in anything and everything we think about verbalizing—each day, all our lives. As our worlds expand over time, consider all the people we talk to, write to, share with, befriend. We take a class and learn the lingo. We embark on a new job and learn all the vernacular we will spout to our customers. We become parents and learn how to speak to our children, their babysitters, their teachers, their friends, their friends' parents, their suitors, their spouses, their children—you get the picture. It is endless!

And that's just about grammar. Then, there's all the rest of it: all the rest of language development and learning and use and exploration.

Vocabulary mushrooms everywhere: new words for new classes; new words for new associations; new words for new books; new words for each stage of our kids' growth; new words for each new change in world affairs. It is truly the stuff of life-long learning.

And social language isn't all grammar and vocabulary either. Think of the dynamics of different conversational modalities: the chatter of teenage girls; the banter of boys; the chat of moms across the playroom; the wisecracks at the baseball game; the high jinks shared on the golf course; the formal Q and A of the chemistry class vs. the lit class; the didactic style of the professor; the style of the letter to the editor; the style of the blog; the style of texting and tweeting. Language use is pragmatic, context-specific, and constantly changing.

It is true that some kinds of social language venues require precise wording and precise words. But that's just some kinds. Others rely on common vernacular and sound stilted if the grammar ante is too high. We set the bar to 'pretty basic' in our street jargon, our commercials, and our neighborly parlance. There are socially-acceptable venues for each of us, and social language dynamically morphs into new forms all the time. Regardless of the level of grammar achieved by any of our students, regardless of whether they can use any grammar outside of the mix-and-match of phrase combinations, social language growth is available to all. It might not reach the same level of complexity in each student, of course, but the fun of using language will grow for the rest of their lives.

I really hate to bring up Barney again, but, some of those old gestalts never die. "The fun and learning never ends!" he chortled.

I couldn't have said it better myself!

Chapter 18
In Conclusion

We have now come to the end of our journey but just the beginning of your child's. You may be reeling from all that natural language acquisition implies—for kids on the spectrum in general and for your child in particular—but please know that all of this information can be considered in due time. You may have taken some first steps already, especially if your child is young. But if your student is older and you really don't know where to start, this final chapter will give you a list of reasonable first steps and help you ease into the process. Once you take those first steps and see how your family can embrace them, you will start to understand how natural language development really is. You definitely know that your child is capable of moving naturally towards more spontaneous, flexible language use, and that is the most important step.

You may not have the time or the resources to start a program for your child today. You may only know that you do not want to invest any more of your child's time in scripted or dead-end language teaching. At least you know what you do not want. And you also know why: because it denies your child's potential, and can actually interfere with real language development.

You now have a viable argument to give your child a chance at language development. That is a valuable start.

First, do no harm

Thirty years ago, SLPs considered ASD kids able to attain natural language development on their own, given time and adequate support. Back then, they were free to initiate the mitigation process by themselves because no one was teaching them language scripts that competed with the natural process. Because they were not being asked to say, repeat, and use scripted language, developmental language was allowed to emerge, albeit more slowly than among their neurotypical peers, but emerge naturally nonetheless.

When ASD kids are not being asked to say, repeat, and use scripted language, developmental language is allowed to emerge.

Our ASD kids today have many wonderful resources, but language development resources have not typically been one of them. If nothing else, you can decide to do no harm with your ASD child and to make sure all well-intended but competing language goals and activities are removed from their programs.

Then, you might want to consider some preliminary steps—easy ones you can take with your family in order to get your feet wet with the concepts and to get your family thinking about your ASD child's language more broadly.

Taking some first steps—with your family

These first steps are some you can take at home. They will get your whole family thinking about the legitimacy of echoed language for your ASD child, for themselves, and for each other.

- Share the illustration on page 59 ("To be or not to be") and discuss the meaning of the comparison to the child quoting from the Disney movie, *Hercules*.

Identify your family's favorite quotes and challenge everyone to use them to communicate.

- Ask everyone in your family to identify their own favorite saying, quote, or other echoed phrase. Then identify one for each other family member. Post them all on the fridge, and challenge each person to use everyone else's in three different ways each day. So, if one person scowls, "Never!" all the time, then everyone tries to communicate with it. If another person cheerfully peppers her conversation with, "You got it!" then everyone tries that.
- Next, ask each person to identify one of your ASD child's favorite quotes, put them all on the fridge, and assign one to each family member to use meaningfully three times a day along with all the other "famous quotes" of your family.
- After a week, have a round-table discussion about what everyone learned about quotes, echolalia, and how they can communicate. See if "movie talk" seems to mean something different to everyone now.

Taking some first steps towards a family sensory diet

Ask everyone in your family to identify his or her sensory diet.

- Now talk with your family about sensory diets and have a round-table discussion in which each person identifies something in his or her own 'diet' and then one thing for each other person. It might be 'scratches chin when thinking' or 'rubs eyes while reading' or 'takes long showers on Sunday morning.' Whatever strikes each person, include it.
- Challenge each person in your family to come up with their own 24/7 sensory diet; post everyone's on the fridge.
- Have everyone contribute to the diet for your ASD child and post it, too.
- Have each person follow his own sensory diet and check off each item during the day—and add more items he or she discovered along the way.
- Have a follow-up conversation about what 'sensory' means and what the idea of a sensory diet is in regard to the ups and downs of a normal day.

Advocate for a focus on natural language development

Taking some next steps—language advocacy

- Request that your child's IEP include a goal to assess his current language development level.

- Eliminate any goals in the IEP or elsewhere that teach your child language outside of a developmental context, no matter how well-intended it is.
- If you are the only one on your child's team who sees your child as capable of developing natural language, seek out someone else to talk to. If you have no one else to talk to, contact our clinic to be connected with a mentor family.
- Provide copies of the *Digest* series, "Finding the Words … To Tell the Whole Story," to everyone on your child's team. Point out sections that will help them understand how you believe your child is capable of developing natural language.
- Request that someone on your child's team read this book; if no one can afford it, apply for a scholarship on our website.
- If your child does not have an SLP who feels able to apply the principles of NLA, look for another one. If you cannot find one, contact our clinic.
- If you are told your child needs to be taught certain phrases and sentences to use for safety, requesting, etc., reply that you want those functional language goals included only as part of an appropriate language development program.

Taking yet more steps—sensorimotor support

- If your child does not have an OT and/or PT who is successfully addressing self-regulation, find someone who can.
- Read books on sensory regulation; check the websites of those who specialize in this service delivery. Make sure it makes sense to you for yourself, your other family members, kids in general, and your ASD child.
- Don't give up. Remember that regulation = teachable moments. If natural language development is a birthright, steps to achieving regulation are, too.

Look for people and resources to support your child's sensory regulation.

Taking more serious steps

- Find someone to work with who will give your child the benefit of the doubt, intellectually. Once you embark on a program for your child, find an ally to work with.
- Find someone who quotes Temple Grandin, and you know you will have a friend. Quote some of Grandin's points and see who nods and smiles. Pick that person. It's always Temple Grandin who says it best. In *The Way I See It* (2008), for instance, she reminded us: "The DSM-IV definition of autism states that 75% of these individuals function at a mentally retarded level based on IQ scores. This sets up a vicious cycle: we expect less from these kids, so they receive fewer opportunities to learn. We don't challenge them to learn because we've already decided they can't. We test these children for IQ, using testing instruments that are largely ill-suited to this population,

Find people to work with who will give your child the benefit of the doubt intellectually and linguistically.

and then point to their low scores as confirmation of impaired mental functioning" (p. 85).

- Find someone to work with who will give your child the benefit of the doubt, linguistically. We have forgotten about the natural language development progression Prizant et al. described in the 1980s and act as if our kids are not capable of achieving natural language development. We have thought that a grammar system must be in place by age six, and when it is not, we have decided that our kids are not capable of developing one.
- Find someone who already knows from experience that this presumption is wrong—or find someone who is willing to listen.

Finally

We have now come full circle and ended where we began: with good intentions and a journey outlined that promises realistic hope for the young children and older students whose language is echolalic. Please feel very real hopefulness that your child is capable of developing and using self-generated language and finding a voice that is uniquely his or her own.

This beginning point is a very exciting place for both of you. Know that your story will be a rich one.

We would love to hear about some of your adventures and some of your child's own words to describe them.

We send along all our best wishes!

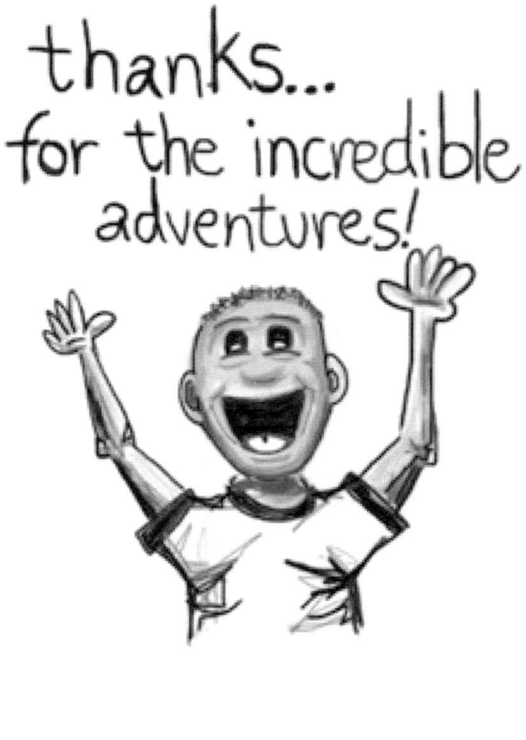

section 6

For Speech Language Pathologists: Language Sampling, Assessment and Intervention

Chapter 19
Collecting and Analyzing a Language Sample

Natural Language Acquisition assessment combines best practices from Speech-Language Pathology with clinical experience using NLA analysis to arrive at a flexible protocol to use in any clinical setting.

Traditional spontaneous language sampling techniques

Speech-Language Pathologists are well-prepared to solicit spontaneous language samples. Whether we are preparing to apply Brown's Stages, Systematic Analysis of Language Transcription (SALT), Developmental Sentence Scoring (DSS), or another measure of language competence, obtaining a representative, spontaneous language sample is well-understood. The elements are: soliciting a conversational sample of a child's spontaneous language by engaging in free play with the child, using materials known to be of interest to him, and matching a child's interest and cognitive level.

Because language analysis is a way of assessing developmental language competence, SLPs attempt to solicit a child's spontaneous use of natural language. "The clinician's main purpose is to keep the child interested, talking, and thinking as creatively as possible" (Lee, 1974, p. 59). In order to facilitate the child's use of his highest-level spontaneous language, the SLP is instructed to positively respond to the child's language, take equal turns (reducing direct questioning once the child is talking freely), and use some higher-level linguistic forms to see if the child will use them as well. An analyzable sample depends on the measure being applied but tends to be either 100 or 50 consecutive, spontaneous utterances (DST vs. DSS) or a 12-minute sample (SALT). Repeated sampling is often encouraged to ensure that the sample is truly representative of the child's linguistic performance.

Traditional spontaneous language analysis

Analysis of spontaneous language has traditionally applied one of several forms of syntactic and/or semantic coding in order to compare a child's use of original language with developmental norms. For example, DSS is a traditional analysis tool that can be used once a child produces 50 consecutive subject + predicate sentences within an hour. Syntax is the main component of analysis, but semantic integrity is included by means of a "sentence point" if the entire utterance is both syntactically and semantically correct. If a child is not producing 50 sentences per hour, Developmental Sentence Types (DST) can be applied to his "pre-sentences."

For DSS analysis, the spontaneous sample is recorded and transcribed, but only 50 consecutive sentences that are original, spontaneous, and analyzable (containing a subject + predicate) are scored and compared with age norms for children two to seven years old. The child's other utterances in the sample can be included in the transcription in order to calculate other measures of linguistic development, particularly Mean Length of Utterance (MLU) and measures of semantic development such as Type-Token Ratio (the ratio of different words to the number of total words).

In DSS, immediate echolalia disqualifies an utterance from analysis. As Lee (1974) stated, "Since the clinician is interested only in a child's self-formulated grammatical structure, sentences which are first formulated by the clinician and then echoed by the child must not be included." Immediate, mitigated echolalia is allowed, however, as Lee noted: "… if a child changes the clinician's sentence in any way and reformulates it into his own grammatical structure, then the child's sentence could be included …" (p. 68).

Language sampling for Natural Language Acquisiton analysis

Natural Language Acquisition (NLA) describes the stages of language development of children who began their development as gestalt language processors. Stage 1 (echolalia) is followed by Stage 2 (mitigated echolalia), when a child discovers the phrase parts of language gestalts and can "mix and match" them to create new wholes. Stage 3 (isolation and recombination of single words) occurs when Stage 2 phrases are further broken down into their component parts (single words), and words are "recombined" to create original, two-word phrases. Stage 4 describes beginning grammar as three- and four-word sentences develop. Stages 5 and 6 continue the development of generative grammar through all the levels and components of a mature grammatical system.

Language sampling techniques for NLA combine traditional methods with what we know about children on the autism spectrum and what we are attempting to ascertain about their use of echolalia, mitigation, word combining, and self-generated grammar. Each child is unique, so the setting for gathering a sample is tailored to each child. Any language sampling for analysis would require at least the following preparation: viewing a spontaneous movie clip taken of the child in his home environment; reading available reports about the child, including OT and PT reports; talking with the child's parents to ascertain the conditions that support his engagement and most spontaneous language use; setting up a clinical environment that considers parent and OT/PT recommendations; and spending at least 1–3 sessions with the child in an appropriate clinical setting.

The setting for gathering a language sample is tailored to each child.

Language sampling itself should include at least these parameters:

1. Physical supports for the child's speech and language access.
2. An attentive communication partner who is experienced in listening to echolalic language.
3. A recording and transcription method that does not interfere with play or spontaneous language production.

Obtain a detailed history of the child's language exposure, linguistic preferences, and language production.

Assessing language with NLA

Language can be assessed at any stage of a child's development using the NLA assessment procedure, as long as adequate linguistic background information has been obtained. Because Stage 1 utterances are echoed from other sources, understanding a child's Stage 1 and 2 utterances typically relies on some cross-referencing with linguistic sources (comments made to the child, favorite movies, songs, games, etc.). Even as a child moves through the stages, the origins of gestalts figure highly into assigning a stage for any particular utterance or utterance part.

For these reasons, an assessment begins by obtaining a detailed history of the child's language exposure, linguistic preferences (favorite stories, etc.), and language production.

Learning the history of language exposure

Depending on the extent of a child's language exposure, the history will be more or less detailed. A pre-school child who has a few favorite movies, books, songs, and games will have a far less complicated history than an elementary-aged student who has listened to many, many stories during his lifetime and might be drawing from any number of them as his Stage 1 comments. If a student is just beginning the NLA process in higher elementary grades or later, the encyclopedia of stories in his mind may be extensive.

Talk to several family members, as each has his or her own insight into the child.

Obtaining an adequate linguistic history also involves learning a child's interests, favorite themes, favorite people, and favorite characters. Discovering a child's most common linguistic themes is also vital to the complete history, even if a child seems minimally communicative. Just knowing which lines a child likes to hear and/or say frequently is a hint about what he might want to communicate.

Talking to several family members is often important. Each will have his or her own understanding of the child. Often siblings will be especially helpful in reporting their brother or sister's favorite themes and which lines the child often says. It is encouraging to find out how much family members often know about the origins of a child's echolalia and to learn that they, too, know the lines, having heard certain movies, stories, or songs dozens of times. Like Bevin and Tori, siblings often engage in the dialogues they find particularly entertaining.

Familiarity with the particular echolalic utterances a child is likely to be using is especially helpful in overcoming the problems inherent in the lack of intelligibility usually presented by children at Stage 1. Long gestalts are hard for young mouths to produce, and most pre-school children have difficulty making themselves understood when they are at Stage 1. Even older children can be quite difficult to understand if they have not mitigated much and are relying on an extensive library of long gestalts.

Obtaining other background material

Before eliciting the language sample to be used for the NLA assessment, it is important that the SLP gather as much information as possible so that the language sample will be analyzable. The following is a guideline for obtaining information:

1. Ask the family to make a home movie of their child in natural situations. Let the family know not to set it up but to simply gather natural footage so a variety of daily situations will be included. An hour's worth of footage often captures several short snippets that prove valuable.

2. Ask the family to compile a complete list of the child's current favorite media and personal language sources as well as past favorites.

3. Ask the family to provide a list of the child's common expressions, their source, and their possible meaning to the child (or at least to the character in the story).

4. Ask the family to provide emails or messages to complete these lists and to keep them current.

Obtain a home movie of the child in natural situations.

Preparing to elicit the language sample

Standard guidelines for obtaining spontaneous language samples are used. Those suggested by Laura Lee in *Developmental Sentence Analysis* (1974) are useful. With children on the spectrum, additional preparation should be made. Among the most important preparatory suggestions are:

1. Provide a setting in which the child's physical and linguistic access could be predicted to be at its best. This means setting up the play room to support the child physically, emotionally, and linguistically. Use of a school "sensory room" or gym with PT/OT recommendations for the child in place might be the most conducive setting. Try out the space during one session and make changes that would help the child feel most safe and supported. If it is evident that the child already talks spontaneously in a particular setting, consider using that one or set up one like it.

2. Provide a linguistic environment that might promote the child's spontaneous use of the language within his developmental competency. Avoid modeling "school language" or known scripted language, avoid asking questions, and avoid giving the impression that there is a "right" thing to say.

3. The language sample can be be taken during the first play session, but it will probably not be the child's best and should be repeated. The first session should be used to establish trust and rapport and to give the child a clear understanding that you are there to listen, not to "teach." The second or third session will probably be the best for eliciting a sample to analyze.

Provide a setting that supports the child's best physical and linguistic access and promotes spontaneous use of language.

4. Try out the audio equipment before the assessment session and determine that the naturalness of the interaction will not be disturbed by its use. If it is interfering, note-taking can be used, but the sample recorded by hand would usually not be complete. Another option would be to have a second, trusted person take notes, but have that person sit well to the side so the child does not think that person will have her own expectations.

Eliciting a spontaneous language sample

General guidelines within the field of Communicative Disorders apply. Language samples should be spontaneous, not prompted, and derived only minimally through question-asking. If you know the child responds spontaneously to question-asking, occasional questions might jump-start conversation, but direct answers to questions would usually not be counted as spontaneous, and would often lack certain grammar.

For children on the spectrum, other guidelines would apply as well. Children's space should be considered so that children feel safe and free to be themselves. Eye contact or other motor responses would not be expected. Toys and materials would be individually selected to match the visual style and interests of the child. Books and videos would not generally be used unless the clinician is confident that they would promote, rather than limit, spontaneous language use.

Generally accepted practices to "keep the conversation going" would be used, including equal turn-taking, using less language than the child, glossing judiciously, and maintaining an accepting and positive demeanor. These practices would be modified to match each child, so an examiner might take very limited turns if they were judged to inhibit the child's use of spontaneous language.

The assessment is of the child's developmental language competence. It is not an assessment of the words, phrases or sentences he has learned to say outside of his language development, e.g. 'scripts' or learned responses, with or without prompting, visual cuing, or other learning strategy. If the child tends to use utterances of this variety, the clinician should continue to try to elicit a segment that is truly spontaneous. This may take more than one session if a child is not used to his spontaneous language being heard, valued, or acknowledged.

Selecting a language sample for assessment

The sample should be long enough to be representative of the child's language competence at the time. It should be at least a 12-minute sample or a 50-utterance sample, but these minimum guidelines do not take into account the highly-variable patterns of children with ASD. A 12-minute sample might have only Stage 1 utterances, when an hour sample reveals Stages 1–4. One 50-utterance sample might contain mostly Stage 2 utterances, while another contains mostly Stage 4. Thus, two samples or one longer one might be needed to capture a more complete sampling of the child's spontaneous language.

The following NLA Scoring Guide is meant for Speech-Language Pathologists' clinical use to assess language levels and to chart language development in their clients. There may be clinician-to-clinician variation in recording styles. One client-clinician dyad might work best with hand-written notes. Another might allow a third person to take notes. Another would be comfortable with audio-taping or even video-taping.

Scoring a language sample with NLA

Samples should be transcribed verbatim. Partner turns, in whole or abbreviated, should be included to provide linguistic context for the conversation. The situation should be noted when important to understanding the linguistic context of the child's comments. All of a child's utterances should be included in the transcript: spontaneous utterances (natural and scripted) and others that were directly elicited (e.g. with a question).

All client utterances from the transcript are transferred to the NLA assessment form, included as Appendix B. Those that are deemed spontaneous (either natural or scripted) and not directly elicited are numbered and scored. An utterance other than a sentence is defined as a "unit of meaning" (series of sounds and words spoken as a unit). Even a long monologue is judged to be one utterance if it is spoken as a unit, as a gestalt.

Scripted utterances that have been specifically taught are numbered on the NLA form but scored 0, even if they are mitigated. NLA scoring reflects natural language development, not the use of learned utterances, even if mitigated. The latter might be valuable to note, however, and comments can be included in the summary.

Scoring guidelines are as follows:

1. Utterances that have been specifically taught are scored 0, both whole learned utterances and mitigated ones.
2. Utterances that are judged to be naturally-acquired whole gestalts, regardless of the length, are scored as Stage 1. Each is a "unit of meaning."
3. Utterances that are judged to be mitigated from natural whole gestalts are scored as Stage 2.
4. Utterances that are single words might be scored as Stage 1 if judged to have been acquired as gestalts; Stage 2 if mitigated from short gestalts as part of a broader Stage 2 process; or Stage 3 if isolated from mitigations as part of a broader Stage 3 process.
5. A two- to three-word utterance could be a Stage 1 gestalt, a Stage 2 mitigation, or a Stage 3 two-word combination. Only knowing the child's linguistic history will tell the examiner which it is.
6. Utterances that are longer than two to three words might be Stage 1 if echoed from elsewhere or Stage 2 if a mitigation. If the child has already successfully negotiated Stage 3, it might be beginning grammar, Stage

4. Again, knowing the child's linguistic history and broader process is imperative to decision-making.

7. Multi-word utterances of any length might be Stage 1 or 2 if they are echolalic in origin. If the child has passed through Stage 3 and it can be determined that the child is generating developmental grammar, they may be more accurately scored as Stage 4–6.

8. Once a child has a large percentage of Stage 4–6 utterances, DSS analysis should follow. Stages 4, 5, and 6 each represent levels within Developmental Sentence Scoring (Stage 4 = DSS 1–3; Stage 5 = DSS 4–6; Stage 6 = DSS 7 and 8). Note that the NLA form groups 4–6 together, however, because assigning Stages 4, 5, or 6 requires a knowledge of DSS. The real value in differentiating Stage 4 from 5 and from 6 is in treatment, because the grammar at each stage can usually be introduced at the same time.

9. Developmental Sentence Scoring is included as Appendix D and should be applied according to the guidelines for DSS.

10. An utterance can be scored as representing more than one Stage if this most accurately describes it. A common occurrence is an utterance that is made up of a mitigation plus an isolated single word, in which case one half point can be tallied in each of the two Stage totals. Another example is a combination of a mitigation plus grammar, in which case half points are tallied in both Stage 2 and Stages 4–6 totals.

11. Total number of points at each Stage are tallied and percentages calculated.

Determining assessment results

Determining the percentage of total utterances at each Stage within an appropriate language sample gives the clinician data to help with clinical decision-making about natural language development.

The following provides basic guidelines:

1. If 80% or more of the utterances in an appropriate sample are at one Stage, the child is likely operating at that Stage developmentally.

2. If 50% or more of the utterances in an appropriate sample are at one Stage, the child is likely operating at that Stage most (or much) of the time.

3. If no single Stage is represented more than 50% of the time, then processes at more than one Stage are being used.

4. The highest Stage that is represented suggests that the child is developing towards that level.

Establishing treatment goals

Treatment goals can be determined from the assessment results.

Stage 1

1. If the child is using Stage 1 language more than 50% of the time, it is important to look more closely at the other smaller percentage(s) and determine the types of language models at Stage 1 that might lead to a larger Stage 2 component by being easily mitigable.

2. If the child is using Stage 1 language 25–50% of the time, it is important to look at the Stage 2 percentage and examples. Looking at the variety and usefulness of Stage 2 mitigations, the clinician can determine what other mitigations might be helpful to move the child solidly to Stage 2 and beyond. The types and variety of Stage 2 mitigations help the clinician assess the types and varieties of models (Stage 1 or Stage 2) that would be the most useful.

3. If the child is using Stage 1 language less than 25% of the time, it may be that Stage 1 language is providing only linguistic "background" for mitigations and providing cross-referencing for Stages 3 and 4.

Stage 2

1. If a child is using Stage 2 language more than 50% of the time, helping to support its functionality and flexibility is important. When people are tuned into the fact that a child is communicating, their feedback helps the child identify what others understand and helps the mitigation process continue. Communicative use of mitigations helps the child to isolate their component parts as well, helping him move some of his language to Stage 3. Ample social language opportunities give the child a feeling of communicative success and helps promote the continuation of natural language development.

2. If a child is using Stage 2 language between 25 and 50% of the time, finer examination of the variety of phrase mitigations is important in order to provide mitigable gestalts and mitigations that will be quickly useful to the child. Social language opportunities are imperative.

3. If the child is using Stage 2 language less than 25% of the time, it is still important to look at those mitigations to see how more examples might help the child isolate the component parts that are yet alluding him.

Stage 3

1. When a child is developmentally ready for Stage 3, his age will likely determine when he tries out his single words and two-word combinations. If he is a pre-schooler, he will probably feel comfortable using them in social situations without feeling pressure to sound more "correct." If he is older, however, and senses how unusual he sounds, he may need encouragement to use this mix-and-match stage in fun practice situations. You will need to set up these situations and play with words (and ideas) with him.

2. If a child is using Stage 3 single words and two-word combinations more than 50% of the time during practice sessions, looking at the variety and flexibility of the combinations is important. Providing opportunities for building a great variety of conceptual combinations will help support the child in getting ready for Stage 4.
3. If the child is using Stage 3 words and combinations between 25 and 50% of the time during practice sessions, it is important to look at Stage 2 and make sure it is comfortable and functional for the child. He may need more Stage 2 language to further break down in order to make a good transition to Stage 3.
4. If a child is using Stage 3 words and combinations less than 25% of the time, it depends on his use of the other levels to determine recommendations. If he is moving out of Stage 1 well and is using Stage 2 flexibly and well, a small percentage of Stage 3 single words provides him with good building materials for Stage 4. This may be just the right combination.

Stage 4

1. If the child is using Stage 4 (or higher) more than 50% of the time, it is important to look at each grammatical utterance to make sure it is developmentally appropriate and foundational to higher-level grammar. It is as important to look at the incorrect sentences as the correct ones, as the former will reflect emerging understanding of the rules of grammar, as well as a child's original thinking. Too many "correct" sentences can be a red flag that the child is trying to sound a certain way, and may undermine the natural developmental process. Too many "correct" sentences increases the possibility that a child will revert to scripted sentences, which he knows are "correct."
2. If the child is using Stages 4–6 between 25 and 50% of the time, it is important to look at Stage 3 to make sure it is rich and varied and supportive of more Stage 4 development. It is also important to look closely at Stage 4 to make sure all structures at each DSS level are represented with a variety of vocabulary and that the child is not trying to move on to higher grammar before he is well-supported with basic grammar.
3. If a child is using Stages 4–6 less than 25% of the time, an examination of the other levels is most important. Grammar should not be promoted before there are adequate building blocks, which need to come from Stage 2 mitigations through Stage 3 single-word isolation.

Repeating the assessment

It is recommended that an assessment be repeated in one to two weeks to help determine if the first assessment reflected the child's true language level. It is also recommended that assessments take place every 3–4 months in order to track longitudinal language development.

In conclusion

To all of you who have read this final chapter and taken it to heart, welcome to the family of those of us who acknowledge the past of our profession and who are ready to pick up the chain of history that we nearly lost two decades ago. Our ASD kids are ready and able to become the language users they have the capacity to be, to be acknowledged as linguistically capable, and to represent themselves as intelligent communicators among their families and peers.

With your help, our ASD kids can attain respect. They are among the half of the population who began their linguistic journey as gestalt language processors, and with our help, they will be able to achieve their rightful status as legitimate language processors. With that elevated status, they can achieve natural language development and flexible use of language to communicate their own personal intentions!

Thank you, and all the best in your worthy endeavor.

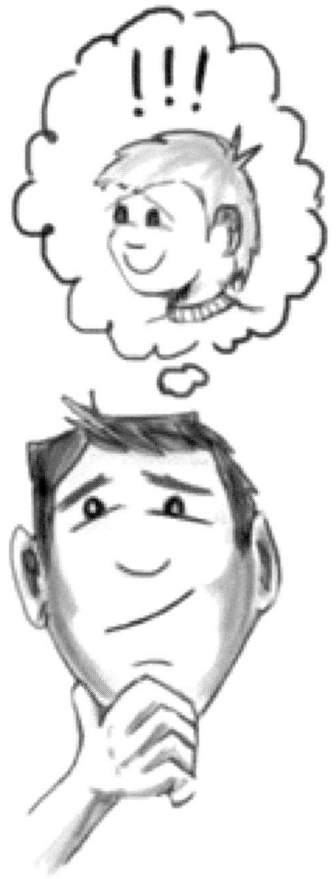

Afterward

In the world of a child with autism, there is no greater power than the combination of pure love, seriously hard work and a bull-dog determination.

Love bends its knees to meet the child on the mat. Love melds itself forward and listens to words spoken from heart to heart. Love stretches up to find and meet inner dreams hidden to most. Love oozes into places in the world of a child and his family that need healing, places that are dry and cracked and in need of the water of hope that love brings.

Love is fearless. Love is research on legs. Love is trying over and over and over. Love sees brilliant when the world sees disability. Love never, ever fails.

Love seeks ways to make it happen, to coax a child to his excellence. Love patiently waits for a child to grow into his world, and love offers stand-by assist as long as it takes.

Love is patient. Love is kind to a mother's heart, and keeps the whole family in mind. Love honors siblings. Love draws excellence into a child's life. Love makes a child irresistible to peers.

Love is never too little; it is never too much. Love oozes hope. When you move in love, you nudge out fear. Love is medicine; love is healing. Love is seriously hard work and love is bull-dog determination.

Love is this book, and love is Marge.

Just this last Friday, Marge accompanied Ben to a school potluck, and Ben came back to the inner sanctum of her clinic bubbling over with joy at sharing his friends with her. After singing about love and wonder for a half hour straight, he selected his oldest, most precious movie to show her—a movie about baby animals. After a while, he shifted the topic to his own babyhood and the years since. With one telling, eye contact, and some pretty nice grammar besides, my Brilliant Ben told "Marge's":

I was a little boy.
Mama's take care of me.

Dreams come true:
My friends are ok.
I'm ok.

Don't worry about me.
I'm perfect this way.

I have determined to frame these words of Ben's and put them on my wall, as a reminder that this young man of mine has an understanding of himself, and of life, that provides a lesson for us all!

And may that lesson resonate with you and your family as it has with mine.

Sincerely,
The Mama

Linda Carter, R.N.
University of Wisconsin Medical Foundation
Madison, Wisconsin

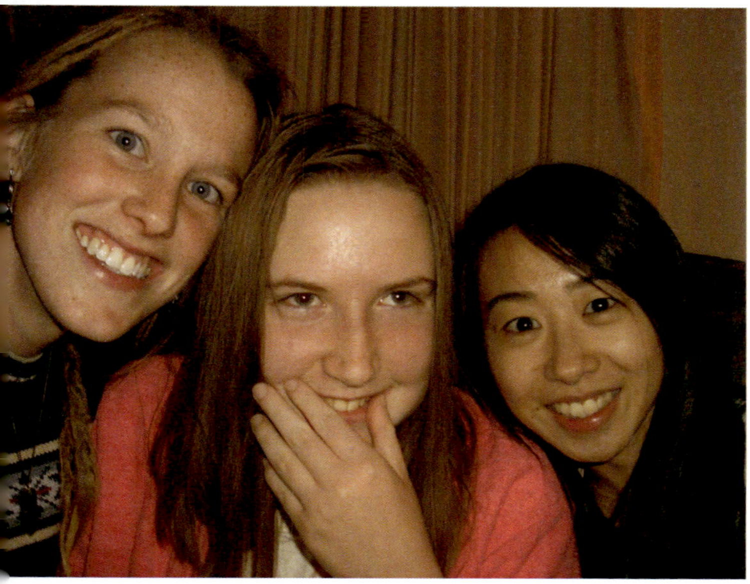

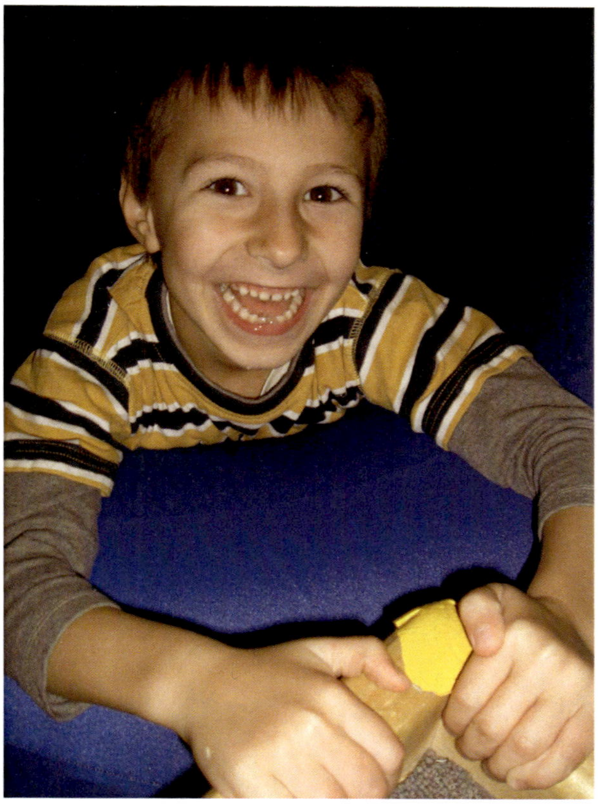

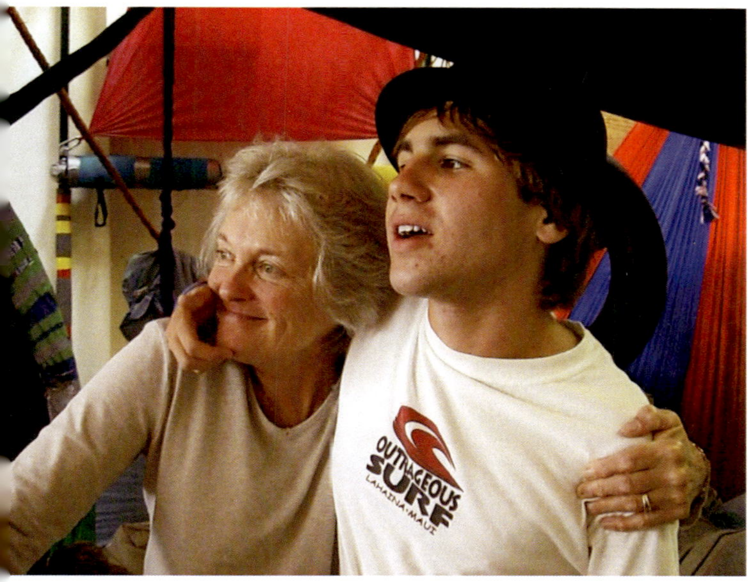

"I feel connected."

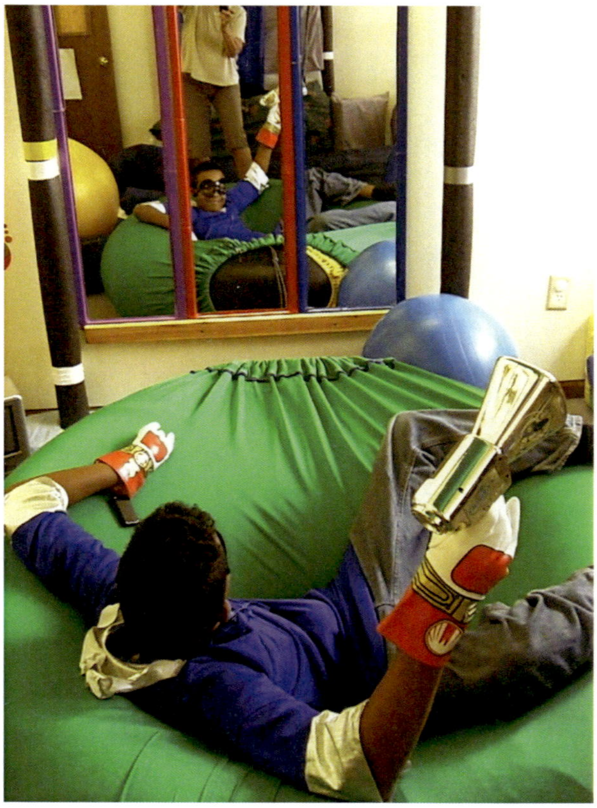

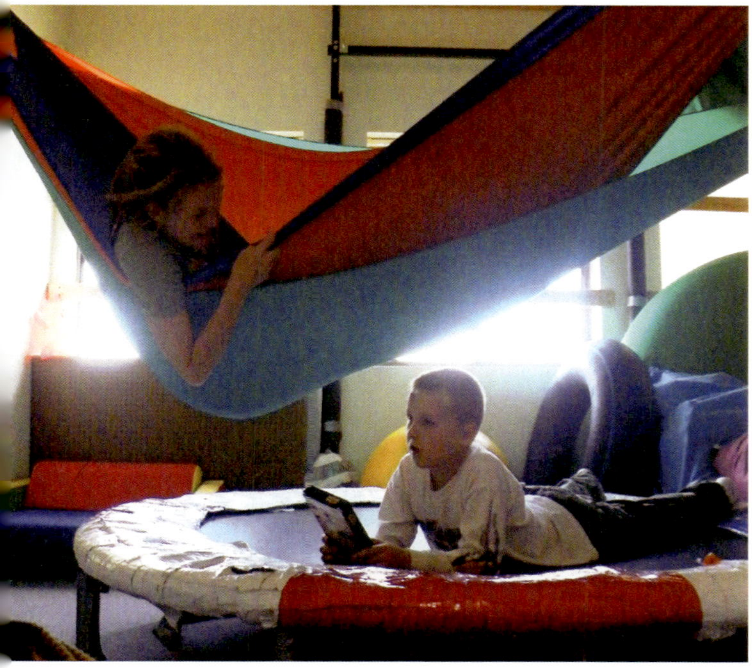

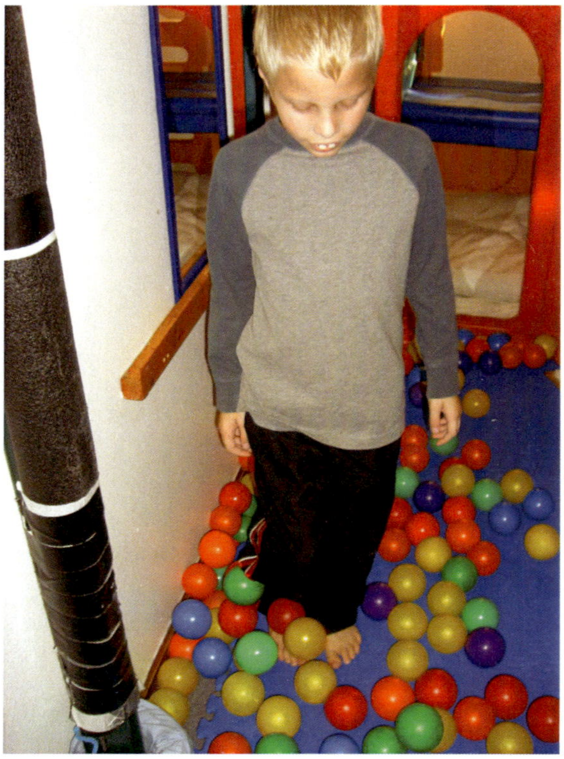

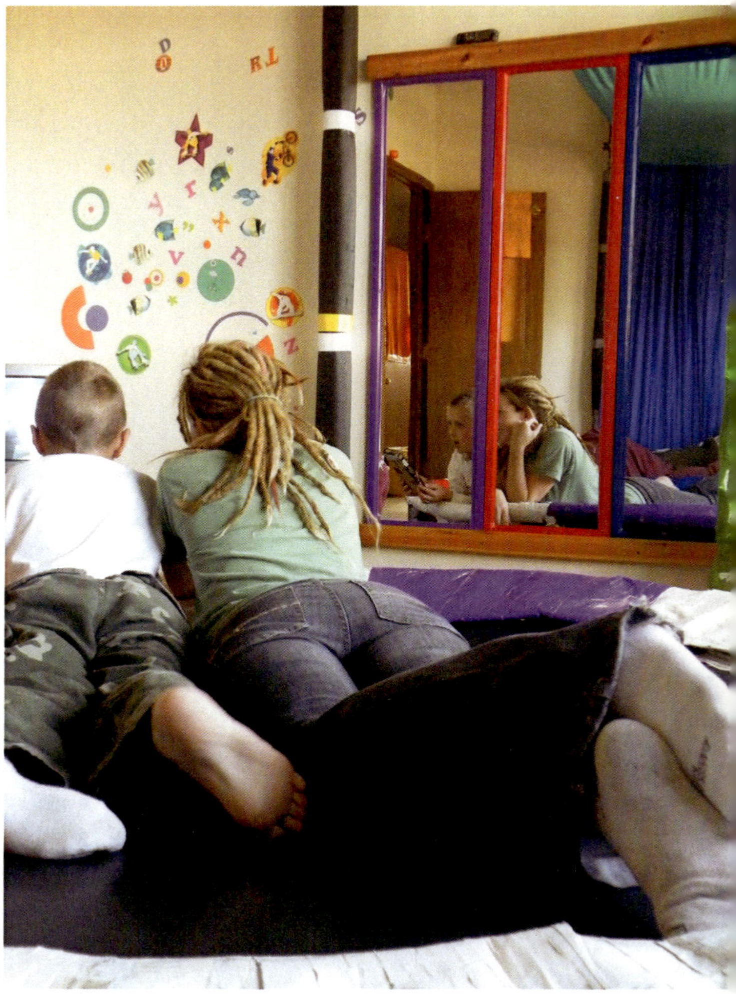

"My friends will take me home."

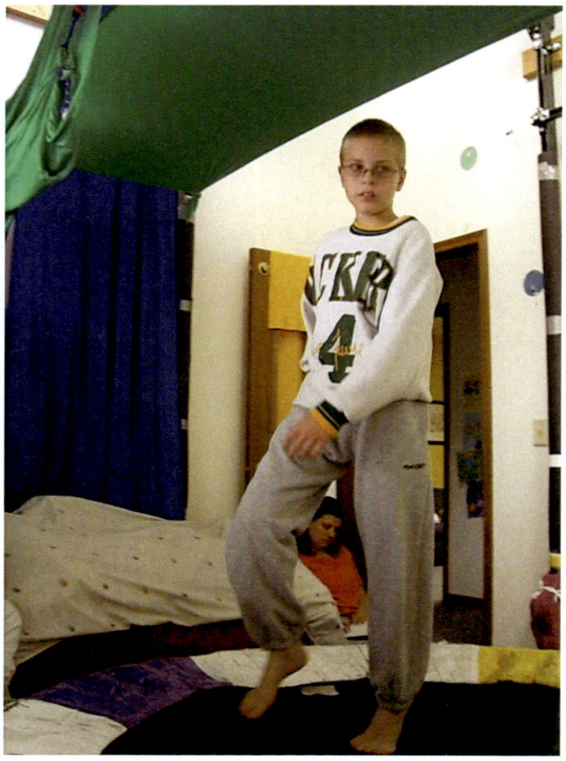

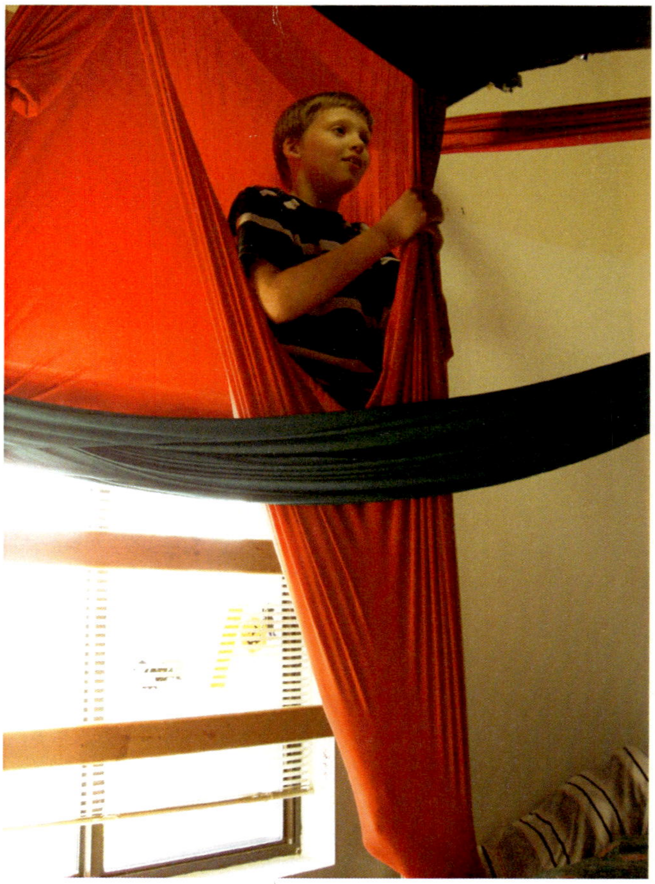

appendices

Appendix A

Natural Language Acquisition Summary

Stage 1	**Echolalia:** Use of complete gestalts: intonational contours, sentences, scenes, episodes, or other wholes processed as single units of sound, taken directly from the environment and used moments, hours, or days later.	**"Good job, Johnny!"** **"Are you OK?"** **"And now, for our feature presentation!"** **"Let's get out of here."** **"Want some more."**
Stage 2	**Mitigated echolalia:** Common parts of gestalts are mitigated from the whole, and a child can mix and match these phrases.	"Let's get" + "some more" = **"Let's get some more!"** "Want" + "out of here" = **"Want out of here."**
Stage 3	**Mitigation of the single word:** Mitigated phrases are further broken down to isolate single words. A "mix-and-match" of single words creates original two-word phrases.	**(1) "Let's—get" + "wanna—get" = "get"** **"Some—more" + "No—more" = "more"** **(2) "Get more!"** and **"More get!"**
Stage 4	**Generation of original sentences with beginning grammar:** The beginning stages of grammar, both correct and incorrect (Development Sentence Scoring levels 1–3)	**I get. Get more no. No get some.** **I wanna get some more toys. He got more toys, and I didn't.**
Stage 5	**Generation of sentences with more advanced grammar:** DSS levels 4–6	**I used to want more toys, but I lost interest.** **How can we get more toys without any more money?**
Stage 6	**Generation of all sentence patterns:** DSS levels 7 and 8	**Why don't we try to buy some more toys with the money we save?**

Appendix B

Assessment Form
Natural Language Acquisition

Student:

Date:

#	Utterance	Stage 1	Stage 2	Stage 3	Stages 4–6

#	Utterance	Stage 1	Stage 2	Stage 3	Stages 4–6

#	Utterance	Stage 1	Stage 2	Stage 3	Stages 4–6
TOTAL:					

Assessment Summary:

Recommendations:

Appendix C

Developmental Sentence Scoring
(L. Lee, 1974)

Name: ____________

Date: ____________

Page: ______

#	Utterance	Indef. Pro.	Pers. Pro.	Main Verb	Sec. Verb	Neg.	Conj.	Inter. Rev.	Wh-Q	Sent. Point	Total

Total # of sentences: ______

DSS score = total points / total sentences: ______

Total # of points: ______

Name: ______________

Date: ______________

Page: ________

#	Utterance	Indef. Pro.	Pers. Pro.	Main Verb	Sec. Verb	Neg.	Conj.	Inter. Rev.	Wh-Q	Sent. Point	Total

Total # of sentences: ______ DSS score = total points / total sentences: ______ Total # of points: ______

Appendix D

Developmental Sentence Analysis: A Grammatical Assessment Procedure for Speech and Langua Clinicians (from Laura Lee, 1974)

Score	Indefinite Pronouns or Noun Modifiers	Personal Pronouns	Main Verbs	Secondary Verbs
1	it, this, that	1st & 2nd person: I, me, my, mine, you, your(s)	A. Uninflected verb: I see you. B: copula, is or 's: It's red. C: is + verb + ing: He is coming.	
2		3rd person: he, him, his, she, her, hers	A. –s and –ed: plays, played B: irregular past: are, saw C: Copula: am, are, was, were D: Auxiliary am, are, was, were	Five early developing infinitives: I wanna see. (want to see) I'm gonna see. (going to see) I gotta see.(got to see) Lemme [to] see. (let me [to] see) Let's [to] play. (let [us to] play)
3	A. no, some, more, all, lot(s), one(s) two (etc.), other(s), another. B. something, somebody, someone	A. Plurals: we, us, our(s), they, them, their B. these, those		Non-complementing infinitives: I stopped to play. I'm afraid to look. It's hard to do that.
4	nothing, nobody, none, no one		A. can, will, may + verb: may go B. Obligatory do + verb: don't go C. Emphatic do + verb: I do see	Participle, present or past: I see a boy running. I found the toy broken.
5		Reflexives: myself, yourself, himself, herself, itself, themselves		A. Early infinitival complements w differing subjects in kernels: I wan to come, Let him [to] see. B. Later infinitival complements: I to go, I told him to go, I tried to g ought to go. C. Obligatory deletions: Make it [t D. Infinitive with wh-word: I know to get, I know how to do it.
6		A. Wh-pronouns: who, which, whose, whom, what, that, how many, how much B. Wh-word + infinitives: I know what to do, I know who(m) to take.	A. could, would, should, might + verb: might come, could be B. Obligatory does, did + verb C. Emphatic does, did + verb	
7	A. any, anything, anybody, anyone B. every, everything, everybody, everyone C. both, few, many, each, several, most, least, much, next, first, last, second (etc.)	(his) own, one, oneself, whichever, whoever, whatever: Take whatever you like.	A. Passive with get, any tense Passive with be, any tense B. must, shall + verb: must come C. have + verb + en: I've eaten. D. have got: I've got it.	Passive infinitival complement: With get; I have to get dressed. I d want to get hurt. With be: I want to be pulled, It's go to be locked.
8			A. have/had been + verb + ing B. modal + have + verb + en: may have eaten C. modal + be + verb + ing: could be playing D. Other auxiliary combinations: should have been sleeping.	Gerund: Swinging is fun. I like fishing. He staring laughing.

Negatives	Conjunctions	Interrogative Reversals	Wh-Questions
it, this, that + copula or auxiliary is, 's, + not: It's not mine., This is not a dog., That is not moving.		Reversal of copula: Isn't it red? Were they there?	
			A. who, what, what + noun: Who am I? What is he eating? What book are you reading? B. where, how many, how much, what…do, what…for: Where did to go? How much do you want? What is he doing? What is a hammer for?
	and		
can't, don't		Reversal of auxiliary be: Is he coming? Isn't he coming? Was he going?	
isn't, won't	A. but B. so, and so, so that C. or, it		When, how, how + adjective: When shall I come? How do you do it? How big is it?
	because	A. Obligatory do, does, did: Do they run? Does it bite? Didn't it hurt? B. Reversal of modal: Can you play? Won't it hurt? Shall I sit down? C. Tag question: It's fun isn't it? It isn't fun, is it?	
All other negatives: A. Uncontracted negatives: I can not go, He has not gone. B. Pronoun-auxiliary or pronoun-copula contraction: I'm not coming, He's not here. C. Auxiliary-negative or copula-negative contraction: He wasn't going, He hasn't been seen, It couldn't be mine, They aren't big.			Why, what if, how come, how about + gerund: Why are you crying? What if I won't do it? How come he is crying? How about coming with me?
	A. where, when, how, while, whether (or not), til, until, unless, since, before, after, for, as, as + adjective + as, as if, like, that, than: I know where you are, Don't come til I call. B. Obligatory deletions: I run faster than you [run], I'm as big as a man [is big], It looks like a dog [looks]. C. Elliptical deletions (score 0): That's why [I took it], I know how [I can do it]. D. Wh-words + infinitive: I know how to do it. I know where to go.	A. Reversal of auxiliary have: Has he seen you? B. Reversal with two or three auxiliaries: Has he been eating? Couldn't he have waited? Could he have been crying? Wouldn't he have been going?	Whose, which, which + noun: Whose car is that? Which book do you want?

Appendix E

Natural Language Acquisition Assessment

Communication Development Center
700 Rayovac Drive, Suite 200
Madison, WI

Student: Dylan

Date: 11/16

#	Utterance	Stage 1	Stage 2	Stage 3	Stages 4–6
1	**Ready, set, go.**	x			
2	**Turn that off.**	x			
3	**Off.**			x	
4	**It's Buzz Lightyear.**		x		
5	**A dinosaur.**			x	
6	**You cut out?**		x		
7	**You cut out Slinky?**		x	x	
8	**No.**			x	
9	**No color.**			x	
10	**Cut out Buzz Lightyear?**		x	x	
11	**Cut out dinosaur?**		x	x	
12	**Cut out Oink Oink?**		x	x	
13	**One, two, three, four, five, six, seven, eight, nine.**	x			
14	**Where's Bouncy?**		x		
15	**Come here.**	x			
16	**Let's go.**	x			
17	**There she is.**	x			
18	**Hide!**			x	

#	Utterance	Stage 1	Stage 2	Stage 3	Stages 4–6
19	**We're in trouble.**	x			
20	**Here she coming.**		x		**x**
21	**Get her.**		x		
22	**Hey, everybody!**	x			
23	**I'm coming.**	x			
24	**You're it.**	x			
25	**That's close.**		x		
26	**Come on, hurry.**		x		
27	**Beth's it.**				**x**
28	**I got it.**	x			
29	**Go outside, Christmas.**		x		
30	**Got it!**		x		
31	**We got it.**		x		
32	**Let's go outside.**		x		
33	**Out the door.**		x		
Sub-totals:		11	13.5	7	1.5
Percentages of Total (33):		33%	41%	21%	5%

Assessment Summary:

This is the sample taken during Dylan's ninth session and excerpted on pages 92 and 93. Movie gestalts had been largely replaced by life gestalts modeled by clinicians during active play, and Dylan used them in a nice variety of similar situations. He could mitigate from them, as demonstrated by his original errors, and was using mitigations more often than short gestalts.

NLA guidelines recommend continuing to introduce a variety of mitigable gestalts in order to solidify progress to Stage 2, making sure there are a variety of communicative opportunities for the Stage 2 mitigations, and refraining from focusing on grammar until there are more building blocks at Stage 3, established by way of Stage 2 mitigation.

Appendix F

Natural Language Acquisition Assessment

Communication Development Center
700 Rayovac Drive, Suite 200
Madison, WI

Student: Bevin

Date: 9/28

#	Utterance	Stage 1	Stage 2	Stage 3	Stages 4–6
1	**Sleep-over.**			x	
2	**Night—play on Halloween night.** [Bevin isolated "night" and "play" and added these to the phrase, "on Halloween night"]		x	x	
3	**Dump it out.**		x		
4	**I'm so glad.** [This may have been a gestalt, but was more likely a mitigation from "I'm so glad I found you" or something similar]		x		
5	**Stop it—** [This was spoken as a mitigated gestalt, not a complete one]		x		
6	**It's scary.** [For Bevin, this was likely a mitigation from "It's so scary!"]		x		
7	**x x sister's x x.** [Mitigated in real-time by "fast-forwarding" through the unwanted parts]		x		
8	**These are stinks.** [The first of a series of "These are …" sentences, suggesting a mitigated sentence-starter]		x		
9	**These are x x x.**		x		
10	**Here, Hulk, here is for you, for you, for you, for you.** [Bevin combined single words and multi-word mitigations]		x		
11	**We are just gonna x x x.** [Likely a mitigation from, "We are just gonna have to get you a new one" or something similar]		x		
12	**I'm gonna just play overnight x x x.** [A nice reworking of the previous mitigation, added to "play" and "overnight," all of it verging on grammar]		x		

#	Utterance	Stage 1	Stage 2	Stage 3	Stages 4–6
13	**It is the only x x x.** [An attempt to mitigate in real time from "It is the only way!"]		x		
14	**And play all night.** ["And" used as an isolated word in a nice combination]		x	x	
15	**And sleep.**			x	
16	**And clean up all the toys.**		x	x	
17	**And wait for Mom and Tori.** [Extending the series of utterances with grammar]				x
18	**How about—**		x		
19	**How about—**		x		
20	**Princess stories.**			x	
21	**No, thank you.** [This could have been a gestalt]		x		
22	**These are—**		x		
23	**Iguanadon, where is it?** [Bevin had isolated Iguanadon and added it to a gestalt phrase he frequently used]	x		x	
24	**Read it.**		x		
25	**No.**			x	
26	**Not yet.**		x		
27	**Read—Euroraptor.**			x	
28	**No.**			x	
29	**No—don't touch it.**		x	x	
30	**OK—I can x x x.**		x	x	
31	**He's so big.** [Only knowing Bevin's linguistic history allowed scoring this accurately]		x		
32	**He's big.** [He then further mitigated Utterance #31]		x		
33	**He's big.**		x		
34	**x x fun to read.**		x		

#	Utterance	Stage 1	Stage 2	Stage 3	Stage 4-6
35	**Oh, look.**	x			
36	x x x x x x x x x x x x x x x x x x [The first of a series of unintelligible story gestalts]	x			
37	x x x x x x x x x x x x x x x x x x	x			
38	x x x x x x x x x x x x x x x x x x	x			
39	x x x x x x x x x x x x x x x x x x	x			
40	x x x x x x x x x x x x x x x x x x	x			
41	**New ones.** [Returning to a series of nice mitigations]		x		
42	**Look inside.**		x		
43	**Years and years.**		x		
44	**Thousands year.**			x	
45	**Millions years.** [This might be more accurately a mitigation from "millions of years," but in this series of mix-and-match phrases, it also seemed like a Stage 3 combination]			x	
46	**You love it—** [Nice extraction from "Don't you love it when..." or something similar]		x		
47	**I love—** [A nice follow-up utterance that changed the pronoun]		x		
48	**Wow!**	x			
49	**Squirrel—**			x	
50	**Girl—**			x	
51	**Victoria.**			x	
52	**The sister, please—**			x	
53	**No.**			x	
54	**Thumper is quiet—quiet.** [There was no reason to consider this a mitigation, and followed a nice series of isolated single words]				x
55	**Don't—don't need it.**		x		

#	Utterance	Stage 1	Stage 2	Stage 3	Stage 4-6
56	**Three sisters come inside.**				x
57	**Thumper, stay inside.**				x
58	**Wait for Tori—**		x		
59	**Thumper's for you.**		x		
60	**Thousand, thousand, million years.**			x	
61	**Fire!** [Spoken like the gestalt exclamation]	x			
62	**Look!** [Same]	x			
63	**Look!**	x			
64	**Look!**	x			
65	**Look!**	x			
66	**Look!**	x			
67	**Look!**	x			
68	**Look!**	x			
69	**Look!**	x			
70	**Look!**	x			
71	**Look!**	x			
72	**Skullasaurus.** [Also spoken like the exclamation from the movie]	x			
73	**Give me a break.**	x			
74	**Say—ghost.** [The first of a nice series of single word combinations]			x	
75	**Say—**			x	
76	**Say—skull.**			x	
77	**Thursday—eat breakfast.** [Scored as single word combinations because of the following utterances]			x	

#	Utterance	Stage 1	Stage 2	Stage 3	Stage 4-6
78	**PBS Kids and eat lunch.**			x	
79	**A little homework and brush teeth and go to bed.** [A wonderful combination of the mitigation "a little homework" with several other single word combos—all verging on Stage 4 grammar]		x	x	
Sub-totals:		20.5	31	23.5	4
Percentages of Total (79):		26%	39%	30%	5%

Assessment Summary:

This is the full sample excerpted on pages 37–39. It was part of a 2-hour session and followed 15 minutes of intense jumping and proprioceptive activity on a large trampoline. Bevin was very excited about planning a sleepover, and was well set up to advocate for himself. He was verbally engaged in short Stage 1 utterances and Stage 2 mitigated phrases for 30 minutes before he used any quiet, gestalt self-talk at all. Bevin demonstrated several strategies for mitigating: fast-forwarding in real time, using phrases in series and changing them, utterance by utterance, and even mitigations of mitigations. He used some nice Stage 3 single word isolating and combined single words with each other and with short mitigated phrases.

Bevin's totals showed that he was not using any one stage a majority of the time, but was processing at each of the first three Stages between 25 and 50 % of the time. Recommendations could be made for each of those Stages:

Stage 1: Since Bevin was using between 25 and 50% Stage 1 gestalts, the guidelines noted that it was important to look at the variety and usefulness of Stage 2 mitigations in order to determine other mitigations that might be helpful to move solidly to Stage 2. Because so many of his gestalts in this sample were single words, longer gestalts would be more useful in providing mitigable language. Bevin's percentage at Stage 1 was just over 25%, but the large number of repeated, single-word gestalts may have skewed these results.

Stage 2: Since Bevin was using between 25 and 50% Stage 2 mitigations, the guidelines noted that finer examination of the variety of phrase mitigations was important in order to provide mitigable gestalts and mitigations that would be useful quickly. Guidelines noted that social language opportunities were imperative.

Stage 3: Since Bevin was using between 25 and 50% Stage 3 single words and combinations, the guidelines noted that it was important to look at Stage 2 and make sure it was comfortable and functional. Guidelines noted that Bevin may need more Stage 2 language to break down.

Stage 4: Since Bevin was using less than 25% of Stage 4 utterances, the guidelines noted that grammar should not be promoted before there were adequate building blocks at Stage 3 (which needed to come from Stage 2 mitigations).

references

Ayres, Jean A. (1979). *Sensory Integration and the Child.* Los Angeles, CA: Western Psychological Services.

Ayres, Jean A. (2005). *Sensory Integration and the Child,* 25th Anniversary Ed., revised and updated by Pediatric Therapy Network. Los Angeles, CA: Western Psychological Services.

Baltaxe, Christiane and Simmons, J. (1981). Disorders of language in childhood psychosis: Current concepts and approaches. In J. Darby (Ed.), *Speech Evaluation in Psychiatry.* New York, NY: Grune and Stratton.

Biel, Lindsey (2010). A sensory diet happens 24/7. *Autism Asperger's Digest,* Mar-Apr and May-June.

Blanc, Marge (2004). Ask the experts: Child-directed language therapy. *Autism Asperger's Digest,* Jan-Feb.

Blanc, Marge (2004). When speech gets stuck: A hierarchy of practical supports for dyspraxia in children with ASD. *Autism Asperger's Digest,* Sep-Oct and Nov-Dec.

Blanc, Marge (2005). Finding the words: To tell the whole story. *Autism Aspergers Digest,* May-June, July-Aug, Sept-Oct, and Nov-Dec.

Blanc, Marge (2006). Finding the words: When it's hard to find your voice! Helping your child with dyspraxia. *Autism Asperger's Digest,* Jan-Feb and Mar-Apr.

Blanc, Marge (2006). Finding the words: When they are pictures! Helping your visual child become verbal. *Autism Asperger's Digest,* May-Jun, Jul-Aug, Sep-Oct, and Nov-Dec.

Blanc, Marge (2007). Echolalia revisited: How to support our kids as they develop language from echolalia to original sentences! Workshop for Minnesota Autism Conference.

Blanc, Marge (2007). Echolalia in context. Workshop for Professional Development Programs, Madison, WI.

Blanc, Marge (2008). Finding the words: With augmented communication, parts 1-4. *Autism Asperger's Digest,* May-June, July-Aug, Sept-Oct, and Nov-Dec.

Blanc, Marge (2010). Communication/more than words: Grammar: How and when to teach it. *Autism Asperger's Digest,* Nov-Dec.

Blanc, Marge and Carter, L. (2007). Echolalia revisited: How to support our kids as they develop language from echolalia to original sentences! Workshop for Minnesota Autism Conference, 2007.

Blanc, Marge (2007). Echolalia in Context. Workshop for Professional Development Programs, Madison, WI.

Blanc, Marge and Carter, L. (2007). Echolalia revisited: The first stage of gestalt language development! Autism Society of Wisconsin Convention.

Bondy, Andrew and Frost, L. (1994). The Picture Exchange Communication System. *Focus on Autistic Behavior,* 9, 1-19.

Brandl, Charlene (1999). *Facilitated Communication-Case Studies: See Us Smart!* Ann Arbor, MI: Robbie Dean Press.

Brown, Roger (1973). *A First Language: The Early Stages.* Cambridge, MA: Harvard University Press.

Cermak, Sharon A. and Larkin, D. (2002). *Developmental Coordination Disorder.* Albany, NY: Delmar.

Chapman, Robin (2002). Personal conversation.

Cropper, Zadock (2000). Personal conversation.

Davis, Ronald D. (1997). *The Gift of Dyslexia.* New York: NY: The Berkeley Publishing Group.

Dennison, Paul E. and Dennison, G. (2010). *Brain Gym Teacher's Edition.* Ventura, CA: Edu-Kinesthetics, Inc.

Develop. (2004). In Frederick C. Mish (Ed.), *Merriam-Webster's Collegiate Dictionary* (p. 341, 11th ed.). Springfield, MA: Merriam-Webster, Inc.

Donnellan, Anne and Leary, M. (1995). *Movement Differences and Diversity in Autism/Mental Retardation.* Madison, WI: DRI Press.

Endow, Judy (2006). *Making Lemonade: Hints for Autism's Helpers.* Cambridge, WI: Cambridge Book Review Press.

Freed, Jeffrey and Parsons, L. (1997). *Right-Brained Children in a Left-Brained World.* New York, NY: Simon and Schuster.

Frick, Sheila M., and Young, S. (2009). *Listening with the Whole Body: Clinical Concepts and Treatment Guidelines for Therapeutic Listening.* Madison, WI: Vital Links.

Gardner, Howard (1983). *Frames of Mind: The Theory of Multiple Intelligences.* New York, NY: Basic Books.

Goldin-Meadow, Susan, So, W. C., Ozyurek, A., and Mylander, C. (2008). The natural order of events: How speakers of different languages represent events nonverbally. *Proceedings of the National Academy of Sciences.* USA 105, 9163-9168.

Grandin, Temple, *The Way I See It,* Arlington, TX: Future Horizons, 2008.

Grandin, Temple (1995). *Thinking in Pictures.* New York, NY: Doubleday.

Grandin, Temple (1997). A personal perspective on Autism. In Donald J. Cohen and F. R. Volkmar (Eds.), *Handbook of Autism and Pervasive Developmental Disorders* (2nd ed). New York, NY: John Wiley and Sons, Inc.

Grandin, Temple (2005). Autism: The way I see it, different types of thinking in Autism. *Autism Asperger's Digest,* Nov-Dec.

Grandin, Temple (2005). Conversations with Kathleen Dunn, #0218D, *Wisconsin Public Radio,* February 18.

Grandin, Temple (2008). *The Way I See It.* Arlington, TX: Future Horizons.

Grandin, Temple and Johnson, C. (2005). *Animals in Translation.* New York, NY: Harcourt, Inc.

Greenspan, Stanley I. and Wiedner, S. (1998). *The Child with Special Needs: Encouraging Intellectual and Emotional Growth.* Cambridge, MA: Perseus Books.

Greenspan, Stanley I. and Wiedner, S. (2006). *Engaging Autism,* Cambridge, MA: Da Capo Press.

Gurian, Michael (1996). *The Wonder of Boys.* New York, NY: Jeremy P. Tarcher/Putnam.

Gurian, Michael and Henley, P. (2001). *Boys and Girls Learn Differently!* San Francisco CA: Jossey-Bass.

Hayden, Deborah A. (2000). *PROMPT Workshop Manual*, Level 1. Santa Fe, NM: The PROMPT Institute.

Kanner, Leo (1943). Autistic disturbances of affective content, *Nervous Child* 2, 217-250.

Kanner, Leo. (1946). Irrelevant and metaphorical language. *American Journal of Psychiatry*, 103, 242–246.

Kientz, Mary A. and Dunn, W. (1997). A comparison of the performance of children with and without Autism on the Sensory Profile. *American Journal of Occupational Therapy*, 51, 530-537.

Koegel, Robert L. and Koegel, L. K. (2006). *Pivotal Response Treatments for Autism*, Baltimore, MD: Paul Brookes Publishing Co.

Leadholm, Barbara J. and Miller, J. F. (1995). *Language Sample Analysis: The Wisconsin Guide*. Madison, WI: Wisconsin Department of Public Instruction.

Lee, Laura L. (1974). *Developmental Sentence Analysis: A Grammatical Assessment Procedure for Speech and Language Clinicians*. Evanston, IL: Northwestern University Press.

Levine, Melvin D (2002). *A Mind at a Time*, New York, NY: Simon and Schuster.

Light, Janice C. and Binger, C. (1998). *Building Communicative Competence with Individuals who use Augmentative and Alternative Communication*. Baltimore, MD: Paul H. Brookes Publishing Company..

Lovaas, O. Ivar (1981). *Teaching Developmentally Disabled Children: The Me Book*. Austin, TX: Pro-Ed, Inc.

Lovaas, O. Ivar, Koegel, R., and Schreibman, L. (1979). Stimulus overselectivity in autism: a review of the research, *Psychological Bulletin*, 86, 1236-1254.

Lyon, Jon G. (1998). *Coping with Aphasia*. San Diego, CA: Singular Publishing Group, Inc.

Marshalla, Pamela (1999). *Imitation*. Temecula, CA: Speech Dynamics, Inc.

MacDonald, James D. (1997). *First Words*. Tallmadge, OH: Family Child Learning Center.

MacDonald, James D. (2004). *Communicating Partners*, Philadelphia: Jessica Kingsley.

MacDonald, James D. and Stoika, P. (2007). *Play to Talk*, Madison, WI: Kiddo Publishing.

McEachin, John J., Smith, T., and Lovaas, O. (1993). Long-term outcome for children with Autism who received early intensive behavioral treatment, *American Journal of Mental Retardation*, 97, 359-372.

McGinnity, Kate, and Negri, N. (2005). *Walk Awhile in My Autism*. Cambridge, WI: Cambridge Book Review Press.

MOM-Not Otherwise Specified (2006). Dr. Strangetalk or: How I Learned to Stop Worrying and Love Echolalia. Retrieved May 30, 2012 from http://momnos.blogspot.com/2006/03/dr-strangetalk-or-how-I-learned-to.html.

Mukhopadhyay, Soma (2008). *Understanding Autism through Rapid Prompting Method*, Denver, CO: Outskirts Press, Inc.

Notbohm, Ellen. (2005). *Ten Things Every Child with Autism Wishes You Knew*, Arlington, TX: Future Horizons.

Notbohm, Ellen and Zysk, V. (2004). *1001 Great Ideas for Teaching and Raising Children with Autism Spectrum Disorders.* Arlington, TX: Future Horizons, Inc.

Peters, Ann, Language learning strategies: Does the whole equal the sum of the parts? *Language*, 1977, 53, 560-573.

Peters, Ann (1983). *The Units of Language Acquisition.* Cambridge, England: Cambridge University Press. 2002 version retrieved from www.ling.hawaii.edu/faculty/ann.

Prizant, Barry M.. (1982). Gestalt processing and gestalt language in Autism. *Topics in Language Disorders*, 3: 16-23.

Prizant, Barry M. (1983). Language acquisition and communicative behavior in Autism: Toward an understanding of the 'whole' of it. *Journal of Speech and Hearing Disorders*, 48, 296-307.

Prizant, Barry M (1983). Echolalia in Autism: Assessment and intervention. *Seminars in Speech and Language*, Vol. 4, No. 1.

Prizant, Barry M.. (1987). Clinical Implications of Echolalic Behavior in Autism. In T. Layton (Ed.), *Language and Treatment of Autistic and Developmentally Disordered Children.* Springfield, IL: Charles Thomas, Inc.

Prizant, Barry M. (1988). Communication problems in the Autistic client. In N. Lass, L. McReynolds, J. Northern, and D. Yoder (Eds.), *Handbook of Speech-Language Pathology.* Toronto, Ontario: BC Decker.

Prizant, Barry M. and Rydell, P. J. (1981). A functional analysis of delayed echolalia of autistic children. Presentation to the American Speech and Hearing Association Convention.

Prizant, Barry M. and Rydell, P. J. (1984). An analysis of the functions of delayed echolalia in autistic children. *Journal of Speech and Hearing Research*, 27.

Prizant, Barry M., and Wetherby, A. M. (1997). Treatment approaches for young children with pervasive developmental disorders: A critical review. Special Session, American Speech-Language-Hearing Association Convention.

Prizant, Barry M., Schuler, A. L., Wetherby, A. M. and Rydell, P. (1997). Enhancing language and communication: Language approaches. In D. Cohen and F. Volkmar (Eds.), *Handbook of Autism and Pervasive Developmental Disorders* (2nd ed.). New York, NY: Wiley.

Prizant, Barry M., Wetherby, A. M., Rubin, E., Laurent, A. C., Rydell, P. J. (2006). *The SCERTS Model: A Comprehensive Educational Approach for Children with Autism Spectrum Disorders*, Vol 1: Assessment; Vol 2: Program Planning and Intervention, Baltimore, MD: Paul M. Brookes Publishing Co.

Ratey, John J. and Johnson C. (1997). *Shadow Syndromes.* New York, NY: Pantheon Books.

Richard, Gail J. (1997). *The Source for Autism.* East Moline, IL: LinguiSystems, Inc.

Rogers, Sally J. and Vismara, L. A. (2007). Evidence Based Comprehensive Treatments for Early Autism. University of California Davis: M.I.N.D. Institute.

Rydell, Patrick J. and Prizant, B. M. (1995). Educational and communicative approaches for children who use echolalia. In K. Quill (Ed.), *Teaching Children with Autism: Methods to Increase Communication and Socialization.* Albany NY: Delmar Publishers.

Sallows, G, and Graupner, T. (2005). Intensive behavioral treatment for children with autism: Four-year outcome and predictors. *American Journal on Mental Retardation*, 110, 417-438.

Schroud, Kathy (1998). Personal conversation.

Science Daily. When using gestures, rules of grammar remain the same. Retrieved June 30, 2008 from www.sciencedaily.com/releases/2008.

Smith, Tristram, Groen, A., and Wynn, J. (2000). Randomized trial of intensive early intervention for children with pervasive developmental disorder. *American Journal on Mental Retardation*. 105, 269-285.

Sunbeck, Deborah (1996). *Infinity Walk: Preparing your mind to learn!* Torrance, CA: Jalmar Press.

Sussman, Fern (1999). *More Than Words*. Toronto, Ontario: The Hanen Center.

Tager-Flusberg, Helen, Rogers, S., Cooper, J., Landa, R., Lord, C., Paul, R., Rice, M., Stoel-Gammon, C., Wetherby, A., and Yoder, P. (2009). Defining spoken language benchmarks and selected measures of expressive language development for young children with autism spectrum disorders. *Journal of Speech, Language, and Hearing Research*. Vol. 52, pp. 643-652.

Tager-Flusberg, Helen, Calkins, S., Nolin, T., Baumberger, T., Anderson, M., and Chadwick-Dias, A. (1990). A longitudinal study of language acquisition in Autistic and Down Syndrome children. *Journal of Autism and Developmental Disorders*, 10, 1-21.

Taylor, Jill Bolte (2008). *My Stroke of Insight*. New York, NY: Viking.

Thordardottir, Elin T., Chapman, R. S., and Wagner, L. (2002). Complex sentence production by adolescents with Down syndrome. *Applied Psycholinguistics*. 23, pp 163-183.

University of Wisconsin-Madison (2002). Kids with down syndrome learn language beyond adolescence. *ScienceDaily*, October 17.

Volkmar, Fred R. and Wiesner, L. A. (2009). *A Practical Guide to Autism: What Every Parent, Family Member, and Teacher Needs to Know*. Hoboken, NJ: John Wiley and Sons.

Wetherby, Amy M. (1992). *Communication and Intervention for Preschool Children*. Buffalo, NY: Educom Associates Inc.

Wetherby, Amy M. and Prizant, B. M. (1999). Enhancing language and communication development in Autism: Assessment and intervention guidelines. In D. Berkell Zager (Ed.), *Autism: Identification, Education, and Treatment*, Chapter 6. Mahwah, NJ: Lawrence Erlbaum Associates.

Wetherby, Amy M., Prizant, B. M., and Huchinson, T. A. (1998). Communicative, social/affective, and symbolic profiles of young children with Autism and pervasive developmental disorders. *American Journal of Speech-Language Pathology*, 7, 79-91.

Wetherby, Amy M., Prizant, B. M., and Schuler, A. (2000). Understanding the nature of the communication and language impairment. In A. Wetherby and B. M. Prizant (Eds.), *Autism Spectrum Disorders: A Transactional Developmental Perspective*. Baltimore, MD: Paul Brooks.

Wilbarger, Patricia and Stackhouse, T. (1999). Sensory defensiveness and related social/emotional and neurological problems. Professional Development Programs, Milwaukee, WI.

Williams, Mary Sue, and Shellenberger, S. (1996). *An Introduction to 'How Does Your Engine Run?' The Alert Program for Self-Regulation.* Albuquerque, NM: TherapyWords, Inc.

Yack, Ellen, Sutton, S., and Aquilla, P. (1996). *Building Bridges through Sensory Integration.* Weston, Ontario: Building Bridges Through Sensory Integration.